MW01100371

FOURTH EDITION

HANDBOOK

OF PAEDIATRICS

FOURTH EDITION

Edited by
H. de V. Heese

Cape Town
Oxford University Press

Oxford University Press
Walton Street, Oxford OX2 6DP, United Kingdom

Oxford New York
Athens Bangkok Bombay
Calcutta Cape Town Dar es Salaam Delhi
Florence Hong Kong Istanbul Karachi
Kuala Lumpur Madras Madrid Melbourne
Mexico City Nairobi Paris Singapore
Taipei Tokyo Toronto

and associated companies in
Berlin Ibadan

OXFORD is a trade mark of Oxford University Press

HANDBOOK OF PAEDIATRICS
Fourth Edition
Second impression 1995
ISBN 0 19 571435 0

First edition published 1975 and later impressions by the department of
Paediatrics and Child health, University of Cape Town
Second edition published 1989 by Haum Educational Publishers, Pretoria
Third edition published 1992 by Oxford University Press Southern Africa
Third edition (second impression) published 1993 by Oxford University
Press Southern Africa
Fourth edition published 1995 by Oxford University Press Southern Africa

© University of Cape Town 1992

Editor: Susan Lawrence
Cover designer: Mara Singer
Medical illustrator: Jeanette Venter
Indexer: Hilary Bassett

Published by Oxford University Press Southern Africa,
Harrington House, Barrack Street, Cape Town 8001, South Africa

Text set in 9.5 on 10.5 pt Times Roman by RHT desktop publishing cc
Reproduction by RHT desktop publishing cc, Durbanville
Printed and bound by SNP Printing Pte Ltd.

FOREWORD

The first edition of *The Paediatric Handbook* was produced by the publications unit of the Department of Paediatrics and Child Health at the University of Cape Town in 1975. Compiled and edited by the late Associate Professor Robert MacDonald and Dr Roy Cooke, the project was made possible by support from the Peninsula Round Table 77 and the Ethical Drug Foundation.

Under the editorship of Dr Roy Cooke, the contents of the 1975 edition were extensively updated and expanded in 1987. The task of its publication had outstripped the resources of the department, and the second edition was published by HAUM Educational Publishers.

The third edition was published by Oxford University Press in 1992 and edited by Professor H de V Heese who was the Head of the Department of Paediatrics and Child Health of the University of Cape Town between 1970 and 1990.

The Paediatric Handbook has aimed at fulfilling the needs of staff of Cape Town's teaching hospitals over the years, as well as the needs of medical practitioners, under- and post-graduate medical students, nursing staff and health personnel in Southern Africa. The fourth edition (renamed: *Handbook of Paediatrics*) has adhered to this philosophy and incorporates numerous revisions and suggestions received from readers.

The handbook is a tribute to the many staff members of the University of Cape Town who are involved with the care of children, and whose contributions over many years have made the *Handbook of Paediatrics* possible.

D W Beatty
Professor and Head of the Department of Paediatrics and Child Health
University of Cape Town

CONTRIBUTORS

C M Adnams BSc (Natal), BSc Hons (*Cape Town*), MB ChB (*Cape Town*), FCP(*SA*) Paed
Lecturer and Paediatrician

A Allie MB ChB (*Cape Town*), FCP(*SA*) Paed
Senior Lecturer and Senior Paediatrician

A C Argent MB BCh, MMed(Paed) (*Witwatersrand*), FCP(*SA*) Paed, DCH(*SA*)
Senior Lecturer and Senior Paediatrician

D H Bass MB ChB, MMed(Surg) (*Cape Town*), FCS(*SA*)
Senior Lecturer and Senior Surgeon

D W Beatty MB ChB, MD (*Cape Town*), FCP(*SA*) Paed
Professor of Paediatrics and Child Health and Head of the Department of Paediatrics and Child Health

E M Bhettay MA (*Madras*), MB BCh, BAO (*NUI*), FRCP (*Edin & Glas*), DCH RCP & S (*Eng*)
Senior Lecturer and Senior Paediatrician

F Bonnici MB ChB, MMed(Paed) (*Cape Town*), FCP(*SA*) Paed
Associate Professor and Principal Paediatrician

M D Bowie BSc (*Natal*), MB ChB, MD (*Cape Town*), FRCP (*Edin*), DCH RCP & S (*Eng*)
Emeritus Associate Professor of Paediatrics and Child Health, University of Cape Town

R A Brown MB ChB (*Cape Town*), FRCS (*Edin*), FCS(*SA*), DCH RCP & S (*Eng*)
Senior Lecturer and Senior Surgeon

A D Butt MB ChB (*Cape Town*), FFA(*SA*)
Senior Lecturer and Principal Anaesthetist, Head of the Department of Anaesthesia at

	Red Cross War Memorial Children's Hospital
B J Cremin	MD (*Cape Town*), MB BS (*London*), MRCS, LRCPD(Obst), DRCOG (*Eng*), FRACR (*Aust*), FRCR (*Eng*) *Associate Professor and Head of the Department of Paediatric Radiology*
S Cywes	MB ChB, MMed(Surg) (*Cape Town*), FACS(Ped), FRCS (*Eng*), FRCS (*Edin*), FRCPS (*Glasg*), FAAP *Charles F M Saint Professor of Paediatric Surgery and Head of the Department of Paediatric Surgery*
M M A de Moor	MB BCh (*Witwatersrand*), FCP(*SA*) Paed *Senior Lecturer and Senior Paediatrician*
R M Fisher	MB ChB (*Cape Town*), DMRD RCP & S (*Eng*) *Senior Lecturer and Senior Radiologist*
S E Franco	MB ChB, MMed(Chem Path) (*Cape Town*) *Lecturer and Clinical Pathologist*
R D Gilbert	MB ChB, MMed(Paed) (*Cape Town*), FCP(*SA*) Paed, DCH (*SA*) *Lecturer and Paediatrician*
A Grobler	B Sc Diet, Dip Thera Diet (*Stell*) *Principal Dietitian, Red Cross War Memorial Children's Hospital*
D H Hanslo	MB ChB, MMed(Path) Microb (*Cape Town*), FF Path(*SA*) Microb , FRC(Path) *Senior Lecturer and Senior Microbiologist*
V C Harrison	MB ChB, MD, MMed(Paed) (*Cape Town*), DCH RCP & S (*Eng*) *Associate Professor and Principal Paediatrician*
P S Hartley	MB ChB (*Cape Town*), FCP(*SA*) Paed *Senior Lecturer and Senior Paediatrician*
H de V Heese	BSc (*Stell*), MB ChB, MD (*Cape Town*), FRCP (*Edin*), DCH RCP & S (*Eng*) *Emeritus Professor of Paediatrics and Child Health, University of Cape Town*

L D Henley	PhD (*Cape Town*) *Lecturer, Department of Paediatrics and Child Health*
E B Hoffman	MB ChB (*Stell*), FCS(*SA*) Orth *Senior Lecturer and Senior Orthopaedic Surgeon*
G D Hussey	MB ChB, MMed(Com Health) (*Cape Town*), FFCH(*SA*), DTM & H RCP & S (*Eng*), MSc CTM (*London*) *Senior Lecturer and Senior Paediatrician*
J D Ireland	MB ChB, MD (*Cape Town*), FCP(*SA*) Paed *Senior Lecturer and Senior Paediatrician*
C D Karabus	MB ChB, MMed(Paed) (*Cape Town*), FRCP (*Edin*), FRCP (*London*), DCH RCP & S (*Eng*) *Associate Professor and Principal Paediatrician*
M A Kibel	MB BCh (*Witwatersrand*), FRCP (*Edin*), DCH RCP & S (*Eng*) *Stella and Paul Loewenstein Professor of Child Health and Head of the Child Health Unit*
M Klein	MB ChB (*Cape Town*), FCP(*SA*) Paed *Associate Professor and Senior Paediatrician*
P I Lachman	BA, MB BCh (*Witwatersrand*), MMed(Paed) (*Cape Town*), DCH, FCP(*SA*) Paed *Senior Lecturer and Senior Paediatrician*
P M Leary	MB ChB, MD (*Cape Town*), FCP(*SA*) Paed, DCH, DA RCP & S (*Eng*), D Obst RCOG *Associate Professor and Principal Paediatrician*
M D Mann	MB ChB, PhD, MMed(NucMed), MMed(Paed) (*Cape Town*) *Associate Professor and Principal Paediatrician*

A J W Millar
MB ChB, FRCS (*Eng*), FRCS (*Edin*), FRACS, DCH RCP & S (*Eng*)
Associate Professor and Principal Paediatric Surgeon

A D N Murray
MB BCh (*Witwatersrand*), FRCS (*Edin*)
Morris Mauerberger Professor of Ophthalmology and Head of the Department of Ophthalmology

J C Peter
MB ChB (*Cape Town*), FRCS (*Edin*)
Helen and Morris Mauerberger Professor and Head of Department of Neurosurgery

A Philotheou
MB ChB, BA Hons (*Cape Town*)
Lecturer and Principal Medical Officer, Department of Paediatrics and Child Health

D J Power
BSc, MB BS (*London*), MD (*Cape Town*), MRCP (*UK*), DCM (*Cape Town*), DCH RCP & S (*Eng*)
Professor of Paediatrics and Child Health

H M Power
BSc Hons, MB BCh (*Witwatersrand*), MD (*Cape Town*), DCH(*SA*)
Lecturer and Paediatrician, Department of Paediatrics and Child Health

C A J Prescott
MB ChB (*St Andrew's*), FRCS (*Eng*)
Senior Lecturer and Principal Ear, Nose and Throat Surgeon

L R Purves
MB BCh, MMed(Path) (*Witwatersrand*)
Associate Professor and Principal Chemical Pathologist

H Rode
MB ChB, MMed(Surg) (*Pretoria*), FCS(*SA*), FRCS (*Edin*)
Associate Professor and Principal Paediatric Surgeon

P Roux
MD (*Cape Town*), FCP(SA) Paed, DCH(*SA*)
Senior Lecturer and Senior Paediatrician

N Saxe
MB ChB (*Cape Town*), FF Derm(*SA*)
Associate Professor and Head of the Department of Dermatology

A A Sive   MB ChB, MD (*Cape Town*), FCP(*SA*)
                        Paed, DCH(*SA*)
                        Senior Lecturer and Senior Paediatrician

L S Smith   MB BCh (*Witwatersrand*), DPH (*Cape
                        Town*), D Bact (*London*), FRC Path (*UK*)
                        *Emeritus Professor of Forensic Medicine
                        and Toxicology and Extraordinarius Pro-
                        fessor of the Law Faculty, UNISA*

**Staff of the Pharmacy, Red Cross War Memorial Children's
                        Hospital**

**Staff of the Poison Reference Centre, Institute of Child
                        Health, Red Cross War Memorial Chil-
                        dren's Hospital**

A J G Thomson   MB ChB, MMed(Paed), MMed(Neuro)
                        (*Cape Town*), FCP(*SA*) Paed
                        *Senior Lecturer and Principal Paediatri-
                        cian*

C W van der Elst   MB ChB, MD (*Cape Town*), FCP(*SA*)
                        Paed, DCH RCP & S (*Eng*)
                        Senior Lecturer and Senior Paediatrician

E G Weinberg   MB ChB (*Cape Town*), FCP(*SA*) Paed
                        *Associate Professor and Principal Paedia-
                        trician*

J Wiggelinkhuizen   MB BCh (*Witwatersrand*), MMed(Paed)
                        (*Cape Town*), FCP(*SA*) Paed
                        *Associate Professor and Principal Paedia-
                        trician*

D L Woods   MB ChB, MD (*Cape Town*), FRCP (*UK*),
                        DCH RCP & S (*Eng*)
                        *Associate Professor and Senior Paediatri-
                        cian*

PREFACE

The principal aim of the *Handbook of Paediatrics* is to provide concise, clear advice which accommodates the needs and time constraints of health-care workers, with an emphasis on the immediate management of life-threatening states, and the early management of common clinical conditions.

The aim of the writers and compilers of the fourth edition of the *Handbook of Paediatrics* has been to produce a handbook which can support medical workers in a wider range of situations in southern Africa.

It is an enormous challenge to achieve a balance between the needs of staff in a tertiary care centre and those in settings with limited facilities. In a developing country, health professionals working in a primary health care facility are often called upon to provide a level of care allocated to secondary levels in developed countries. Bearing this in mind, we have added a number of sections and chapters that are aimed at helping those who do not have quick access to library facilities or expert opinion.

The development of the *Handbook of Paediatrics* since 1975 is the product of contributions from past editors, authors and users. Suggestions and criticism from the latter have played a major role in influencing changes to successive editions and impressions of the *Handbook*. The task of the editor was considerably eased by Professor David Beatty and his colleagues who gave their full support; Ms Diane du Toit, who typed the manuscript; and Professor Mike Mann who provided welcome advice.

H de V Heese
Editor

CONTENTS

EMERGENCY REFERENCES

1 RESUSCITATION

A C Argent and D H Bass

Cardiorespiratory arrest is most frequently the result of:

♦ hypoxia related to respiratory infections or a foreign body;
♦ shock from hypovolaemia or of cardiogenic origin;
♦ convulsions; or
♦ a combination of the above.

Cardiac arrythmias are an unusual cause of arrest in children unless severe electrolyte abnormalities (particularly potassium) are present, or if drug overdose (especially tricyclic antidepressants) has occurred.

If at all possible, respiratory and cardiorespiratory arrests should be prevented by early and vigorous treatment of hypoxia and shock. An 'unexpected arrest' in hospital should always be regarded as a possible failure of medical management.

Children at risk of cardiorespiratory arrest should ideally be managed where monitoring facilities are available, and the equipment for resuscitation is readily at hand.

Areas where children may need resuscitation must be provided with appropriate equipment of the right size for a range of ages.

Although resuscitation of the collapsed child is the immediate priority, care must be taken to screen other patients from unpleasant scenes. If parents are present it is important to keep them informed of progress and, if possible, the anticipated outcome.

If there is any doubt as to whether cardiopulmonary resuscitation (CPR) should be attempted then begin the process, and review the decision as soon as more information is available.

Basic cardiopulmonary resuscitation

Note the time of onset of resuscitation. If possible, have someone available to document medication and progress, otherwise collect all the ampoules that are used and total them at the end.

The standard approach of A (airway), B (breathing), C (circulation) should be employed. The ABC should be completed using basic measures, after which additional support measures should be implemented.

Airway

◆ **Clear** the airway by removing debris or vomitus by suction, or if suction is not available, by tipping the head to one side and wiping debris away with a finger.
◆ **Extend** the neck slightly and lift the jaw by pulling the angle of the mandible forward. (Do not overextend. If the child is injured, take care with neck movement.)
◆ **Consider** the possibility of a **foreign body**. If likely:
  ◇ Child older than five years: **Apply Heimlich manoeuvre**. Make a fist with one hand immediately below the xiphisternum, grasp it with the other hand and apply force (one to six times) in the direction of the upper thoracic spine.
  ◇ Child under five years: **Place the child face down** on your arm and deliver one to four sharp blows to the lower thoracic back with the other hand.

Warning

Do not blindly insert objects into the mouth in order to remove a foreign body, as this may lodge an object more firmly.

Breathing

◆ **Check** if any respiratory effort is present.
◆ **Apply** artificial ventilation if no respiratory effort is present.

Method of artificial ventilation

Bag and facemask preferable if available.
Mouth to mouth ventilation. (CDC guidelines suggest that HIV transmission is only a risk if blood is present, MMWR 1988; 37:377-388.)

◆ **Maintain** the position of airway patency.
◆ **Place** your mouth over the patient's nose and mouth in the smaller child. In the older child cover only the mouth and **obstruct** the nose with fingers. (Alternatively, cover the nose and close the mouth.)

◆ **Administer** slow breaths of 0,5-1 second duration.
◆ **Apply** enough pressure to visibly move the chest. If inordinate pressure is required, then check the position of the head, insert an oral airway and exclude a foreign body by inspecting the oropharynx and laryngeal inlet with the aid of a laryngoscope.
◆ **Rate:** In a small child give 20-25 breaths/minute. In the older child, 15 breaths/minute.
◆ **Provide** 100% oxygen to the mouth of the patient as soon as possible at a rate of at least 2-5 litres/minute.

Cardiac action

◆ **Check** the carotid (in an older child), femoral or the brachial pulse.
◆ **Apply** cardiac compression if a pulse is not palpable or very slow.

Method of cardiac compression

◆ Small child: **grasp both sides of the chest with the hands. Compress** the lower third of the sternum with thumbs.
◆ Older child: **place the child in the supine position. Apply pressure** to the lower third of the sternum with the heel of the hand.
◆ The **force of the compression** should depress the chest by approximately one third of the antero-posterior diameter.
◆ **Rate**: 80-100 beats per minute.
◆ **Continue** with ventilation between chest compressions.
◆ **Continue** cardiac compression until pulses are again palpable or a decision is made to discontinue resuscitation. See page 7.

Advanced cardiopulmonary resuscitation

Airway

Intubation

Adequate ventilation can usually be achieved by using a face-mask and bag. Intubation is indicated if there is: difficulty with face mask ventilation, inadequate oxygenation, gastric distension with high risk of regurgitation and aspiration, or if ongoing ventilation will be necessary.

Method

- **Provide** oxygen during the procedure.
- **Place** the child on its back with the head in a neutral position (do not overextend the neck).
- **Use** the largest laryngoscope blade that can be easily accommodated in the child's mouth.
- **Use** the smallest endotracheal tube (ETT) recommended. See chart inside front cover and on page 8. If there is not a leak past the endotracheal tube at pressures of >25 cm H_2O then the endotracheal tube should be replaced with a smaller tube as soon as possible.

Breathing

Check if the ETT position is appropriate.

- **Insert** a large nasogastric tube to decompress the stomach.
- If the ETT position is appropriate and the chest is difficult to ventilate, **consider a possible pneumothorax**. Insert bilateral intercostal drains if there is any doubt.

Cardiac

Cardiac output

Assess the cardiac output by feeling peripheral pulses and checking the capillary refill time (CRT). Easily palpable peripheral pulses and a CRT similar to that of the observer indicate good cardiac output and further management can be directed to the underlying cause of the arrest.

Poorly palpable or absent peripheral pulses, together with a prolonged CRT indicate inadequate cardiac output and the need for further support.

Check the venous pressure (neck veins and liver size).

- Collapsed neck veins and a normal size liver indicate hypovolaemia (see pages 7 and 10 for management): 20 ml/kg of fluid should be given rapidly.
- Distended neck veins and an enlarged liver indicate volume overload or cardiac malfunction. Exclude a pneumothorax. If there is no pneumothorax, check for pericardial effusion (barely audible heart sounds, poor to absent cardiac impulse) and if necessary perform pericardiocentesis. If there is no pericardial collection, treat with diuretics and inotropic support (see page 12).

Method of pericardiocentesis

♦ Attach a 10 ml syringe to a narrow gauge needle (21 or 22 gauge).

♦ Insert subxiphoid and advance slowly under the ribs towards the left midclavicle while aspirating constantly (if available, an ECG electrode should be attached to the needle with an alligator clip to identify myocardial activity).

♦ Withdraw any fluid. Withdrawal of pericardial blood should be associated with rapid improvement. Pericardial blood does not clot in the syringe.

Check an ECG trace

♦ Abnormally wide QRS complex: give calcium and sodium bicarbonate intravenously and get electrolyte results as quickly as possible.

♦ Asystole: repeat ADRENALINE.

♦ Bradycardia: repeat ADRENALINE and add ATROPINE if no response.

♦ Ventricular tachycardia: treat with intravenous LIGNO-CAINE.

♦ Ventricular fibrillation: defibrillate.

♦ Normal QRS complex and no heart sounds: give calcium and ADRENALINE for electromechanical dissociation.

Drugs

While cardiopulmonary resuscitation is being carried out, another person should attempt to obtain vascular access (see Table 1.1).

Route of administration

♦ **Intravenous**: via a free-running drip. Ensure that excessive amounts of fluid do not run into the patient during the resuscitation. Mini-droppers (60 drops per ml) should be used on all drips unless hypovolaemia (see page 10) is thought to be responsible for the arrest. If the patient is hypovolaemic then 5 or 15 drops/ml-giving sets should be used.

Table 1.1: Vascular access

Route	Sites	Comment
Intra-osseus	Medial aspect of upper tibia	Insert 15-18 gauge needle until 'give' indicates marrow cavity. Dilute any irritant solutions very well.
Peripheral vein	Dorsum of hands, scalp in younger children, feet and cubital fossa	Can almost always use if experienced. Can also be used as cut-down sites. Cut-down on the saphenous vein at the ankle may provide rapid venous access.
Central vein	Cubital fossa cut-down	Ideal for CVP monitoring and fluid administration. Do not use jugular or subclavian push-ins.
	Femoral vein	Probably safest site for the insertion of a central line by Seldinger technique.

Note: Drugs should be injected into the drip-giving set as close to the patient as possible. With slow drip rates and long extension sets it may take a long time for the drugs to reach the patient.

Specific agents

See Paediatric Resuscitation Chart (page 8).
- ◆ ADRENALINE: given in all cases of cardiac arrest. Respiratory arrest does not usually require drugs if the heart rate picks up rapidly.
- ◆ SODIUM BICARBONATE: provides no benefit during acute resuscitation unless hyperkalaemia is thought to have precipitated the cardiac arrest or there is an underlying severe metabolic acidosis secondary to bicarbonate loss.

Note

ADRENALINE is not effective intratracheally in standard doses. ATROPINE is effective when given intratracheally.

Hypothermia

The patient should be covered while resuscitation continues. If the patient appears cold on arrival then warming should be instituted, using heating blankets and overhead lamps.

Electrolyte, acid base and glucose status

◆ **Collect a blood specimen** for estimation of blood gases and electrolyte concentrations. This may help provide an explanation of the arrest and will provide a basis for further electrolyte and acid base management. (See pages 212-3.)
◆ **Check** blood glucose immediately at the bedside.

Treat any underlying problems

Detailed discussion of the management of underlying problems will be found in the appropriate chapters of this book.

If the aetiology of the arrest is not clear, consider convulsions and treat with anticonvulsants. See page 340.

Termination of resuscitation

Indications

◆ Review of records reveals clinical decision not to resuscitate.
◆ No heart beat after ten minutes of CPR.
◆ Exclusion of treatable causes such as pneumothorax, cardiac tamponade, hypovolaemia, hypothermia (<34 °C), hypoglycaemia and electrolyte problems.
◆ No spontaneous respiration after one hour of resuscitation and correction of all possible abnormalities.

Treatment of shock

Shock is a state in which there is inadequate perfusion of the tissues.

Pathogenesis

Shock is the result of:

◆ **Absolute hypovolaemia**
   Examples: gastroenteritis, trauma with haemorrhage, burns. These are the most common causes of shock. The extent of fluid loss may be concealed in serous cavities, tissue interstitium, or the gastrointestinal tract.

Figure 1.1 Paediatric resuscitation chart[†]

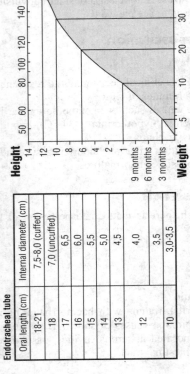

To use this chart, select the smallest endotracheal tube appropriate to a specific age. An estimate of age can be made from either the weight or the height of the child.

Endotracheal tube

Oral length (cm)	Internal diameter (cm)
18-21	7,5-8,0 (cuffed)
18	7,0 (uncuffed)
17	6,5
16	6,0
15	5,5
14	5,0
13	4,5
12	4,0
	3,5
10	3,0-3,5

	5	10	20	30	40	50 kg	Indications
ADRENALINE (ml of 1 in 10 000) *initial* intravenous or intra-osseous	0,5	1	2	3	4	5	Bradycardia (after adequate ventilation) Asystole
ADRENALINE (ml of 1 in 1 000) *subsequent* intravenous or intra-osseous (or *initial* endotracheal)	0,5	1	2	3	4	5	
* ATROPINE (ml of 100 µg/ml) intravenous or intra-osseous (or double if endotracheal)	1	2	4	6	6	6	Bradycardia
Sodium bicarbonate (ml of 8,4%) intravenous or intra-osseous (dilute to 4,2% in infants)	5	10	20	30	40	50	Hyperkalaemia with ECG changes

Height

14
12
10
8
6
4
2
1
9 months
6 months
3 months

Weight

*Calcium chloride (ml of 10%) intravenous or intra-osseous	0,5	1	2	3	4	5	Hyperkalaemia Hypocalcaemia
DIAZEPAM (ml of 5 mg/ml emulsion) intravenous or rectal	0,4	0,8	1,6	2	2	2	Convulsions
Glucose (ml of 50%) intravenous or intra-osseous (dilute to 25% in infants)	5	10	20	30	40	50	Hypoglycaemia
*LIGNOCAINE (ml of 1%)(without ADRENALINE) intravenous or intra-osseous	0,5	1	2	3	4	5	Ventricular tachycardia
NALOXONE *neonatal* (ml of 20 µg/ml) intravenous or intra-osseous	2,5	5	—	—	—	—	Opiate overdose
NALOXONE *adult* (ml of 400 µg/ml)	—	0,25	0,5	0,75	1	1,25	
Initial DC defibrillation (J) for ventricular fibrillation or pulseless ventricular tachycardia	10	20	40	60	80	100	
Initial DC cardioversion (J) for supraventricular tachycardia with shock (synchronous) or ventricular tachycardia with shock (non-synchronous)	5	5	10	15	20	25	
Initial fluid bolus in shock (ml) crystalloid or colloid	100	200	400	600	800	1000	

* Caution! Non-standard drug concentrations may be available:
Use ATROPINE 100 µg/ml or prepare by diluting 1 mg to 10 ml or 500 µg to 5 ml in physiological saline.
Note that 1 ml of calcium chloride 10% is equivalent to 3 ml of calcium gluconate 10%
† Modified from Oakley PA. *Br Med J* 1993; 306: 1613.

◆ **Relative hypovolaemia**
Examples: spinal injury or disturbance of peripheral vascular tone.
◆ **Decreased myocardial contractability**
Examples: myocarditis, myocardial contusion. Included in this category is mechanical disturbance, as in cardiac tamponade or tension pneumothorax.
◆ **Septic shock**
Example: a combination of the above mechanisms.

Clinical presentation

◆ Cold peripheries with poorly palpable peripheral pulses, tachycardia and hypertension.
◆ Respiratory distress, an altered level of consciousness and a diminished urinary output.

Note: homeostatic mechanisms will defend the blood pressure until late in the process. **Hypotension is a very late manifestation of shock.**

Assessment

Check neck veins, liver size, heart sounds, bleeding points and blood pressure.

◆ If the veins in the neck are not distended, or the liver is not enlarged: hypovolaemia.
◆ Distended veins, audible gallop rhythm on auscultation or poorly-heard heart sounds: poor myocardial contractability.
◆ Heart sounds poorly audible on auscultation: exclude pneumothorax and cardiac tamponade.
◆ If there is doubt as to whether or not the shock is hypovolaemic, give a fluid challenge of 5 ml/kg rapidly, using a syringe and three-way tap. Assess response.

Management

Patients in shock should not be moved until an adequate circulatory volume has been established. If adequate cardiac output has not been established, the patient should be intubated prior to any transfer.

Assessed as hypovolaemic from blood loss

Secure and control active bleeding site(s) as rapidly as possible.

Improve oxygenation

◆ Provide oxygen supplementation to all patients with shock, initially with a face mask or a nasal catheter or head box.

◆ **Intubate** and provide ventilatory support if a depressed or altered level of consciousness persists, $PaCO_2 > 5$ kPa (37,5 mmHg) in the face of acidosis (pH <7,25), increasing respiratory distress, or inadequate oxygenation (saturation <90%) despite above measures.

Ensure adequate circulatory volume

Vascular access — see Table 1.1.

Assessed as hypovolaemic

Give 20 ml/kg fluid IV immediately. Colloids such as plasma or Haemaccel may be used; crystalloids such as Ringer's lactate or normal saline (i.e. electrolyte concentration approximates that of serum) are also appropriate, although these move out of the intravascular compartment more rapidly than do colloids. Syringes attached to three-way taps should be used to give fluid as rapidly as possible.

Note: the use of microdroppers for hypovolaemic patients is inappropriate, as adequate fluid volumes cannot be administered rapidly.

Assessed as possibly hypovolaemic

Give fluid challenge of 5 ml/kg rapidly (see fluids noted under "Assessed as hypovolaemic"). Re-assess. If there is still no evidence of venous distension and perfusion is not adequate, keep giving fluid boluses of 5 ml/kg rapidly until a response is obtained.

Failure of fluid challenge

◆ Venous pressure can be measured using a peripheral venous line if it is free-flowing.

◆ If lower than 10-12 cm H_2O: give more fluid.

◆ If higher than 10-12 cm H_2O: reassess as to whether the reading is an accurate reflection or an over-reading. Insert a central venous line to measure central venous pressure (CVP). See Table 1.1 for venous access.

Table 1.2 Drugs for cardiogenic shock

Drug	Dose
Inotropes:	
DOPAMINE	5-20 mcg/kg/min
DOBUTAMINE	5-20 mcg/kg/min
ADRENALINE	0,05 - 1 mcg/kg/min
After-load reduction:	
NITROPRUSSIDE	0,5 - 9 mcg/kg/min

DOPAMINE and DOBUTAMINE can be mixed together in 5% dextrose solution.

To prepare solution:

$$\frac{\text{Required dose of drug (µg/kg/min) x 6 x weight (kg)}}{\text{Drip rate (ml/min)}}$$

= number of mg of drug to be added to each 100 ml of fluid to give the desired dose.

◆ Institute inotropic support if the CVP is >10 cm H_2O and perfusion is not adequate. See 'drug infusion' below.

Improve myocardial contractability

Electrolytes

See pages 213-4.

◆ Correct electrolytic abnormalities. Calcium and potassium concentrations are the most critical.
◆ Correct hypokalaemia before correction of hypocalcaemia is attempted.

Drug infusion

◆ Start with inotropic support, using DOPAMINE and/or DOBUTAMINE (see Table 1.2 for dosage).
◆ If the heart rate is not appropriately rapid i.e. (<120/m in child under one year, or <100/m in an older child) use ADRENALINE for chronotropic activity.

♦ Use NITROPRUSSIDE to decrease afterload only if there is an adequate pre-load, i.e. CVP >10 cm H_2O and blood pressure is higher than 90 mmHg systolic.

Aim to maintain a systolic blood pressure of more than 90 mmHg.

Warning

Long-acting cardiac drugs such as DIGOXIN are contra-indicated in the acute management of shock.

Monitoring

Monitor vital signs and response to treatment

Heart rate, capillary-filling time and blood pressure. Respiratory rate. Level of consciousness.

Monitor oxygenation

Pulse oximeter (if available). Blood gases. Maintain PaO_2 11-16 kPa (80-120 mmHg) with adequate ventilatory support. Correct pH of <7,1 with sodium bicarbonate if ventilation is adequate.

Monitor urine output

Check volume, specific gravity and pH. A urinary catheter should be inserted.

Treat underlying condition(s)

For details see the chapter appropriate to the condition.

2 ALLERGIC DISORDERS

E G Weinberg

It is estimated that 20% of all South African children are affected by allergy, and the statistic is increasing. The reason for the increase is unknown but it may be associated with socio-economic factors and rapid urbanization.

Many environmental factors probably contribute to the sensitization of an allergy-prone subject in early life. The season of the year when the child is born; parental smoking; residence in damp homes, or homes with high housedust mite and mould exposure, and increasing industrial pollution are all associated with an increased risk of allergy development.

Recent genetic studies suggest that atopy (the ability of a child to produce high concentrations of IgE directed against common allergens) may be inherited and is carried on chromosome 11 as an autosomal dominant with variable penetrance. Most allergic children have a strong family history of allergy.

An allergic reaction is an altered response to an antigen or allergen. Once an allergic individual has been sensitized to an allergen, specific IgE antibodies develop. The combination of allergen and IgE located on the surface of mast cells in the respiratory and gastrointestinal tracts or the skin, results in the release of potent chemical mediators from the cell granules. Among these are histamine, serotonin, eosinophil chemotactic factor (ECF) and neutrophil chemotactic factor (NCF). Metabolic products of arachidonic acid metabolism in the mast cell membrane release potent smooth muscle constrictors and inflammatory agents, including leukotrienes and prostaglandins. An early and late phase inflammatory action occurs, resulting in the characteristic clinical features associated with common allergic disorders.

Asthma, allergic rhinitis, food allergy and anaphylaxis are covered in this chapter. Atopic eczema and urticaria are discussed in Chapter 44.

Allergic disorders tend to develop at different ages in children – the so-called 'allergic march'. Atopic eczema often presents in early infancy. Food allergy is also more common at this stage. Asthma and allergic rhinitis usually present between the ages of two and five years, although there is always much individual variation. It is common for two or more allergic disorders, e.g. rhinitis and asthma, to be present in the same child.

Asthma

Definition

Asthma is a difficult condition to define but should be diagnosed whenever a child has recurrent wheezing or cough which responds to a bronchodilator. Of note is that about 5-10% of children with asthma present with a chronic cough without wheezing.

Pathophysiology

There have been many changes in the concepts held about the mechanisms and mediators involved in asthma. Inflammation plays a very important role in most cases, as do bronchospasm and airway hyperreactivity to physical and environmental stimuli. None of these mechanisms occur in all cases of asthma, which remains a complex disease with various degrees of severity.

Diagnosis

Childhood asthma often presents with sudden acute attacks usually initiated by viral infections. The diagnostic problem is often made more difficult in young children because of their inability to perform simple pulmonary function tests.

The initial approach to diagnosis is to take an adequate history followed by the physical examination. The history includes the family history and the patient's symptoms. This helps to exclude conditions which mimic asthma, e.g. inhaled foreign body, cystic fibrosis, bronchiolitis.

Investigations should include simple pulmonary function studies, either peak flow or FEV_1, to establish a baseline prior to treatment. If airflow obstruction is present the diagnosis can be confirmed by showing significant improvement of >15% in peak flow or FEV_1 after an inhaled β_2 agonist. Most children from about five or six years are able to perform these studies very well. Unfortunately this technique cannot be used in younger children.

A therapeutic trial with a bronchodilator may confirm the

diagnosis of asthma much more efficiently. A record of the changes in peak flow rates measured at home, especially if entered in a carefully kept diary, will show response to medication. This approach yields as much definitive information as an exercise or histamine challenge.

Skin tests

Most asthmatic children are atopic and limited skin testing to determine possible sensitivity to environmental allergens is useful. Once the offending allergen has been identified, parents can be counselled on ways to limit exposure. The recommended skin prick tests are to housedust mites (*Dermatophagoides pteronyssinus*), cats, dogs and South African grasses. A saline-negative control and histamine-positive control should always be included in the test series in case the patient has dermatographism or has received antihistamines prior to the test. CAPRAST tests, although more expensive, are a useful alternative if skin prick tests cannot be performed for any reason.

Education

Parent education and, where appropriate, child education as to the nature of asthma is essential. Careful explanation is required regarding the role and use of various medications. It is preferable to provide written instructions on the use of medicines and especially the treatment of acute attacks. Parents need to know when they should seek medical assistance.

Environmental control

Avoidance measures may be effective in lessening the symptoms of asthma as long as they are carried out correctly. Clear written instructions should be provided for parents. It is especially important to advise on ways of reducing housedust mite or pet exposure in the child's bedroom. The need to prevent the exposure of the asthmatic child to cigarette smoke cannot be overemphasized.

Psychological factors

These do not actually cause asthma, but can have a significant effect on the frequency and severity of attacks. Stress and anxiety may result in acute asthma attacks. If a child does not respond to treatment as anticipated, the possibility of underlying psychological or family problems or poor use of medications should be considered. Teachers should be aware of a child's asthma and treatment and they should also know how to handle emergencies.

The acute attack

Clinical presentation

Do not underestimate the severity of an asthma attack. Signs of a severe attack include anxiety, restlessness, tachycardia and intense wheezing on auscultation. Whispering speech and pulsus paradoxus indicate severe airway obstruction. Measurement of the peak flow is the most useful objective assessment of the degree of airway obstruction.

Treatment with bronchodilators

Inhalation

◆ β_2 agonist bronchodilators in inhaled form are the most useful drugs for treating acute attacks of asthma. Metered dose inhaler (MDI) bronchodilators, such as SALBUTAMOL (Ventolin) or FENOTEROL (Berotec) 2 puffs (200 µg), may be administered every two or three hours. The powder forms of these inhalers require active inhalation which may be beyond the ability of a child with a bad attack of asthma.
◆ For young children, a paper cup may be used, with a hole large enough to take the mouthpiece of a MDI cut in it. The cup is held over the child's mouth and three or four puffs of the MDI fired into it. The cup usually fits snugly over the face and little medication is lost. Excellent bronchodilatation results when this method is used.
◆ If there is no response to the inhaler, either initially or after a second dose 30 minutes later, the child should be treated as for acute severe asthma. See pages 18-20.

Nebulization

Several home nebulizers are available. They are simple air compressors which nebulize SALBUTAMOL or FENOTEROL respirator solution via a facemask nebulizer. It should be remembered that air and not oxygen is being used to nebulize the bronchodilator, and this may be a disadvantage.

In infants and children under two years

Add 0,5 ml IPRATROPIUM BROMIDE SOLUTION to 1 ml of

normal saline and nebulize three to four hourly. SALBUTA-
MOL or FENOTEROL SOLUTION 0,5 ml may be combined
with the IPRATROPIUM BROMIDE.

Over two years of age

Add 1 ml SALBUTAMOL or FENOTEROL SOLUTION to
1 ml normal saline and administer three to four-hourly. IPRA-
TROPIUM BROMIDE SOLUTION 1 ml may be added to this
mixture.

If there is no response to two nebulizations given 30 minutes
apart then the child must be managed as for acute severe
asthma.

Acute severe asthma (status asthmaticus)

This is diagnosed when:

◆ there is no response to two puffs of a β_2 agonist bronchodilator given 30 minutes apart; or
◆ there is no response to two nebulizations with a β_2 agonist
  bronchodilator.

Acute severe asthma may occur in any asthmatic child, usually
quite suddenly. There is no response to the usual methods of
treatment, probably because of severe inflammation of the airway mucosa and plugging caused by thick tenacious mucus
plugs. Precipitating factors include allergen exposure, viral
infections, weather changes or emotional upsets. It is quite common for no cause to be found.

**Acute severe asthma must be regarded as a medical emer-
gency.**

Clinical presentation

◆ An anxious patient with laboured breathing, audible wheeze
  and tachypnoea which interfere with speech and feeding.
◆ Marked hyperinflation of the chest with use of the accessory
  muscles of respiration.
◆ Markedly diminished breath sounds with intense wheezing
  noted on auscultation.
◆ Pulsus paradoxus >10 mmHg during inspiration.

Management of acute severe asthma

A simple way to remember which treatment is required is to
use the '4H's': **Hospitalize,** treat **Hypoxaemia,** administer

HYDROCORTISONE (or other IV corticosteroid) and **hydrate** the child adequately.

Hospital

The child must be admitted to hospital, preferably to an intensive care unit.

Oxygen

Give oxygen by facemask or nasal prongs.

Hydration

Set up IV drip with 5% dextrose water at 60-80 ml/kg/24 hours.

Medications

♦ Nebulize with β_2 agonist preparations. Give: 1 ml of SALBUTAMOL or FENOTEROL respirator solution diluted with 1 ml of normal saline in the nebulizer. Repeat two to three-hourly.

♦ HYDROCORTISONE 2 mg/kg IV or METHYLPREDNISOLONE or DEXAMETHASONE, irrespective of whether the child has previously had steroid therapy or not. The dose is repeated every six hours except for DEXAMETHASONE which is given once. The majority of children improve by this time. Convert to an oral PREDNISONE course for five to ten days after an episode of acute severe asthma. Improvement should be monitored with a peak flow meter.

♦ AMINOPHYLLIN must be used with caution as severe side-effects may occur in children. It should only be used where facilities for measuring the serum levels are available and the child is in a high care unit or ICU.

Doses to be used are as follows:

Loading dose: AMINOPHYLLIN 6 mg/kg IV over ten minutes (if the child has not had any theophyllin therapy in the previous 24 hours). If the child has had theophyllin previously, a constant infusion of 0,5 mg/kg/hour is used following measurement of the serum level. This infusion rate can be achieved by using the following guide:

◇ Add 2 ml of AMINOPHYLLIN (250 mg/10 ml) to 100 ml 5% dextrose water.

◇ Select a 60 drops/ml drip administration set.

◇ Weight of patient in kg.

◇ Set the drip rate per minute to correspond with the patient's weight in kg.

Note

♦ If the patient responds poorly to therapy, arterial blood gases should be monitored as necessary.
♦ ECG monitoring is essential if IV AMINOPHYLLIN is being given.
♦ Continuous low flow oxygen to keep the PaO_2 above 8 kPa (60 mmHg) must be administered via nasal prongs.
♦ Do not overhydrate the patient.
♦ Monitor peak flow levels at least every six hours.

Danger signs in acute severe asthma

Restlessness
Peak flow <60% of predicted
Rising pulse rate
Rising $PaCO_2$ >4,7 kPa (>35 mmHg)
'Silent chest' on auscultation
PaO_2 of 7 kPa (50 mmHg) or less
Chest pain (intrathoracic air leak)
Disturbance in level of consciousness

Table 2.1 Classification of asthma

	Frequency of wheezing or coughing	Night cough or wheeze	Hospital admissions for asthma	PEFR % predicted
Mild	Not more than once per month	No	None	>80
Moderate	Not more than once per week	Infrequent	One admission	60-80
Severe	More than once per week or daily	Frequent	More than one admission	<60

Asthma maintenance treatment programme

Maintenance treatments for asthma fall into two main categories: bronchodilators which include β_2 agonists, methylxanthines and anticholinergics; and anti-inflammatory or prophylactic agents such as SODIUM CROMOGLYCATE, KETOTIFEN and corticosteriods (inhaled or oral).

Modes of delivery

Delivery of the drug by inhalation is always preferable. Dry powder or metered dose inhalers (MDI) are usually used. Much lower doses may be used when there is direct delivery of medication to the airways, and this reduces the likelihood of side-effects.

DRY POWDER INHALERS AND MDI's: these are simple devices ideal for use in children aged five years or older. Many younger children can also use them effectively. However, for younger children and older ones with poor inhalation technique, a spacer device should be attached to the MDI, e.g. an Aerochamber with soft facemask or volumatic spacer.

Nebulizers

These are used both at home and in hospitals. They are beneficial for children with severe chronic asthma, who are experiencing acute attacks or for very young children. Careful instruction must always be given as to the limitations of these devices, and parents must be cautioned to seek medical help when the child fails to respond to this form of therapy. These devices should be considered dangerous unless the parents have been adequately educated as to their limitations and disadvantages.

Treatment schedules

Asthma therapy aims at achieving as normal a quality of life as possible for the child. The child should be able to grow and develop normally, participate in sport, attend school regularly and to sleep well at night. Treatment programmes vary according to the frequency and severity of the child's symptoms. Careful monitoring of the child's growth and attention to possible side-effects of treatment are essential.

Mild infrequent asthma

Most children with asthma experience only mild and infrequent episodes of wheezing and coughing in the course of a year. Their quality of life is unaffected and their symptoms are easily controlled by the intermittent use of β_2 agonist therapy. Prophylactic agents, such as SODIUM CROMOGLYCATE, are only indicated in anticipation of possible precipitating events like exercise, cold air or exposure to animals or pollen.

Frequent episodic asthma

Approximately 20% of asthmatic children have more frequent symptoms (>six episodes per year) to the extent that schooling and sleep are affected. These children require daily prophylactic therapy. SODIUM CROMOGLYCATE is usually highly effective and safe for children. Alternatively, a trial of KETOTIFEN may be attempted. Although inhaled steroids are highly effective, they are not first-line prophylactic agents in this context as their effect on growth may be a problem, especially if doses >400 µg/day are required.

If there is no therapeutic effect after a six-week trial of SODIUM CROMOGLYCATE or an eight to twelve-week trial of KETOTIFEN, inhaled steroids should be introduced and the other agents discontinued.

Low doses of inhaled steroids appear safe. Initially doses of 400 µg/day (200 µg twice-daily to encourage compliance) may be administered in conjunction with a β_2 agonist. Inhaled steroids should be administered in powder form or via a spacer to increase their effectiveness and to minimize the incidence of oropharyngeal candidiasis.

Severe chronic asthma

Children with severe chronic asthma form a small minority of childhood asthmatics. Aggressive therapy is required in these children to alleviate daily symptoms, chronic airway obstruction, sleep disturbance and poor exercise tolerance. Larger doses of inhaled steroids (>600 µg/day; upper limit 1 000 µg/day) are often indicated. Side-effects may occur at these levels and should be carefully monitored. If larger doses are required, consideration should be given to the use of FLUTICASONE (Flixotide) by MDI or diskhaler. This has been shown to have fewer systemic effects. If bronchodilatation is poor with β_2 agonist therapy, sustained-release theophyllins or IPRATROPIUM BROMIDE should be used.

If oral steroids are needed, alternate-day PREDNISONE is best, using the lowest dose possible.

Common problems in asthma management
Infants and small children

Treatment may be difficult for various reasons. Drugs may be delivered by using a MDI attached to an aerochamber with a soft facemask or a simple paper or plastic cup spacer. A face-mask nebulizer is probably the most effective way of delivering drugs effectively. In mild cases oral β_2 agonists may be tried.

Inhaled β_2 agonists constitute the first line of therapy in more severe cases. If there is no clinical improvement IPRAT-ROPIUM BROMIDE may be added. Should symptoms persist, nebulized SODIUM CROMOGLYCATE or oral KETOTIFEN are used. If there is still poor control, sustained-release theo-phyllin products may be tried. Oral steroids using the alternate-day regimen particularly may be required in severe cases. Nebu-lized or inhaled steroid preparations should also be useful in this difficult group.

Exercise-induced asthma (EIA)

Exercise-induced asthma is best controlled with an inhaled β_2 agonist used for three to five minutes before exercise. SODIUM CROMOGLYCATE administered 20 minutes prior to exercise is also very effective. Lack of response to these measures implies poor asthma control.

Nocturnal asthma

Regular episodes of coughing and wheezing at night (usually in the early hours of the morning) indicate poor asthma control and the need for more effective therapy. Once appropriate daytime therapy has been prescribed, then attention should be paid to any possible nocturnal symptoms. The new long-acting β_2 ago-nists SALMETEROL (Serevent) and FOMOTEROL or long-acting theophyllins taken at bedtime are often effective.

Attention to environmental control in those children with sen-sitivity to household allergens should be recommended.

Allergic rhinitis

There are two forms of allergic rhinitis: the seasonal form known as hay fever and the perennial form with persistent symptoms. Intense sneezing, watery rhinitis, nasal congestion and conjunctivitis are the main symptoms. Itching is especially found in the seasonal form. Symptoms may often mimic a cold but the persistence of symptoms or their seasonal nature helps to make a diagnosis.

Seasonal allergic rhinitis or hay fever

Symptoms are usually precipitated by exposure to seasonal windborne pollens, e.g. grass and tree pollens or fungal spores. It usually occurs in spring, early summer and at the change of seasons. There is intense sneezing, watery nasal discharge and itching. Not only the nose itches but also the palate and the ear canals. The diagnosis is usually easily made.

The allergen is identified by means of a history, skin testing or CAPRAST. Clumping of eosinophils will be seen on smears of nasal mucus stained with Hansel's stain.

Treatment

Environmental control

It is usually impossible to avoid the allergens that cause seasonal allergic rhinitis.

Antihistamines

The older antihistamine preparations with their sedative side-effects are no longer recommended. Very successful results may be obtained by using the new short-acting non-sedating antihistamines, such as CETIRIZINE (Zyrtec) and LORATADINE (Clarityne).

Mast cell stabilizers

SODIUM CROMOGLYCATE (Rynacrom) nasal spray or drops may be effective in the seasonal form of allergic rhinitis.

Topical steroids

BECLOMETHASONE (Beconase), BUDESONIDE (Rhinocort) or FLUTICASONE (Flixonase) nasal sprays are also effective. Children often prefer the aqueous form of these preparations.

Immunotherapy

This is very effective, and especially for grass pollen allergy where virtually all children will benefit.

Note

Depot steroid injection or oral steroids are not necessary for the control of symptoms.

Perennial allergic rhinitis

Symptoms are persistent throughout the year in this form of rhinitis. Nasal itching is usually not a feature, but obstruction and watery nasal discharge are troublesome. Children usually have the typical pale allergic faces with blue discolouration of the lower eyelids ('allergic shiners'). A nasal crease is often noted. Repeated upward rubbing of the nose (the allergic salute) produces the crease. Allergic mannerisms, such as pulling the face and the salute, are common. The nasal mucous membrane is swollen and paler than normal. The turbinates appear wet and a watery nasal discharge may be present. Secondary complications result from the mucosal swelling, including maxillary sinusitis and serous otitis media.

Perennial allergic rhinitis is usually the result of sensitivity to allergens that are present in the environment throughout the year, e.g. housedust mite, pet allergens or fungal spores.

Treatment

♦ Environmental control: this is an essential component of treatment. Simple schemes to reduce exposure to indoor mite, mould and pet allergens are often very effective.
♦ Antihistamines: the newer non-sedating antihistamines such as CETIRIZINE, LORATIDINE or the longer-acting ASTEMIZOLE (Hismanal) may be effective in controlling symptoms.
♦ SODIUM CROMOGLYCATE nasal spray or drops are not very effective in perennial allergic rhinitis but younger children may respond well.
♦ BECLOMETHASONE, BUDESONIDE or FLUTICASONE nasal spray: highly effective in this form of rhinitis.
♦ **Immunotherapy**: this is often very successful – especially if the child is sensitive to a single unavoidable allergen. The procedure is ineffective when more than two allergens are combined in the vaccine. It is not intended as a substitute for removal of avoidable allergens, e.g. allergy to dogs and cats.

Note

Oral steroids are not recommended unless symptoms are

particularly severe and response to therapy is poor. This is becoming unlikely with the range of treatments now available.

Nasal decongestant drops of any type should not be used for prolonged periods. Even though the danger of rebound chemical rhinitis is unlikely with some preparations, their prolonged use is not recommended.

Food allergy

Food allergy is thought to affect between 1 and 4% of the paediatric population, and especially infants and young children. It becomes less common beyond the age of two or three years. True food allergy always involves an immune mechanism and should not be confused with the many cases of intolerance to foods, such as tyramine in cheeses or the toxins contained in contaminated foods.

Clinical presentation

There is often a family history of food allergy or other atopic disorders which is useful in diagnosis.

Gastrointestinal symptoms such as vomiting and diarrhoea are the most common manifestation of food allergy but skin reactions like urticaria, atopic dermatitis, angio-oedema, respiratory symptoms (including nasal obstruction or wheezing) may occur.

Few foods have been implicated in true food allergy in infants. Those that have been include egg white, cows' milk, soya, peanuts, wheat and fish. Later, sensitivity to shellfish, berries and nuts may occur and persist throughout life.

Diagnosis

A careful history, skin test or CAPRAST may be of some help in establishing the diagnosis and the offending food. Where there is any difficulty, elimination diets, oligo-allergenic diets or rarely double-blind placebo-controlled food challenge tests may be indicated. The latter is used only in special units.

Treatment

Treatment is usually effective if the offending food is eliminated from the diet, e.g. a milk or egg-free diet. Where the food cannot be identified, good results have been obtained in some cases by using SODIUM CROMOGLYCATE powder (Nalcrom) administered in a small amount of warm water ten to 20 minutes before feeds. Alternatively, KETOTIFEN given twice daily has been reported to be of some use.

Anaphylaxis

Anaphylaxis is an acute hypersensitivity reaction caused by the administration of an allergen or antigen to which the patient is sensitive. These may include many drugs, antibiotics (especially PENICILLIN), vaccines, sera, insect bites and stings, especially bee-stings. Some food (especially egg whites, peanuts and shell-fish) have caused anaphylaxis when eaten by children.

The onset is usually unexpected and may occur within seconds to minutes after exposure to the allergen. The child will collapse and rapidly enter a state of shock and, possibly, respiratory arrest. In general, reactions which occur immediately are the most severe and may well be fatal.

Treatment

A successful outcome depends on IMMEDIATE therapy.
In the following order give immediately:

1 **Adrenaline** 1:1 000 0,3-0,5 ml IM. May be repeated at intervals of 20 minutes if necessary.
2 **Antihistamine** e.g. PROMETHAZINE (Phenergan) 0,25-0,5 mg/kg IM.
3 **IV fluids**: shock is due to hypovolaemia secondary to massive exudation of intravascular fluid. Maintenance of normal intravascular volume by IV fluids is essential. Initiate fluid at 20 ml/kg immediately. Colloids such as plasma or Haemaccel or crystalloids such as Ringer's Lactate or normal saline are recommended.
4 **Oxygen**: given by facemask or nasal catheter to prevent hypoxaemia.
5 **AMINOPHYLLIN** is administered if bronchospasm develops in spite of ADRENALINE therapy. It must be given slowly IV in a dose of 4 mg/kg.
6 **Steroids**: administered after the immediate and urgent steps outlined in 1, 2 and 3. Steroids have a slow onset of action. Administer HYDROCORTISONE 100-200 mg IV four to six-hourly for 24 hours or longer if required. Alternatively DEXAMETHASONE may be given.

Additional steps

1 Intubation if there is airway obstruction as a result of angio-oedema.
2 DOPAMINE 5-15 µg/kg/minute is infused if cardiovascular collapse occurs.

Note

1 Try to identify the offending allergen.
2 Provide a Medic Alert disc once the patient has recovered.
3 Provide an injectable adrenaline device for patients e.g. Ana-guard or Epipen.
4 Educate the patient on the risk of re-exposure to allergen.
5 In bee-sting-allergic patients, immunotherapy to bee venom should be considered.

3 ANAESTHESIA

A D Butt

Preparation for surgery

Psychological support and consent

The parents should be given a clear explanation of the procedure(s) involved and should give their written consent (see pages 311-2). A child who is old enough to understand should be told why he or she is in hospital by the doctor or parent in a compassionate and encouraging manner.

Clinical state

Elective anaesthesia is contra-indicated in the presence of active infections that result in systemic effects. These include colds, which may be diagnosed by the presence of symptoms or signs from any two of the following:

♦ mild sore or scratchy throat or malaise;
♦ temperature >38 °C;
♦ dry cough, congestion, stuffiness; or
♦ sneezing, rhinorrhoea.

It is recommended that, if possible, surgery be postponed until the patient has been symptom-free for ten to 14 days. Small patients, i.e. those less than six months old or those requiring endotracheal intubation, are particularly at risk.

Major system disease, e.g. diabetes or asthma, must be adequately treated or controlled. A patient receiving steroids (including extensive topical application) for more than ten days in the three months prior to anaesthesia, requires steroid supplementation peri-operatively.

For emergency surgery the patient's condition must be made as optimal as time permits. Correction of acid base and electrolyte disorders and adequate hydration are essential pre-operative requirements.

Haemoglobin levels and blood transfusion

A minimum haemoglobin level of 10 g/dl was generally accepted in the past. At present unnecessary transfusion should be avoided but blood should be on standby or crossmatched, depending on the nature and extent of the surgery, current haemoglobin level and toxicity of the patient. A haemoglobin of 9 g/dl is adequate for a minor procedure in a healthy patient.

Oral intake

Hypoglycaemia and dehydration must be avoided in the pre-operative period when food intake has to be restricted. The following are practical guidelines:

◆ Feed until six hours before operation.
◆ Four hours before the operation, offer as much **clear fluid** by mouth as the patient wants. Half-strength Darrow's with 5% dextrose water, flavoured with orange, is recommended. Nil per mouth thereafter. If urgent, it is almost certainly safe to anaesthetise a patient $2\frac{1}{2}$ hours after the intake of clear fluid.

Anaesthesia

See Table 3.1 for drugs used in paediatric anaesthesia.

Premedication

◆ Oral fluids only if less than six months old.
◆ See Table 3.1 for those over six months.
◆ The child is best left undisturbed after receiving the pre-medication.

Administration and technique

General anaesthesia (including KETAMINE) should not be administered by inexperienced personnel, and especially to infants and small children. Uncuffed endotracheal tubes should be used in patients under seven years old. A leak **must** be present on inflation of pressures greater than 20 cm water.

Management of postoperative pain
Nonsteroidal anti-inflammatories

Nonsteroidal anti-inflammatory drugs given orally or per rectum have proven to be most effective for the control of

Table 3.1: Drugs used in paediatric anaesthesia

		Paediatric dose	Route	Availability and remarks
PREMEDICATION (over 6 months)	TRIMEPRAZINE (Vallergan)	3–4 mg/kg/dose	Oral 2 hours pre-operatively	Syrup Forte: 30 mg/5 ml Tabs: 10 mg Maximum dose: 90 mg
	Plus			
	DROPERIDOL (Inapsin)	0,1–0,2 mg/kg/dose	Oral 2 hours pre-operatively	Maximum dose: 5 mg
	ATROPINE	0,03 mg/kg/dose	Oral	Inj.: 0,5 mg/ml (1 ml/amp.) Given prior to KETAMINE anaesthesia
	MIDAZOLAM (Dormicum)	0,5 mg/kg/dose	Oral 30 min. pre-operatively	For outpatients. Tabs: 15 mg Maximum dose: 15 mg
ANAESTHETIC AGENTS induction	THIOPENTAL SODIUM	3–4 mg/kg/dose	Slow IV	Use 2,5% solution. Titrate until effect obtained

		Paediatric dose	Route	Availability and remarks
Induction and maintenance	HALOTHANE	0–2% (max)	Inhalation	Use calibrated vaporizer only
	KETAMINE (Ketalar)	1–2 mg/kg/dose 5–10 mg/kg/dose	Slow IV IM	Inj. IV: 10 mg/ml (20 ml vial) Inj. IM: 50 and 100 mg/ml (10 ml vials) Supplement with other agents e.g. NITROUS OXIDE or FENTANYL
Maintenance	ENFLURANE or ISOFLURANE	0–3% (max)	Inhalation	Specialist use only
Relaxants (IPPV essential)	SUXAMETHONIUM (Scoline)	1 mg/kg/dose 2–4 mg/kg/dose	IV IM	Inj.: 50 mg/ml (2 ml vial) Give ATROPINE first
	TUBOCURARINE	0,6 mg/kg Neonate: 1/3 dose	IV	Inj.: 10 mg/ml (1,5 ml amp.)
	ALCURONIUM (Alloferin)	0,3 mg/kg	IV	Inj.: 5 mg/ml (2 ml amp.)

		Paediatric dose	Route	Availability and remarks
	PANCURONIUM (Pavulon)	0,08-0,10 mg/kg	IV	Inj.: 2 mg/ml (2 ml amp.)
	ATRACURIUM (Tracrium)	0,3-0,5 mg/kg	IV	Inj.: 10 mg/ml (2,5 ml amp.)
	VECURONIUM (Norcuron)	0,08-0,1 mg/kg	IV	Inj.: 4 mg powder per amp. Prolonged effect in neonates
Relaxant reversal	ATROPINE +	0,03 mg/kg	IV	Inj.: 0,5 mg/ml (1 ml amp.)
	NEOSTIGMINE (Prostigmin)	0,05 mg/kg Given together	IV	Inj.: 0,5 mg/ml (1 ml amp.) Inj.: 2,5 mg/ml (1 ml amp.) 2,5 mg/ml (5 ml multiple dose vial)
	or			
	GLYCOPYRROLATE (Instead of ATROPINE)	0,015 mg/kg	IV	0,2 mg/ml (1 or 2 ml amp.)

		Paediatric dose	Route	Availability and remarks
Analgesia (Opiates) (IPPV advised)	FENTANYL (Sublimaze)	1-2 µg/kg/dose	IV	Inj.: 50 µg/ml (2 ml amp.)
	MORPHINE	0,1-0,15 mg/kg/dose	IV or IM	Inj.: 10 mg/ml (1 ml amp.)
Nonsteroidal anti-inflammatories	DICLOFENAC (Voltaren)	1-2 mg/kg	Oral or suppositories Single dose	Tab: 25 mg Suppos.: 12,5 mg, 25 mg and 100 mg
	IBUPROFEN (Brufen)	5 mg/kg	Oral, six-hourly	Susp.: 100 mg/5 ml
Local anaesthetics	lignocaine (Xylocaine 1 or 2%)	Local anaesthetic: maximum dose: 3 mg/kg without vasoconstriction	By infiltration	Inj.: multiple dose vial (5, 10 and 20 mg/ml)
		7 mg/kg, with vasoconstriction	Never to digits or penis	Plus adrenaline: for vasoconstriction 1:200 000 for reducing toxicity or prolonging effect: 1:500 000

	Paediatric dose	Route	Availability and remarks
REMICAINE 2% (Remicard)	For ventricular arrhythmia: 1 mg/kg dose	IV	Inj.: 20 mg/ml (5 and 20 ml amp.) 100 mg/ml (5 ml amp.)
BUPIVACAINE (Macaine 0,5%)	Maximum dose: 2,5 mg/kg	By infiltration Never IV	Inj.: 10 ml amp.

post-operative pain and swelling, especially after orthopaedic, maxillo-facial and oral surgery (including tonsillectomy). The oral dose should be given with the premedication, or a suppository should be inserted as soon as possible after the patient has been anaesthetised. See Table 3.1. **Note: These drugs may cause increased bleeding.**

Local anaesthesia

Children of all ages (including neonates) feel pain. Where possible the use of intra-operative local anaesthetic is the safest and most effective means of providing post-operative analgesia. BUPIVACAINE (Macaine) is preferred because of its longer duration (max. dose 2,5 mg/kg, length of action four to six hours). Wound infiltration, intercostal blocks, inguinal, penile and caudal blocks are easily performed. The exact technique should be learned from standard texts on anaesthesia but brief descriptions of inguinal and caudal block are given.

Inguinal block

Inguinal block may be used for herniotomy or orchidopexy. A blunted 23 gauge needle is inserted 1 cm medial and 1 cm inferior to the anterior superior iliac spine. Three 'pops' may be felt as the skin, the external oblique and internal oblique are penetrated. Three fanned-out injections are made at right angles to the inguinal ligament while withdrawing the needle. A skin wheal in the direction of the skin incision is also made. BUPIVACAINE 0,5% up to 2 mg/kg is used.

Caudal block

Analgesia up to the umbilicus is easily obtained without interfering with motor function. Upper abdominal levels may be reached, but large doses are necessary. The sacral hiatus has a bony prominence on each side (cornu) and is easily palpable. It lies absolutely in the spinal midline, although in the recommended lateral 'knees and hips fully flexed' position it is found above the soft tissue midline cleft. It is identified at the apex of an equilateral triangle formed by the posterior superior iliac spines and the prominences.

An aseptic technique must be used. A 22 gauge needle (preferably short-bevelled) is introduced at 45° to the spine and directed cephaladwards in the midline. A distinct pop is usually felt as the sacrococcygeal membrane is perforated. At this stage the needle direction is altered to run parallel to the back directly up the spine. It is advanced two or three more millimetres. The injection is made after checking that the CSF does not leak from the needle. Frequent aspirations should be made while injecting, in order to exclude intravascular injection. Furthermore, very little pressure should be required using a 10 ml syringe. The recommended dose is 1 ml/kg of 0,25% BUPIVACAINE.

Intravenous and intramuscular morphine

Children under the age of three months and prematurely born infants up to 60 weeks post-gestational age are sensitive to the respiratory depressant effects of all opiates.

Recommended doses

IV infusion

♦ 10-30 µg/kg/hr (0,2 mg/kg in 20 ml 5% dextrose water at 1-3 ml/hr).

An infusion is preferred and should be started before the child is in pain. A syringe driver is needed. If pain is already present a bolus IV loading dose of 0,025 mg/kg (six months to one year) to 0,05 mg/kg (>one year) is needed. IV bolus doses are contra-indicated in unventilated infants up to the age of six months, but MORPHINE may be given as an infusion to neonates in an intensive care setting at a rate of 10-15 µg/kg/hour.

IM injection

♦ Four to six-hourly.
♦ >One year: 0,1 to 0,15 mg/kg.
♦ Six months to one year: 0,025 to 0,05 mg/kg.
♦ <Six months: 0,025 mg/kg plus ICU setting preferred.

Caudal MORPHINE (specialists only)

A dose of 0,05 mg/kg diluted with BUPIVACAINE or 0,5 ml/kg of saline provides prolonged pain relief (12-24 hours) for any operations from the thorax down. However, these patients will be at risk from severe respiratory depression and must be in an ICU for the next 24 hours with OXYGEN and NALOXONE (see page 619) at the bedside.

Oral and sublingual analgesics

Oral

◆ PARACETAMOL (Panado) 10 mg/kg/dose four to six-hourly.
◆ MEFENAMIC ACID (Ponstan) 6,5 mg/kg/dose eight-hourly.

Sublingual

TILIDINE (Valoron) 1 drop/year of age eight to 12-hourly. Not recommended if under one year old.

Sedation and analgesia for procedures outside the operating theatre

The goals of using these agents must be defined.

Anxiolysis

Reassurance and explanation are most important.

◆ Oral MIDAZOLAM (Dormicum) 0,5-0,7 mg/kg (short-acting) is most useful. DIAZEPAM (Valium) 0,2 mg/kg may also be used and is effective. Give 30 minutes prior to the procedure.

Sedation

If the child is too young to communicate but must lie still:

◆ CHLORAL HYDRATE 50 mg/kg by mouth one hour prior to procedure.

Sedation and analgesia [1]

For more painful and uncomfortable procedures, e.g. cardiac catheterization, the following scheme is recommended:

◆ Local infiltration of LIGNOCAINE 1% (short-acting) or BUPIVACAINE 0,5% should be performed where possible if pain is anticipated.
◆ Up to one month: CHLORAL 50 mg/kg by mouth (depending on the child's condition).

---

[1] For principles of pain management in malignant diseases see page 303.

♦ One to six months: PETHIDINE 1 mg/kg/IM plus CHLO-RAL 50 mg/kg oral.

♦ >Six months: PETHIDINE 1 mg/kg IM plus SPARINE 0,5 mg/kg IM plus PHENERGAN 0,5 mg/kg IM.
Never exceed 50 mg PETHIDINE in total (one single injection).

♦ >Three years: VALLERGAN 3 mg/kg oral, DROPERIDOL 0,2 mg/kg oral, plus VALORON 1 drop per year of age given 45 minutes before.

These drugs should be given 45 minutes before the procedure with the exception of VALLERGAN and DROPERIDOL which are given two hours before.

4 ARTHRITIS

E M Bhettay

If symptoms point to musculoskeletal disease then take a history, do a clinical examination, laboratory studies and radio-imaging examinations.

Definitions

◆ **Arthralgia** means joint pain.
◆ **Arthritis** implies joint inflammation.
◆ **Enthesitis** means inflammation at the insertions of ligaments and tendons into bone.
◆ **Rheumatism** refers to musculoskeletal pain or discomfort.

History

Specific information should be obtained so that you can form a clear understanding of the nature of a symptom or a sign.

Pain

Where? When? Mode of onset? Duration? Severity? Aggravating or relieving factors? Radiation? Associated features? Referred: pain from the hip is often felt in the knee.

Stiffness

Worse in the morning and aggravated by inactivity. It is relieved by activity.

Swelling

Ask about swelling. Deformity, limp, loss of function, interference with activities of daily living.

Aetiological factors

Direct trauma (including thorn). Exposure to tuberculosis, injections (hepatitis, HIV), tick bite, infection (viral, dysentery), jaundice, vaccination (rubella), school (activities, sports, punishment).

Systems

Symptoms relating to other systems, and especially the skin, eye, cardiac, respiratory, renal and central nervous systems.

Family history

Arthritis, spondylitis, haemophilia, jaundice.

Examination

If indicated, record temperature daily or four-hourly over a matter of days to determine a pattern.

Musculoskeletal

Completely expose and examine all joints for signs of inflammation on inspection, palpation, and active and passive range of movements. Swelling may be diffuse (synovial hypertrophy, effusion, cellulitis, oedema), or localized (Baker's cyst, synovial blow-out, ganglion, fibroma, lipoma, osteoma, exostosis). The capsular pattern involvement will be shown by a characteristic set of impaired movements for each joint.

◆ Pain on passive movement in only one direction indicates ligamentous pathology.
◆ Soft crepitus demonstrates synovial inflammation, and coarse crepitus worn joint surfaces.
◆ Painful resisted movement indicates contractile structure pathology (except bursitis, tender lymph node, fracture), and inability to move a joint ankylosis.

Palpate entheses and look for tender points (fibromyalgia). Do not omit axial skeleton or functional assessment, e.g. grip, gait. Examine footwear.

Skin

Look for rashes, e.g. bruises, exanthems, erythema nodosum, erythema marginatum and other manifestations of rheumatic fever, bacterial endocarditis, morphoea, keratoderma blenorrhagica, psoriasis, Kawasaki disease, eyelid heliotrope, photosensitivity, butterfly, facial rash, Raynaud's phenomenon; alopecia, clubbing, anaemia, nodules, splinter haemorrhages, vasculitis, spider naevi, telangiectasia, sclerodactyly, nailfold infarcts, nodules; and for Gottron's sign (vasculitic rash on the knuckles of the fingers and toes).

Table 4.1 Localization of involved anatomical structure(s)

Movement	Painful	Painless
Active movement	Problem at joint.	No arthritis, pain is referred.
Passive movement	Painful in one direction: problem of ligament, tendon, muscle. Painful in several directions: joint capsule i.e. arthritis.	No arthritis.
Resisted movement	Contractile structure i.e. tendon or muscle disease.	No arthritis.

In systemic onset juvenile chronic arthritis, a characteristic evanescent salmon-pink macular erythema may occur, and the Koebner phenomenon may be elicited (erythematous rash produced by stroking of the skin with a fingernail).

Mouth

Tonsillitis, mucosal ulcerations, reduced opening (mouth or temporomandibular joint).

Lymph nodes

All groups including epitrochlear nodes.

Respiratory

Pulmonary tuberculosis (PTB), diffuse interstitial pulmonary fibrosis (DIPF), pleurisy, chronic fibrosing alveolitis (CFA).

Cardiovascular system

Pulses, hypertension, pericarditis, murmurs, congestive cardiac failure.

Abdomen

Hepatomegaly, splenomegaly, lymph nodes, renal tenderness or enlargement, ascites.

Genito-urinary tract

Urethral discharge (gonorrhoea), balanitis (Reiter's syndrome), scrotal ulcers (Behcet syndrome).

Eye

Conjunctivitis, phlycten, band keratopathy, irregular pupil (synechiae), hypopyon, cataract.

Central nervous system

Psyche, involuntary movement, muscle-wasting or weakness, sensory deficit, entrapment neuropathy.

Diagnosis

Causes of arthritis may be congenital, traumatic, infective, inflammatory, mechanical, neoplastic, haematological, or degenerative. A number of factors should be considered when making a diagnosis:

Age

Infancy: congenital (arthrogyposis), neonatal-onset multisystem inflammatory disease (NOMID), fetal alcohol syndrome, sepsis. Toddler and school-going: trauma, hypermobility, child abuse, growing pains, sepsis, tuberculosis (TB), Henoch's purpura, Kawasaki disease, viral infections, rheumatic fever.

Sex

Male: haemophilia, enthesopathy related arthritis (ERA), juvenile ankylosing spondylitis (JAS).
Female: systemic lupus erythematosus (SLE), polyarticular and early-onset pauci-articular juvenile chronic arthritis (JCA).

Number of joints

Monarticular: sepsis, trauma, haematological, mechanical, JCA, tumours.
Oligo-articular: reactive, growing pains, JCA, inflammatory bowel disease, infection.
Polyarticular: JCA, acute rheumatic fever (ARF), SLE, JAS.

Pattern of joint involvement

Age

Infancy: sepsis, CDH, contractures.
Child: trauma, oligo-articular arthritis with uveitis.

Sex

Male: ERA, AS, haemophilia.
Female: SLE, gonococcal.

Number of joints

Monarticular: sepsis, TB, trauma, tumours, ARF, JCA.
Pauci-articular: reactive, ERA, JCA with uveitis, ARF, hypo-
gammaglobulinaemia.
Polyarticular: SLE, dermatomyositis, JCA, ARF.

Region

Hands and feet: hypertrophic pulmonary osteo-arthropathy
(HPO), dactylitis.
Small joints: viruses (rubella, hepatitis B).
Large joints: viruses (mumps, varicella), ARF.
Lower limbs: spondylarthropathies, ERA, JAS, reactive.
Axial: spondylarthropathies, ERA, JAS, reactive.

Investigations

These are determined by the clinical presentation. For example:
if infection is suspected — blood for Hb, WCC, platelets.
Obtain material for culture, e.g. throat swab, discharges from
skin, ear, eye, urethra, stool, blood, synovial fluid. Include
Mantoux, antistreptolysin O titre, ECG and chest X-ray.

If non-infective, and arthritis persists for several weeks:
collagen screen, immunoglobulins, renal and liver function
tests. Later: test for Lyme disease antibodies, factor VIII-related
antigen, ferritin, coagulation studies, histocompatibility, serological tests for syphilis, human immune deficiency virus. Refer
for an ophthalmological opinion. Electromyography, muscle/
synovial biopsy, arthroscopy, ultrasound, scintigraphy, com-
puted axial tomography scanning, or magnetic resonance imaging may be indicated.

Management

Drug therapy

◆ Appropriate antibiotics for infective and reactive arthro-
   pathies.
◆ Simple analgesics for mechanical conditions, e.g. Perthe's.

Anti-inflammatory drugs

◆ Nonsteroidal (NSAID), e.g. INDOMETHACIN, KETO-PROFEN.
◆ Steroids
   ◇ Systemic:
   oral, e.g. PREDNISOLONE
   pulse IV, e.g. METHYLPREDNISOLONE.
   ◇ Local:
   ocular, e.g. BETAMETHASONE
   ◇ Intra-articular TRIAMCINOLONE is used when only one or two joints are troublesome.
◆ Refer to a rheumatologist should these measures fail. Disease-modifying anti-rheumatic drugs (DMARD) may have to be employed under the supervision of a specialized clinic.

Referral

Where indicated refer to:

Physiotherapist

Assessment. Exercise programme and pool therapy to maintain range of movement, muscle tone and strength. Treatment for pain relief.

Occupational therapist

Evaluation

Activities of daily living, work-place. Sensory, motor, perceptual and functional development.

Provision of, and training with, supportive devices

Splints, pressure garments, crutches, wheelchair.

Support

Psychosocial.

Education

Disease, principles of joint protection, back care techniques.

Advice

Disability, activities of daily living, emotional/mental problems.

Social Worker

Assisting with re-integration into the community.

Rehabilitation

Assistance through community agencies such as the Juvenile Arthritis Organization and the Association for the Physically Disabled (see Appendix 5, page 688).

5 ARTIFICIAL FEEDING

H de V Heese and A Grobler

Breast-feeding is best for babies. Artificial feeding may at times be necessary as breast-feeding is not always possible.

General notes on milk
Components of milk
Proteins

♦ Lactalbumin, lactoferrin and a small proportion of casein form the bulk of protein in breast milk.
♦ The protein source of most commercial formulas is cow milk or soya protein isolate.
♦ There is four to five times more casein in cow milk than in breast milk, and this is responsible for the coarse curds in a baby fed with cow milk.
♦ Bovine albumin may irritate bowel mucosa, leading to gastrointestinal bleeding and iron-deficiency anaemia.

Carbohydrate

♦ Breast milk and modified cow milk formulas are sweeter than fresh cow milk because of their higher carbohydrate content (7% against 5%).
♦ Milk-based formulas contain mainly lactose, sucrose or maize (corn) syrup, or malto dextrin. See pages 52 and 53.

Fat

♦ Breast milk fat is easier to digest because of its small globule size.
♦ Cow milk fat contains a much higher proportion of low molecular weight (butyric and caproic) and high molecular weight (palmitic and stearic) saturated fatty acids, than does human milk.
♦ The fat content of both breast and cow milk is subject to wide variations.

◆ The body cannot synthesize essential fatty acids, e.g. linoleic acid and α-linolenic acid. Conversion of these fatty acids to their long-chain derivatives may be slow in preterm infants and in disease states.

◆ Deficiency of linoleic acid in preterm infants on cow milk formulas may result in dryness of the skin, weakness, hair loss, growth retardation and failure to thrive.

Electrolytes and minerals

◆ Fresh cow milk's total electrolyte load is approximately 235 mmol/l as against 70 mmol/l for breast or modified cow milk.

◆ Calcium and phosphorus load in cow milk is respectively four and five times greater than in breast milk.

◆ Iron and zinc concentrations in cow milk are lower and have a lower bio-availability than in breast milk.

Vitamins

◆ Essential micronutrients such as niacin and ascorbic acid in fresh cow milk are relatively low.

See pages 55-6 for the requirements of infants on breast milk substitutes.

Methods of bottle-feeding

Breast and bottle

If the supply of breast milk is insufficient, the breast-feed may have to be complemented (i.e. followed) by a bottle-feed. A supplementary feed, i.e. replacing an entire breast-feed by a bottle-feed, is given if the mother has insufficient milk at times or where the mother has to leave the infant at home without a supply of expressed breast milk while she is at work. Neither complemented nor supplemental feeds should be sweetened or thickened unless specifically indicated, (i.e. to increase calories or to prevent reflux/aspiration respectively).

Bottle only

Most artificial feeds are based on cow milk which has been modified. In deciding on a particular preparation, consideration must be given to the gestational age of the neonate and the maturation, age and weight of the infant to be fed. Factors such as the energy, type and amount of protein, fat, carbohydrate, vitamin, iron and mineral content of the milk, as well as its price and availability from a local clinic, have to be considered.

Available milk

Some of the varieties of formulas available in South Africa are given in Table 5.2 on pages 52-3. Information is also provided on their content, general uses and other characteristics. Manufacturers supply more information about a specific brand of milk on the tin or as an insert.

Liquid milk

Cow milk: fresh or pasteurized or sterilized. Fresh untreated cow milk should always be simmered for 15 to 20 minutes as it alters casein and bovine albumin and will also destroy microorganisms and decrease the risk of infection.

Evaporated milks

Fifty per cent of the water is removed from cow milk in the manufacturing process. To reconstitute to the equivalent value of full-strength milk, an equivalent quantity of water is added. The milk may require the addition of sugar. Evaporated milks are available in tins as Ideal Milk. For further dilution see page 54.

Powdered formulas

These are commercial preparations which are convenient and have a composition which approximates that of human milk. In this type of formula there is a varying degree of modification by the manufacturer to the type and content of protein, fat, carbohydrate, electrolytes and minerals; so too for the addition of essential amino acids, fatty acids, vitamins, iron and minerals.

The less significantly modified formulas are available as skimmed, low fat or full cream powdered milk, depending on the relative amount of butter fat. Skimmed milk and low fat milk both contain 3,5 g protein, 5,0 g carbohydrate (lactose) and 0,5 g and 2,1 g fat respectively per 100 ml. Full cream milks are commonly used because of their lower prices, but are not very suitable for neonates and infants under six months because of their higher protein and sodium content, contributing to an increased renal solute load. Full cream milks therefore require dilution if used for these infants. The resulting energy deficit must be made good with added sugar and or oil and the infant should be provided with iron and vitamins. Skimmed milk is not an adequate feed as the sole source of nutrition in the growing infant below the age of one year.

To approximate breast milk more closely in more significantly modified formulas:

♦ protein has been reduced;
♦ casein partly replaced by whey;
♦ fat made more unsaturated;
♦ carbohydrate increased;
♦ sodium and calcium reduced; and
♦ essential amino acids, fatty acids, vitamins, iron and minerals have been added.

They are simple to prepare and may be given in full strength – even to low birthweight infants. Special formulas further adapted for very low birthweight and low birthweight infants are also available (see Table 5.2 on pages 52-3). Some preparations for term infants are acidified, e.g. Pelargon. Acidified milks have antibacterial properties. They are also supplied by agencies for the nutrition of infants in poor areas as their taste discourages older individuals from taking such milks.

Special milks

♦ Prevention of atopic disease, e.g. sensitivity to cow milk protein: soya bean preparations, e.g. Isomil, Infasoy and goat milk.
♦ For lactose intolerance: soya preparations as above or AL-110.

Constituents of, and energy supplied by, available milk

General approximate values for protein, carbohydrate, fat, and mineral content and energy supplied by milks are given in Table 5.1. Always refer to the manufacturer's information supplied with the tin for specific values.

In calculating the energy supplied by a particular milk refer to Table 5.2.

The protein, fat and essential fatty acid, and carbohydrate content of any artificial feed should approximate breast milk in that it should supply:

Table 5.1 Constituents of milk

	Protein	Carbo-hydrate	Fat	Minerals	Calories	Kilo-joules
	g/l	g/l	g/l	g/l	kcal/l	kJ/l
Breast milk (average)	12	70	38	2,1	710	2 840
Cow milk (fresh)	33	48	37	7,0	690	2 780
More significantly modified cow milk[1,2]	15-24	69-91	26-38	2,0-6,5	650-810	2 730-3 400
Less significantly modified cow milk[2]	33	48	37 (varies)	8,0	650	2 600
Evaporated cow milk[2]	27	48	29	7,0	650-700	2 600
Low fat milk	35	50	21	7,1	530	2 226
Skimmed cow milk[2]	35	48	5	7,25	350	1 200

[1] The range is relatively wide depending on how closely the composition of the milk approximates that of breast milk.

[2] Values given are for reconstituted milk according to the manufacturer's instructions, including the addition of sugar where indicated.

♦ 7-10% of calories as protein;
♦ 45-50% of calories as fat with a minimum of fat calories made up as essential fatty acid (300 mg linoleic acid);
♦ 40-45% of the calories as carbohydrates.

Practice and techniques of bottle feeding

Every infant requires individual handling. Infants may vary their energy intake in the amount of fluids they drink per individual feed, from day to day, or under different environmental circumstances.

Most infants thrive on cow milk if certain general principles are adhered to. Basic steps in advising a mother about bottle-feeding are listed below.

Table 5.2 Some varieties of milk available in RSA

General uses	Comments and indications	Formulas available	Protein	fat	CHO	Type of CHO	Cal/100ml
Preterm infant, low birthweight infant	Increased protein, fat, carbohydrate, energy, sodium, calcium, phosphorus content	Pre-Nan – Nestlé	2	3,4	7,9	L+MD	70
		S26-Preemie – Akromed	2	4,4	8,6	L+MD	81
Early infancy	Produces a soft curd in the stomach. Like breast milk it is whey-predominant and contains cystine	S26 – Akromed	1,5	3,6	7,2	L	67
		Nan – Nestlé	1,5	3,4	7,6	L	67
		Similac 60/40 – Ross	1,5	3,8	7,3	L	67
Early infancy	Casein-predominant. Produces firm curd in the stomach. Ensures longer satiety. Suitable for the 'Hungry Baby'. Cheaper than whey-predominant milks	Similac – Ross	1,5	3,6	7,3	L	67
		SMA – Akromed	1,5	3,5	7,0	L	67
		Lactogen No.1 – Nestlé	1,7	3,4	7,4	L+S+MD	67
Early infancy	Acidified casein-predominant. Useful under poor hygienic circumstances	Pelargon – Nestlé	2	3,1	8,1	L+S+MD +MS	68
Weaning or follow-on	Older infants, from the age of six months. Higher protein and sodium content. Fortified with vitamins, iron and trace metals. More unsaturated than saturated fat	Lactogen No.2 – Nestlé	3,1	2,8	7,5	L+S+MD	66
		Infagro – Akromed	2,5	2,8	8	L+S	67

General uses	Comments and indications	Formulas available	g/100ml			Type of CHO	Cal/100ml
			Protein	fat	CHO		
Cow milk allergy Lactose intolerance	Soya formulas. Cheapest milk substitute. 30% of cow milk-intolerant children develop soya intolerance. Mineral bio-availability reduced	Infasoy – Akromed	1,8	3,6	6,9	S+MS	67
		Isomil – Ross	1,8	3,6	6,9	S+MS	67
Lactose & sucrose intolerance	Disaccharide-free	AL110 – Nestlé	1,9	3,3	7,4	MD	67
Non-specific maldigestion or malabsorption	Altered fat content. MCT predominant. May cause essential fatty acid deficiency in chronic liver disease. Supplement with fatty acids	Portagen – BMS	2,2	3	7,4	MS+S	67
	Hydrolysed casein, lactose, sucrose and soya free	Nutramigen – BMS	1,9	2,6	9,1	MS+MSS	67
	Semi-elemental. Disaccharide free. Hypo-allergenic. Contains 40–50% MCT	Pregestimil – BMS	1,9	2,7	9,3	See literature	67
		Alfare – Nestlé	2,2	3,3	7	See literature	65

CHO – Carbohydrate
MD – Maltodextrin
MS – Maize starch
MSS – Maize syrup solids
MCT – Medium chain triglycerides
S – Sucrose
L – Lactose

Choice of milk

This is determined by factors such as:

♦ the age and maturity of the infant;
♦ the socio-economic status of the family unit;
♦ the availability of the milk product in the area or at the health clinic.

Reconstitution of milks

Powdered milks

Always refer to the manufacturer's instructions. Most modified milk powders have measures provided.

♦ One measure is added to every 25 ml water or multiples of these according to the manufacturer's instructions.
♦ Milk powder must **not be packed down** in the measure as an overconcentrated feed will result, with possible hazards such as hypernatraemia.

Evaporated milks

One part milk to one part water.

Dilution of milks

In the first six months of life for term infants:

♦ more significantly modified powdered reconstituted milk – undiluted;
♦ less significantly modified powdered reconstituted milk – three parts milk : one part water;
♦ fresh cow milk – three parts milk : one part water; and
♦ evaporated – two parts milk : three parts water.

Fluid requirements

Calculate the infant's fluid requirements according to weight in kilograms (weight to two decimal places, e.g. 3,75 kg). See page 209.

Energy requirements

Calculate the infant's energy requirements according to his or her actual or expected weight (if underweight) in kilograms (weight to two decimal places, e.g. 3,75 kg). See page 376.

Adjustment of energy content

The energy content of certain feeds is less than full strength breast or cow milk. Examples are diluted fresh cow milk and overdiluted evaporated milk. Some children, due to their illness, and especially respiratory patients, have higher requirements for energy.

The following can be used to increase the energy content of feeds:

◆ to make up the shortfall, one rounded 5 ml teaspoonful (5 g) of sugar is added per 100 ml of milk, providing approximately 85 kJ (20 kcal) of energy;
◆ in the event of weight gain not being satisfactory, further supplementation with 2-3 ml of sunflower seed oil per 100 ml of milk may be indicated. One ml oil provides 38 kJ (9 kcal).

Frequency of feeds

Term babies are fed

◆ on demand, i.e. when he or she shows signs of hunger, provided the intervals between feeds are not less than two to three hours;
◆ according to fixed times, e.g. four-hourly, i.e. five or six feeds per day; and
◆ from the age of three or four months the infant commonly drops the night feed and should sleep through.

Note

It is important to distinguish a hunger cry from other causes of crying, e.g. thirst, discomfort, or pain.

Addition of vitamins, iron and fluoride

Bottle-fed infants require:

◆ vitamins C and D (supplied in a multivitamin syrup) from the first week of life;
◆ iron from one month of age;
  ◇ Many artificial milks have additional vitamins and iron to make up their deficiency in cow milk. The amounts added may be insufficient to supply the daily requirements of the infant, e.g. preterm. Vitamin and iron supplements are usually necessary for the first year of life. See page 85.

◆ breast- and artificially-fed infants require fluoride to protect their teeth against caries in most areas in South Africa. The need depends on the
  ◇ fluoride content of the water in the area. See page 377.
  ◇ The optimal amount is 1 ppm and where fluoride concentrations are less than 0,7 ppm, additional fluoride should be given. See page 377.

Introduction of mixed feeding

As a general rule, solids may be introduced after 12 weeks. Though early weaning does not generally influence weight gain or growth in length, it may be to the disadvantage of infants with a predisposition to allergic or coeliac disease to do so even at 12-16 weeks.

◆ Every infant, however, is an individual in his or her own right, and the decision to introduce solids depends more on the mother's interpretation of her baby's needs than on age alone, e.g. if the infant is dissatisfied after a feed, demands more frequent feeds, or is not interested in more milk.
◆ Solids should be introduced one at a time in small amounts (not more than a teaspoonful to start with) and they should be smooth and fine in consistency.
  ◇ It is normal for an infant to apparently attempt to push the teaspoon away with the tongue when first introduced to solids.
  ◇ The addition of cereal to the bottle feed is not favoured unless done under supervision in the event of, for example, reflux, laryngeal incompetence or incoordinate swallowing.
◆ Solids are usually given before a bottle feed, but a thirsty infant may prefer to have a drink first. Offer the infant cereals, puréed fruits and vegetables as a start and gradually introduce a full mixed diet in mashed form.
◆ **Introduce one new taste at a time.**
◆ After the age of nine months, 600 ml of milk per day is sufficient and the child should thrive on this and his or her mixed diet.
  ◇ A monotonous single-source diet like mealie meal porridge, without a supplement of milk or another protein source, will lead to protein energy malnutrition even if the quantity of food is adequate.

Note

◆ Mothers should be discouraged from imparting their sense of taste to their infants.
  ◇ They should be refrained from adding salt, sugar, margarine or butter for 'taste' reasons.
◆ Care should be taken not to give excessive amounts of cereals during infancy. Home-cooked meat, chicken and fish should be finely minced. When egg is introduced, start with the yolk. Egg white should only form part of the diet after one year of age.

Assessment of satisfactory feeding

Weight gain should be monitored every four to six weeks and recorded on a growth chart. If weight does not follow the centile for the individual child he or she is probably underweight. **Always ascertain the cause.** Signs of correct feeding include

◆ a satisfactory gain in weight;
◆ a contented infant;
◆ six to eight wet napkins per day.

Unsatisfactory weight gain

◆ Carry out a full examination to exclude congenital or acquired disease.
◆ Check fluid and energy intake against requirements. Calculate this from **the volume and type of milk feed and solids intake over a 24 hour period.**
  ◇ **The approximate energy value of food** including cereal preparations which contain on the average:

protein	5-10%
carbohydrate	70-80%
fat	2-10%

  ◇ Note that cereals are a good source of energy but a poor source of protein. A portion (30 g dry weight) of baby starter-cereal contains approximately 3 g protein and 470 kJ (112 kcal).
◆ If the energy and fluid intake are satisfactory exclude
  ◇ abnormal losses;
  ◇ acidosis;
  ◇ congenital or acquired conditions;
  ◇ emotional deprivation;

◇ infection;
◇ metabolic disturbance.

Advice on technique and utensils

The mother or caregiver should be given advice on:

◆ the necessity of the bottle and teat being clean, and on sterilization of materials;
◆ the storage of reconstituted milk and on its temperature when feeding the baby.
  ◇ Before offering a feed, the mother (or whoever feeds the baby) should allow a few drops of milk to fall on the back of her or his hand to ensure that it is not too hot for the baby to drink.

Warning

◆ The baby should **never** be left to feed from a bottle propped against the pillow, because of the danger of the inhalation of milk and the risk of otitis media. The infant must be held semi-erect and the bottle held in the hand of the individual feeding him or her.
◆ The temperature of milk may not be evenly distributed when a microwave oven is used to warm it.

General advice

Mothers should be warned about common mistakes such as:

◆ making artificial feeds too strong (hypernatraemia) or too weak (failure to thrive, hunger stools);
◆ believing that a normal stool is abnormal;
◆ failure to differentiate between thirst and hunger;
  ◇ A thirsty baby needs a drink of cooled, boiled water, not milk.
◆ in the second six months, milk and other liquids can be given from a cup.

Stools

◆ Normal stool patterns vary with age and dietary intake. The unsure mother (and inexperienced medical practitioner or nurse) often calls a normal stool abnormal.
◆ Constipated stools are hard and painful to pass.

◆ Meconium stools are passed during the first three or four days of life. They are greenish-black, odourless and thick and sticky.

◆ Transitional stools are thin and stringy, varying from green to brown. They follow the meconium stool stage and are passed up to eight or more times per day.

◆ Milk stools are passed after the first week and their character is influenced by the type of milk feed.

◇ Breast milk stools during early weeks may be loose and explosive, or from the start they may be homogenous, pasty and mushy and clinging to the nappy. They vary from orange to green and have a slightly sour smell. Stools may be passed with every feed, but the occasional infant may pass a stool of normal consistancy every three to five days.

◇ Modified cow milk formula stools are firm and putty-like, pale and do not cling to the nappy. They may contain curds, turn green or brown on exposure to air, and have a typical odour.

◇ Soya formula stools are of varying consistency, colour and smell. In some infants, stools are a greyish mush with a distinctive unpleasant smell (rotten beans or vegetables).

◆ Vegetables may appear almost unchanged in the stool when first introduced.

◆ Black or very dark stools are often due to altered blood in the neonate or to iron-containing medications.

◆ Starvation stools of underfed infants are small, dark green and frequently passed.

◆ Infants with respiratory infection may have stools with stringy mucus.

◆ Stool frequency decreases with an increase in age until there are only one or two stools per day, but there is a wide individual variation.

Feeding preterm and underweight-for-gestational age infants

Preterm and underweight-for-gestational age infants <1,5 kg

◆ Give IV fluids for the first 48 hours after birth.

◇ If this is not possible, give a similar solution by continuous intragastric drip (see Table 21.1, page 209 and page 206).

◇ A continuous flow is tolerated better than if the fluid is given intermittently.

◇ Start with expressed breast milk, a low birth weight infant formula or a significantly modified milk.

◇ Expressed breast milk and a significantly modified milk may be fortified with the addition of one 5 ml teaspoonful (5 g of a malto dextrin e.g. FRN-glycolode, Polycose (1g = 4kCal)) and/or 1-3 ml MCT oil, e.g. Liproçil, Lipofactor (1ml = 1g = 9kCal) to 100 ml of milk.

◆ Tube feeding is necessary until the baby is able to suck. This will depend on the gestational age, but sucking is usually possible after the weight has reached 1,8 kg.

◇ The length of nasogastric tubing to be passed is twice the distance from the suprasternal notch to the xyphoid plus 2,5 cm. See page 451.

Preterm and underweight-for-gestational age infants over 1,5 kg

◆ Start feeding at three to six hours after birth. Commence with fortified expressed breast or modified cow milk.

◇ Diluted evaporated milk (two parts milk to three parts water) with one rounded 5 ml teaspoonful of sugar added to 100 ml of milk may be offered if breast milk or modified milk is not available.

◇ Preterm infants, if bottle-fed, can be given diluted full cream milk when they reach 2,25 kg if modified milks are not available.

◆ Suggested feeds per day:

◆ under 1,75 kg   three-hourly x 8

◆ 1,75 to 2,25 kg   three-hourly x 7

◆ over 2,25 kg   four-hourly x 5.

6 BEHAVIOUR DISORDERS

P M Leary

Introduction

Beauty is said to lie in the eye of the beholder and the same can be said for behaviour disorders in childhood. Actions regarded as acceptable or even praiseworthy by one set of parents may represent serious misconduct to another couple. Complaints of disordered behaviour often reflect parental ignorance of the stages through which the child passes in the course of normal social, emotional and intellectual development. Thus, shyness towards strangers and considerable negativism in the home are normal manifestations between the ages of one and three years.

Table 6.1 Social and emotional development

Age	Stage	Characteristics
1st year	Oral stage	Infant totally dependent. No demands made on him or her. Needs one-to-one relationship with mother or care giver.
2nd year	Anal stage	More mobile. Early need to conform and comply with mother's requests. Control acquired over eliminations. Parallel play.
2-6	Genital stage	Sex awareness. Involvement in cooperative play and group activities. First stirrings of conscience.
6-12	Latency	Establishment of peer relationships. Formal learning with vast expansion of knowledge.
12-25	Puberty and adolescence	Independent identity formation. Social attitudes and opinions established. Emotional separation from parents. Sexual role. Need to experiment.

Table 6.2 Intellectual development

Age	Stage	Characteristics
0-2 years	Adualism to dualism	Distinction between self and non-self developed. Initial non-selective smiling gives way to stranger response and separation anxiety. Inability to hold memory images of absent objects and people.
2-7 years	Animism	Egocentric – demands immediate gratification. Unwilling to defer to needs of others.
		Animistic – credits inanimate objects with human motives and emotions.
		Pre-operational logic – unable to recognize obvious incongruities, e.g. multiplicity of Father Christmases in December.
		Authoritarian morality – accepts statements and rules made by parents as incontravertible.
7-16 years	Realism	Gradual development of ability to think in logical fashion.
		Initial approach is concrete but increasing ability in teens to think and reason in the abstract.

The doctor requires detailed knowledge of the normal developmental stages if he or she is to help in individual cases. Approximate delineations and the principal behavioural features of each stage are set out in Tables 6.1 and 6.2.

Behaviour disorders are more likely when certain situations and factors prevail in the child's life. The absence of a consistent and effective mother-figure in the early years produces various manifestations of anxiety and antisocial behaviour in later childhood. Serious marital disharmony may induce attention-seeking behaviour and aggression, while emotional disturbances are common in children from single-parent households. Frequent changes of residence and school may induce anxiety symptoms and social withdrawal. School failure may lead to loss of self-esteem, depression, attention-seeking and even conversion hysteria.

Specific problems

Aggression

Unprovoked aggression and violence in a child with a normal IQ may reflect anxiety, depression or unresolved anger. Aggressive outbursts should evoke a consistently neutral response and a short period of isolation from peer and adult company. Detailed history-taking is necessary in order to ascertain underlying causes.

Encopresis

Faecal soiling may represent overflow-incontinence in the presence of severe constipation and faecal impaction. This situation responds to the management of the constipation and the establishment of a regular bowel habit. (See pages 218-20.) Persistent soiling in the absence of constipation may reflect serious psychopathology and it is advisable to refer the child to a child psychiatry unit.

Enuresis

In the absence of organic disorders (urinary tract infection, spina bifida), enuresis reflects immaturity of bladder function or emotional disturbance. Thus it is important to establish the type of enuresis before instituting investigations and treatment.

Ten per cent of normal six-year olds still wet their beds. When a child has never had a prolonged period of sustained night-time dryness (years or many months), bedwetting is due to immaturity. Routine urine testing should be carried out in every case. Further investigation is not indicated in the absence of daytime urinary symptoms. When enuresis develops after a prolonged interval of nocturnal continence, anxiety-provoking circumstances should be considered. The symptom is quite common after the birth of a sibling, change of school, or divorce. Child abuse should also be kept in mind. See Chapter 14, page 146.

Treatment for the preschool child entails simple measures such as late-afternoon fluid restriction and lifting the child to pass urine in the late evening. There is no place for the early use of potentially dangerous tricyclic drugs. School-age children respond well to the electronic buzzer. Treatment with IMIPRAMINE 10-25 mg or OXYBUTYNIN 5-10 mg at supper may be considered in resistant cases. When enuresis is due to emotional disturbance, steps must be taken to reduce tension and anxiety in the child's life.

Fire-setting

This may be accidental, but when recurrent it represents aggressive attention-seeking usually in response to a hostile, repressive or disruptive background. Extensive inquiry into the child's domestic situation is indicated.

Head-banging and rocking

Usually a harmless bed-time routine but it may cause the parents to fear injury. Occasionally reflects deprivation or anxiety. Usually outgrown by three years. Padding of cot sides may be indicated.

Hyperactivity

A subjective and arbitrary diagnostic label. Restlessness and distractability have many causes in childhood (see Table 6.3). Intervention is necessary when a sustained level of motor activity, short attention span and impulsiveness prevent a child from developing age-appropriate skills and abilities. An analytic approach is necessary in every case and management must be individually tailored.

Table 6.3 Causes of 'hyperactive' behaviour

Preschool activity pattern – normal for age group.
Fatigue – due to late nights; noisy sleeping environment.
Hunger – no breakfast; chronic undernutrition.
Personality trait – 'Type A' – often hereditary.
Developmental delay – child not mature enough for formal schooling.
Emotional disturbance – usually relates to domestic disharmony.
Adolescence – restlessness and aimless exertion are common at this age.
Chronic illness – asthma; congenital heart disease.
Drugs – notably PHENOBARBITONE, CLONAZEPAM and some bronchodilators.
Mental retardation – behaviour in keeping with mental rather than chronological age.
Brain damage – certain children with cerebral palsy and following severe head trauma, meningitis and encephalitis.
Psychosis and autism – uncommon–evidence of loss of contact with reality.
Attention deficit hyperactivity disorder (ADHD).

The summary prescription of METHYLPHENIDATE (Ritalin), without examination and the taking of a detailed history, is to be deplored. The drug is effective when restlessness and limited attention span reflect relative immaturity for age and personality traits. It is also effective in genuine cases of attention deficit hyperactivity disorder. The drug is administered after breakfast on school mornings in a dosage of 0,3-0,5 mg/kg. At this level side-effects, other than slight appetite suppression, are unusual. Duration of action is four to five hours, effectively covering the school morning. The drug should not be administered over weekends or during school holidays. Daily dosage in excess of 20 mg is no more effective than lower levels and is likely to be attended by adverse effects. No child receiving METHYL-PHENIDATE should continue the therapy for more than six months without a trial period off medication. If the child's teacher reports no fall-off in classroom performance it may be assumed that maturation has occurred and that drug therapy is no longer necessary.

METHYLPHENIDATE is ineffective when restlessness and distractability are due to emotional disturbance, low intelligence or an undiagnosed physical complaint. The drug should never be prescribed for preschool children.

Learning disabilities

A child with learning disability is one who fails to make acceptable scholastic progress despite average or above-average intelligence, normal vision and hearing, good physical health and satisfactory emotional adjustment. The doctor's role is to identify and treat physical conditions such as organic disease, visual impairment, deafness and epilepsy, which may impair the child's ability to function in the classroom. In the absence of gross signs, examination of the neurological system is directed towards the elicitation of 'soft signs'. Most of these are indicators of functional immaturity for age rather than focal pathology. The principal consulting room tests are listed in Table 6.4, together with norms. EEG abnormalities, when found in children with learning disability, are of a non-specific nature and the investigation is not recommended unless the history suggests a seizure disorder. The management of learning disability falls in the province of the remedial teacher and school psychologist.

Table 6.4 Learning disability: principal tests used

Function tested	Test	Normal
Gross motor	Hop repetitively on one foot on the spot.	Achieved by fifth birthday. 20 times with no associated movement by seventh birthday.
	Heel and toe (tandem) straight line walking.	No deviations or associated arm movements by seventh birthday.
	Sit up from supine position keeping arms folded across chest.	From eighth birthday heels do not leave the ground.
Fine motor	Thread 0,5 cm diameter beads without significant tremor.	Achieved before fourth birthday.
	Move protruded tongue rapidly from side to side.	From seventh birthday with no associated movements of face or jaw.
	Both hands held up in suppliant gesture with fingers slightly flexed.	From seventh birthday no mirror movements in opposite hand.
	Fingertips of one hand touched rapidly in succession to thumb five times.	
	Rapid pronation/supernation of hand and forearm with elbow bent at 90°.	From eighth birthday no mirror movements in opposite hand.
Copying	See 'Visual'.	
Visual motor	Catch tennis ball thrown from three metres with both hands.	Achieved by sixth birthday.

Function tested	Test	Normal
Visual	Copy △	Achieved by 5,5 years.
	Copy ▨	Achieved by sixth birthday.
	Copy ◇	Achieved by seventh birthday.
	Copy ○ ◇ ⊲	Achieved by eighth birthday.
Body image	Carry out verbal instruction to touch left thumb to right ear etc. on self and tester.	Correct on self by seventh birthday. Correct on tester by eighth birthday.

Reprinted with the kind permission of *Modern Medicine of SA. MMSA* 1984; 10:9:54.

Lying

In preschool children 'tall stories' are often an expression of their inability to distinguish between fact and fantasy. In such cases rebuke is inappropriate. Older children may tell transparent lies in imitation of their parents, in order to avoid punishment or as an attention-seeking device.

Masturbation

Infantile masturbation is uncommon and may be mistaken for a seizure. Most toddlers and young children play with their genitalia from time to time. This should be regarded as a normal act of self-exploration and never as cause for rebuke. Persistent masturbation in public by an older child may reflect psychopathology and referral to a psychologist or child psychiatrist is advisable.

Sibling rivalry

This is a normal feature of family dynamics. The first child frequently shows some reversions to more infantile behaviour on the birth of a second child. The situation calls for parental understanding and suitable periods during which the 'displaced' toddler receives undivided attention. Animosity between older siblings often represents limit-testing within the safety of the family bond. Parental insight, together with fair dispensation of praise and tokens of approval, will usually serve to contain the situation.

Sleep disorders

Sleep-refusal distresses parents far more than the child. Underlying infection or other disease must be excluded and errors of feeding technique eliminated in the infant who cries endlessly and will not go to sleep. The mother requires reassurance so that guilt feelings about her mothering ability can be counteracted. CHLORAL HYDRATE 50 mg/kg in the evening for one or two weeks often serves to establish a satisfactory sleep pattern. The toddler's sleep refusal may be due to separation anxiety, fear of the dark or excessive daytime sleep. Sleep in the parental bed should be firmly discouraged. Night terrors and nightmares may reflect daytime tensions. The child's lifestyle should be examined for sources of stress, and unsuitable television avoided.

Stealing

Theft must be classed as a survival technique when perpetrated by underprivileged children. Children who do not lack material possessions steal as an attention-seeking device and thefts often occur only in their own homes. A child who desires popularity may steal in order to finance a supply of sweets or cakes for distribution amongst his or her peers.

Temper tantrums

These occur when a toddler is checked or fails to secure immediate desires. Characteristically the child will throw him- or herself to the ground and scream and kick. Such behaviour should evoke the immediate withdrawal of the parent or care-giver from the child's presence. He or she should be left alone until in a more acceptable frame of mind. Consistently applied, this management will soon bring an end to temper tantrums.

Thumb-sucking and nail-biting

Thumb-sucking in children under three years of age demands no special management. Older children suck their thumbs when they are feeling tired or insecure. The symptom calls for attention to the underlying cause rather than reproach. Nail-biting is practised at some time by at least one third of all children. The habit may reflect underlying tension and is self-limited. Reproach and nail-painting with distasteful substances are contra-indicated.

Tics

Repetitive facial grimaces, head-shaking and shrugging of the shoulders are seen fairly frequently in children of school age. The child is aware of his or her actions but has no control over them. He or she is usually manifestly anxious and the victim of inner conflicts. Tics of recent onset may respond to adjustments in lifestyle. Long-standing tics call for skilled psychotherapy.

7 POISONOUS BITES AND STINGS

Staff of the Poison Reference Centre

Additional advice may be obtained by phoning a Poisons Information Centre. (See Appendix 5, page 692.)

Snake bite

Identify the snake if possible. Fang marks may not be visible even in severe envenomations.

Antivenom (1 ampoule = 10 ml) is obtainable from the South African Institute for Medical Research (SAIMR), Johannesburg.

First aid

♦ **Reassure** the patient. Stress that few bites result in serious envenomation.
♦ **Wipe** the venom off the skin.
♦ **Place** a clean pad over the bite site.
♦ **Apply** a broad compressive bandage (crêpe or similar) over the pad as soon as possible. Pressure should be similar to that used when binding a sprained ankle and should not act as a venous tourniquet. Extend the bandage to the whole limb if possible.
♦ **Immobilize** the bitten limb with a splint.
♦ **Antivenom** is given intramuscularly (2 amps/20 ml) as a first aid measure in proven bites by mambas, cobras, puff adders and gaboon adders.

Warning

♦ DO NOT INCISE THE WOUND.
♦ Tourniquets are only used for proven bites by dangerous elapids (e.g. cobras and mambas) where antivenom treatment is several hours away.
♦ Wash the eye(s) with copious clean water for 20-30 minutes in eye envenomation (rinkhals and m'fezi). Antivenom diluted 1:10 in water may be used as an eyewash if water is ineffective.

Specific management
Antivenom

♦ **Evidence of systemic envenomation** is an indication for IV administration of **adequate amounts** of antivenom (6-10 amps.).
♦ **Children** need the same doses as adults (see package insert for details).
♦ **Anaphylaxis may occur.** Be prepared for it: have ADRENALINE etc. at hand. See page 27.

Adders and spitting cobra
Clinical presentation

Venom locally cytotoxic. Severe local pain, swelling and ecchymoses, bullous haemorrhagic skin lesions.

Treatment

♦ **Polyvalent antivenom** intravenously (6-10 amps.) if systemic signs are evident or if there is spreading of local damage and swelling.
♦ **Antivenom not required:** small adder species and ineffective for berg adder. The latter has neurotoxic venom causing ptosis, bulbar palsy, anosmia and mydriasis lasting two to three weeks. Treatment is symptomatic.
♦ **Replace** fluid loss and observe for hypovolaemic shock.
♦ **Surgical intervention** is indicated for the relief of pressure when tissue swelling threatens to compromise blood supply.

Boomslang
Clinical features

Bite rare. Venom haemotoxic. Ragged wound may ooze from the outset. Disseminated intravascular coagulation within 12-36 hours.

Treatment

♦ Order specific serum from SAIMR, Johannesburg (see Appendix 5, page 688) if boomslang bite is suspected.
♦ **Administer** specific serum intravenously at the first sign of a coagulation defect, i.e. clinical manifestation and/or prolonged partial thromboplastin time (PTT) = >45 sec. or clotting time >9 min. if PTT unavailable.

◆ **Treat disseminated intravascular coagulation.** See page 242.

Cobra and mamba

Clinical features

Venom rapidly neurotoxic. Ptosis and visual disturbance lead on to a general flaccid paralysis.

Treatment

◆ **Polyvalent antivenom in large doses** (10 or more amps.) IV if systemic symptoms develop.
◆ **Maintain** airway and prepare to assist respiration.

General management

◆ **Antitetanus** prophylaxis for all bites: tetanus toxoid. See pages 272-3.
◆ **Antibiotics** for wound sepsis.
◆ **Analgesics** for pain.

Scorpion sting

The sting of all scorpions is painful.

Dangerous scorpions belong to the family *Buthidae* and are distinguished by small pincers and prominent thick tails. (See Figure 7.1). Of these, Uroplectes is the most common but least venomous. Parabuthus and Buthotus can cause severe neurotoxic envenomation. It is extremely difficult to distinguish between Uroplectes and other Buthids. It is suggested that all

Figure 7.1 Non-buthid and buthid scorpions

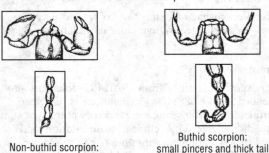

Non-buthid scorpion:
large pincers and thin tail

Buthid scorpion:
small pincers and thick tail

Buthid scorpion stings be managed similarly. Non-buthid scorpions have a minimal haemolytic and local cytotoxic effect. See Figure 7.1.

Scorpion antivenom is obtainable from the SAIMR, Johannesburg (See Appendix 5, page 688).

Buthid scorpion sting

The bite is usually painful but with little local reaction. It may be invisible.

Clinical features

Coarse involuntary movements, tremor, ataxia, muscle cramps and weakness, dysphagia and dysarthria. Paraesthesiae, hyperaesthesiae, pyrexia, increased sweating, respiratory depression.

A hyperactivity syndrome, similar to that seen in PHENOTHIAZINE overdose, is common in children and indicates serious envenomation.

First aid (all scorpion stings)

♦ **Infiltration** with local anaesthetic around the sting site is the most effective pain control measure.
♦ **Application** of cold packs, crepe bandaging and immobilizing the affected limb with splints can be useful in retarding the spread of venom via the lymphatics.
♦ **Anti-inflammatory** agents are more effective than analgesics.

Warning

MORPHINE derivatives for pain are contra-indicated as the neurotoxic action of the venom may be potentiated.

Specific management

♦ **Admit** all patients stung by these scorpions for at least 12 hours' observation.
♦ **Administer** scorpion antivenom 5 ml IM to all children under 12 years with a confirmed history of Buthid scorpion bite. For children over 12 years and adults administer antivenom 5 ml IM if systemic signs are present.
♦ **Eye envenomation** is treated by washing out with copious water or saline over 20-30 min. Antivenom diluted 1:10 with

water may be instilled into the eye. Local anaesthetic eye drops such as OXYBUPROCAINE or PROPARACAINE may be useful.
◆ **Antitetanus** prophylaxis for all stings. See pages 272-3.

Warning

◆ Anaphylaxis or allergy to antivenom is a risk. See page 27.
◆ Prepare for assisted ventilation.
◆ **Avoid narcotic analgesics and barbiturates** which may potentiate the respiratory depressant effect of the venom.

Spider bite

Many spiders are capable of inflicting a painful bite with the potential for local secondary infection. Genuinely poisonous bites may be neurotoxic or cytotoxic.

Spider antivenom is obtainable from the SAIMR, Johannesburg (See Appendix 5, page 688).

Neurotoxic spiders

Latrodectus indistinctus, formerly L. mactans (black widow, black button spider)

Widespread, natural fynbos habitat. Black globular abdomen,

Figure 7.2 *Latrodectus sp.* (neurotoxic)

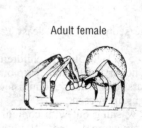

Adult female

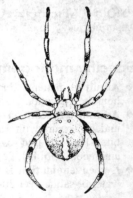

typically with bright red streak or dot on dorsal surface and no ventral markings.

Clinical features

Bites can cause serious morbidity.

Black widow bite causes rapid onset of severe cramping muscular pain that is initially localized but which spreads to limbs, chest and abdomen. Muscle fasciculations, tremor, coarse involuntary movements and increased muscle tone. Abdominal rigidity may simulate peritonitis. Profuse sweating, paraesthesiae, pyrexia and restlessness may lead on to respiratory paralysis or sudden cardiac arrest.

Latrodectus geometricus (brown widow)

Widespread, prefers built-up areas. Brown globular abdomen mottled on the dorsal surface with a geometric pattern. Red-orange hourglass-shaped ventral marking.

Figure 7.3 *Latrodectus indistinctus*

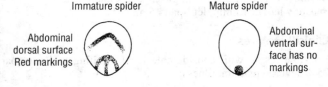

Immature spider

Abdominal dorsal surface Red markings

Mature spider

Abdominal ventral surface has no markings

Figure 7.4 *Latrodectus geometricus*

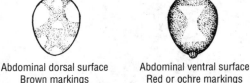

Abdominal dorsal surface
Brown markings

Abdominal ventral surface
Red or ochre markings

Clinical features

Capable of producing serious illness in children. Its bite is however, less serious than that of *L. indistinctus*. A bite results in pain, and paraesthesiae is localized to the bite region. Children may experience increased sweating, restlessness and agitation.

Treatment

The effect of antivenom administration is usually dramatic and will reverse symptoms and signs.

◆ **Ice pack** to bite area to delay absorption.
◆ **Spider antiserum**: 5 ml IM if systemic symptoms are present. Repeat if no relief of symptoms within two to four hours (risk of allergic reaction or anaphylaxis). If there is a delay in obtaining antiserum, muscle cramps may be controlled with 10% calcium gluconate IV 50 mg or 0,5 ml/kg/dose up to 1 g or 10 ml in children over 12 years (adults) at a maximum rate of 50-100 mg or 0,5-1 ml/min. This may be repeated after 30 minutes and once more after a further 60 minutes. The effect is short-lived.

Cytotoxic spiders
Chiracanthium (sac spider)

◆ Free-ranging hunter. Found in foliage, fast-moving species.
◆ Medium-sized.
◆ Straw-coloured body with glossy black chelicerae.
◆ Body length 13 mm, leg span 35 mm.

Clinical features

Boil-like lesion with considerable local swelling and oedema. 25% develop pyrexial illness.

Figure 7.5 *Chiracanthium sp*

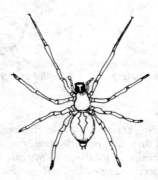

Treatment

Apply GENTIAN VIOLET to the bite site to prevent secondary infection.

Loxosceles (violin spider)

♦ Free-ranging hunter, found beneath rocks in caves or dark corners of houses.
♦ Small and delicate with long thin legs.
♦ Brownish or dark brown with black markings.
♦ Violin-shaped marking on carapace.
♦ Body length 9 mm, leg span 50 mm.

Clinical features

Bites are initially painless with intense pain developing in two to eight hours. Central necrotic area sloughs after ten days leaving a deep ulcer which heals very slowly.

Treatment

Analgesia as required. See page 34. Apply GENTIAN VIOLET to prevent secondary infection.

Figure 7.6 *Loxosceles sp*

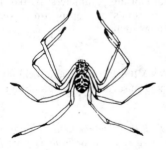

Sicarius (six-eyed crab spider)

♦ Lives buried in sand beneath stones, in caves, animal burrows etc.
♦ Large robust spider, dorso-ventrally compressed.
♦ Body covered with sand particles from habitat, lodged amongst body setae.

Figure 7.7 *Sicarius sp*

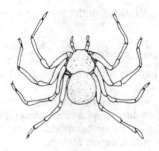

◆ Freshly moulted colour is yellowish or reddish brown.
◆ Very small eyes.
◆ Body length 15 mm, leg span 50 mm.

Clinical features

Bites are surrounded by a haemorrhagic zone with little oedema. Disseminated intravascular coagulation has been described in animal work but no reports have been substantiated in humans.

Investigations

Check for abnormal clotting parameters: partial thromboplastin time (PTT) = >45 seconds or clotting time greater than nine minutes, if PTT is unavailable.

Treatment

◆ Apply GENTIAN VIOLET to prevent local infection.
◆ Treat disseminated intravascular coagulation as described on page 242.

The help of Dr GJ Muller, Department of Pharmacology, University of Stellenbosch Medical School, is gratefully acknowledged.

8 BREAKING BAD NEWS

L D Henley

Breaking bad news is never easy. It is emotionally demanding, it takes time and you will feel ill-equipped.

Preparing for the interview

Your attitude may be more important than the words you use.

- You cannot change the diagnosis but you can try to ease the burden of it. It helps if you can put yourself in the parents' position. Think how you might feel in a similar situation.
- Anticipate the kind of information parents need and might want to know. Find out more about the condition and available community resources.
- If appropriate, include another team member in the interview (e.g. a social worker or a nursing sister who is known to the parents).
- Be gentle and sympathetic. Maintain eye contact and use touch appropriately. A cold, business-like approach is never warranted.

Conducting the interview

Pace rather than protect from bad news.

- Unless absolutely unavoidable, don't give bad news over the telephone. Privacy and lack of interruption are essential. Don't break news in a busy clinic or on a ward round. Sit down. It suggests you are there to stay — at least for a while.
- Check that parents know who you are and what you do. It may not be self-evident, especially in a large hospital.
- Speak to both parents together. Information transmitted from one spouse to another can easily be distorted. It also places an unfair burden on the spouse who has to convey the information. Single parents may want a relative or close friend present.

♦ The baby should be present at the first interview and held by one of the parents. Refer to the patient by name, not as 'it'. This focuses the meeting on a person rather than a medical problem.

  ◊ Do not include an older child in the initial interview. Parents have the right to be the first to give their own child bad news. If the parents are reluctant, then ask if they would like you to do so.

♦ Parents want to be told the diagnosis as soon as possible. If there is a delay in reaching a definitive diagnosis, explain why and keep the parents informed about ongoing investigations. Never be afraid to say you don't know. But always add that you will either find out or find someone who does know.

♦ Ask parents what they think caused the condition. Parents often blame themselves, especially if the disease has a genetic basis or can be related to pregnancy or birth. Stress to parents that they are in no way 'responsible' for their child's condition. Cultural beliefs can also influence parents' understanding of causation. For example, they may blame the condition on ancestral wrath incurred because they might have failed to observe an important cultural tradition or ritual.

♦ Use simple language that parents can understand. Avoid jargon and offensive words (e.g. mongol, idiot). Explain the meaning of medical terms. Use diagrams to simplify and clarify your explanation. In general, leave technical details for later interviews. Before introducing a new piece of information check that what you are saying is being understood: 'Am I making sense?', 'Do you see what I mean?'. Ideally parents should be given explanations in their home language. Use an interpreter if necessary.

♦ Parents may forget much of what you tell them at the initial interview. You may have to explain the diagnosis many times. Some parents may raise the same questions repeatedly as if these had never been answered before. Other parents may be reluctant to ask too many questions as they feel that the doctor is too busy. Unanswered questions or evasive replies may lead to dissatisfaction and suspicion that information is being withheld.

♦ Provide parents with simple literature on the condition (if available). Pamphlets can be read and reread at home. They can be given to relatives, teachers and friends. Tell parents to write down whatever they don't understand, no matter how trivial, for discussion at the next appointment.

◆ Parents may be given conflicting information, particularly in a hospital setting. One way to reduce confusion is to have a checklist in the folder of what parents are told (aetiology, diagnosis, prognosis etc.) and when. See page 483.

Where there is hope, be hopeful.

◆ If parents ask a question, it is assumed they want a truthful answer. However, not all parents are equally adept at handling the truth. Do not destroy hope. Concentrate on the positive aspects of recovery and retained function, rather than on the negative aspects of what may be lost.

Being truthful is not the same as being blunt.

◆ Parents may deny or question the diagnosis of a serious illness or handicap. This is normal and understandable. Listen but gently stress the reality of the situation: 'I wish it were otherwise, but sadly there is no question about the diagnosis'. If parents request a second opinion, cooperate by helping to arrange an appointment or by sending records.

Learn to listen more and talk less.

◆ Although you can offer no anaesthetics to ease the pain of hearing bad news, you can share it by listening and responding to parents' concerns and feelings. One of the most common mistakes doctors make is not to let parents talk.

◆ Anger and extreme distress are common reactions to hearing bad news. Anger is probably the most difficult to manage, especially if it is directed at some aspect of nursing or medical care: 'the diagnosis was made too late' or 'the treatment was inadequate'. Try to identify the source of the anger. If necessary, offer an apology for any insensitivity or error. Any attempt to refute an allegation or defend a colleague usually makes matters worse. Anger is most quickly defused by allowing its expression.

◆ It is natural to feel uncomfortable if a parent starts to cry. Allow the parent to cry. Crying tells you that what you are discussing is important, albeit painful, to the parent. Don't introduce a new subject until the parent has regained control. People don't handle factual material well when they are experiencing strong emotions. It is important not to suddenly change the subject because you are feeling helpless. Don't be afraid of silences. Parents need to digest what they are being told.

◆ Be kind to yourself. You're going to make mistakes and you may feel a sense of failure, but remember that it is the news, not the bearer of the news, that is bad and causing distress.

Closing the interview

◆ Ask parents to repeat in their own words what you have told them. This allows you to identify gaps in their knowledge, gauge their level of understanding and correct any misconceptions.

◆ Don't leave parents with a feeling of no future. Talking to parents should not end after breaking the news. Outline a plan of management. If necessary arrange another appointment. Tell parents if and when you are available. If possible give a contact telephone number. It provides a lifeline and is unlikely to be abused. Mention sources of support, e.g. social workers, ward back-up and parent support groups.

When a child dies the following guidelines may be helpful:

◆ Don't avoid the parents because **you** are feeling uncomfortable. Allow them to express their grief. Don't say 'I know how you must feel' (unless you have lost a child yourself). Parents are often plagued by feelings of doubt and guilt. Reassure them that they did everything they could for their child. Where death is due to an accident (e.g. drowning or burns) it is natural for parents to blame themselves. Allow them to express these feelings.

◆ Don't offer pacifications like 'It happened for the best' or 'It's God's will'. Don't suggest that they can always have another child or they can be thankful they have other healthy children at home.

◆ Don't suddenly change the subject when parents mention their dead child. Allow them to talk about the child as often as they wish.

◆ Anticipate the kind of practical information parents may want to know such as 'What must we do about the body?' Suggest they contact an undertaker who can advise about funeral arrangements. Muslim families make their own burial arrangements.

◆ Make yourself available. Parents often feel 'cut off' from the close ties they develop at the hospital. Where practical, plan several phone calls or surgery visits with the parents during the following year. This lets parents know that they and the patient are not forgotten. It also offers an opportunity to answer any lingering questions or ease any remaining guilt.

The worse the news, the greater the effort in communicating it.

Further Reading

Buckman R. *How to Break Bad News: A Guide for Health Care Professionals.* Baltimore: The John Hopkins University Press; 1992.

Jellinek MS, Catlin EA, Todres ID and Cassem EH. Facing tragic decisions with parents in the neonatal intensive care unit: clinical perspectives. *Pediatrics* 1992; 89: 119-122.

9 BREAST-FEEDING

C W van der Elst and D L Woods

Successful breast-feeding is the single most effective factor in lowering infant mortality.

A mother who breast-feeds offers many advantages to both herself and her baby. These include convenience, a financial saving and a lower incidence of diarrhoeal disease, allergy and obesity. Breast-feeding promotes mother-baby bonding and hence the well-being of the child.

Before breast-feeding begins

Successful breast-feeding depends largely on maternal motivation. The decision to breast-feed should be made before, or early in, pregnancy. During the antenatal period the mother should be taught the physiology and method of breast-feeding. A well-informed midwife or doctor should be available to discuss breast-feeding and answer any questions. The best preparation is for the mother to watch another mother breast-feeding.

Careful attention should be paid to the technique of feeding. The nursing mother should be warm and comfortable, preferably sitting up with the infant cradled in one arm across her body and facing her breast. The nipple and breast are supported by the thumb above and the fingers below. The rooting reflex is evoked to prompt the baby to search for and latch onto the areola and nipple together.

Massaging the nipples before delivery is not recommended as it may stimulate uterine contractions that can be stressful to the fetus. Exposure to sunlight for three to five minutes each day lessens the possibility that the nipples will crack during the first week of lactation. Flat nipples must be corrected before delivery. Using the thumb and forefinger and commencing at the nipple base, the skin is gently stretched away from the nipple. This exercise is to be repeated five times daily.

Getting started

If the mother and baby are well, the infant should be put to the breast immediately at birth. This practice results in a higher incidence of prolonged breast-feeding. Demand-feeding should be encouraged so that the mother and baby set up their own routine. However, for the first few days the infant should not be allowed to suck for more than five minutes at each breast per feed. The breast is usually emptied in this time and prolonged sucking may result in sore nipples. Only small amounts of milk are produced at first, and the infant may lose up to 10% of its birthweight. This is common and is no cause for alarm. In most cases complementary feeding is not necessary and may even be harmful. Many mothers give water to their babies between feeds but this also is not recommended. By the fifth day the mother's milk supply can be expected to have increased and most infants will be gaining weight by one week of age. It may occasionally take a few weeks for adequate lactation to be established. The infant should suckle both breasts at each feed. Offer alternate breasts first at successive feeds.

It is essential that the mother and the infant room-in together after delivery in order to strengthen bonding and encourage demand feeding. Encouragement and advice from other mothers who are successfully breast-feeding is invaluable. Most urban communities have breast-feeding counsellors who help mothers with problems, but very little professional help is available in rural areas. Health care providers should offer support, encouragement and education on the process of lactation. For example, a mother needs support after caesarean section, with twins, with a preterm neonate, or if her baby is unwell. She may need help in the initiation of lactation, the position for nursing and latching on. Careful explanation that it may take up to three weeks for full volume lactation to be achieved may prevent early feeding failure.

Breast-fed babies should be given additional VITAMIN D (400 IU/day) if they have limited exposure to sunlight or were preterm at birth. Vitamin D is available in multivite syrups, which are obtainable from most clinics. Fluoride should be given in areas where there is a deficiency in the water supply. See page 377. Iron supplementation is recommended from three months. See page 240.

Too little milk

Inadequate lactation in the early stages may be the result of rigid feeding schedules, emotional stress, anxiety, sore nipples or fatigue.

Many mothers stop breast-feeding because they believe that they have insufficient or 'weak' milk. The initial milk (colostrum) is thin and watery but it is rich in protective immunoglobulins. Later, foremilk and hindmilk are produced. Foremilk appears dilute but this is normal. Hindmilk is thicker and rich in fat and is obtained only when the breast has been partially emptied.

Useful indicators of adequate lactation are that the baby tends to fall asleep on the breast, starts to gain weight by the fifth day, the mother's breast feels full before the feed and empty afterwards and there are six or more wet nappies per day. Alternatively, if a scale is available, the baby is shown to gain 25-30 g per day when test weighed after each feed, averaged over a 12-24 hour period.

Appropriate steps should be taken to identify and treat the cause of inadequate lactation. The best way to enhance milk production is to put the infant to the breast at regular intervals, as frequently as two-hourly during the day. The mother should be encouraged to relax when feeding and to drink adequate fluids.

In general, complementary feeds are not advised for breast-feeding babies. They decrease the production of breast milk and confuse the infant. However, the working mother should express her milk into a bottle for missed feeds. Expressed milk will stay fresh for 48 hours in a refrigerator and is best given to the infant using a cup. Supplementary feeds may be offered where refrigeration is not available. See pages 52-3.

If lactation remains inadequate a doctor may prescribe SULPIRIDE (Eglonyl) 50 mg (one capsule) or METOCLO-PRAMIDE (Maxolon) 10 mg (one tablet) orally three times daily for ten days. The manufacturers do not comment on the use of these drugs during lactation and they are not a substitute for good guidance by breast-feeding clinics.

Engorgement

With generalized engorgement the whole breast feels hard and tender. Either sucking or expression should be used to empty the breast.

A blocked milk duct results in hard swelling and tenderness of a segment of the breast. The overlying skin may be erythematous but the mother does not feel ill. The obstruction can usually be resolved by allowing the baby to empty the breast, by providing local heat (a warm compress), and by gently massaging the breast towards the nipple. Analgesics are seldom necessary.

Mastitis and breast abscess

With simple engorgement the mother feels well, but with mastitis she becomes ill and pyrexial, and the breast is swollen, painful and inflamed. Treatment consists of antibiotics (ERYTHROMYCIN, CLOXACILLIN or an oral CEPHALOSPORIN), local heat and analgesics. It is usually not necessary to stop breast-feeding and it is essential to empty the infected breast. A breast abscess presents as a painful fluctuant mass which remains palpable after the breast has been emptied. There is often skin induration and oedema over the infected area. The abscess must be drained surgically and the infant should be temporarily taken off that breast.

Nipple problems

Careful antenatal preparation, correct feeding and fixing techniques and demand feeding all help prevent damaged nipples. Ensure that the nipples are dried after feeds, then allow a little colostrum or hindmilk to be left to dry on the nipples after each feed. The anti-infective properties and fat protect the nipples. Exposure to sunlight or ultraviolet light for short spells assists in healing sore nipples. Nipple shields may also be of use during this time. If the nipple is very painful, breast feeding should be temporarily stopped and the milk expressed into a cup or bottle for the infant. Breast-feeding can gradually be restarted after a few days. Treat monilial infection, if present, in both mother and infant.

Maternal illness

Acute maternal illness rarely warrants stopping breast-feeding. Mothers with a cold or flu should continue to breast-feed, as should a mother with food poisoning, malaria or syphilis. Tuberculosis is not a contra-indication to breast-feeding but the infant should be placed on prophylactic ISONIAZID, PYRAZINAMIDE and RIFAMPICIN. BCG should not be given and should be referred to the local tuberculosis clinic. See page 566. Mothers with 'cold sores' (Herpes simplex type I) can breast-feed but care must be taken not to expose the baby to open sores. Advice for mothers who are HIV positive or who have

AIDS and wish to breast-feed, is controversial. In a developed country it is advisable not to breast-feed, but in a developing country it is in the best interests of the baby to breast-feed.

Maternal drugs and breast-feeding

Most drugs are excreted in the breast milk but usually not in pharmacological amounts.

The following medications are contra-indications to breast-feeding:

◆ ACE inhibitors;
◆ cytotoxic drugs;
◆ iodine;
◆ radioactive medications; and
◆ TETRACYCLINE.

The following are **not** contra-indications to breast-feeding:

◆ analgesics (e.g. PARACETAMOL);
◆ anticoagulants (WARFARIN);
◆ anti-asthmatic medications (not containing iodine);
◆ antibiotics (except TETRACYCLINE);
◆ anti-epileptic medications e.g. PHENOBARBITONE, PHENYTOIN;
◆ antithyroid medications;
◆ anti-depressants; or
◆ cortisone.

Most childhood vaccines, including the oral polio vaccine, can be given while the mother is breast-feeding.

10 BURNS

H Rode and A J W Millar

A burn is the result of energy transfer to the skin. The local effect will be determined by the source and duration of energy transfer. Principles of management are: relief of pain, accurate assessment of the nature and extent of injury, fluid resuscitation, early burn wound closure, support and rehabilitation.

Burns are divided into minor or major burns. A minor burn is a partial thickness burn of less than 10% surface area in a child older than one year. A major burn is a partial thickness burn of more than 10% surface area, a full thickness burn of more than 3% surface area and any burn that involves the head and face, hands, feet, or perineum. Inhalation burns present with respiratory distress. Inhalation injuries, circumferential burns, electrical injuries, neonatal burns, infected burns and burns in patients with serious pre-existing or concomitant injuries are also classified as major burns. A patient with a major burn should be admitted to hospital.

Assessment

Important factors must be considered when assessing the seriousness of a burn. They are:

♦ the nature and time of the burn;
♦ the age of the patient;
♦ the site of the burn wound;
♦ the estimated body surface area (BSA) burnt;
♦ the depth of the injury;
♦ the general physical status of the child; and
♦ the nature of concomitant injuries.

The extent of the injury is expressed as the BSA involved according to age (see Table 10.1). The open hand of the patient represents approximately 1% of the BSA.

The depth of a burn wound is expressed in terms of a partial thickness or full-thickness injury. (See Table 10.2)

Table 10.1 Body surface area percentages according to age

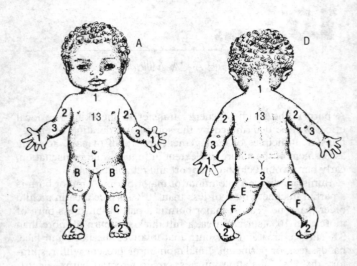

	Age (years)				
	<1	**1**	**5**	**10**	**15**
A/D Head	10	9	7	6	5
B/E Thigh	3	3	4	5	5
C/F Leg	2	3	3	3	3

Table 10.2 Assessment of the severity of a burn

Clinical presentation	Partial thickness burn	Full thickness burn
Pain	Painful	Usually painless
Blisters	Large, growing	Absent or small
Colour	Red, hyperaemic	Black, white No circulation evident
Texture	Can be normal	Leathery
Healing	Within three weeks	Not healed at three weeks

Emergency management

◆ **Remove** smouldering or hot clothing. **Ensure** an adequate airway. **Immerse** small burns in cold water (18 °C). **Cover** the burn wound with a clean, dry dressing.
◆ **Chemical burns:** copious irrigation with water.
◆ **Electrical burns:** evaluate circulation and ventilation.
◆ **Inhalation injury:** administer 100% oxygen with a face-mask.

Transport of a patient with a major burn

The patient is usually stable immediately after the injury. Prior to transport, commence resuscitation (see Table 10.3), pass a nasogastric tube, cover the wound with a clean dressing or poly-thene cling-film (from the kitchen) and keep the patient warm.

Definitive management of a minor burn

Treat as an outpatient.

Initial therapy

◆ Administer analgesics. See page 38.
◆ Clean the wound(s) with water (shower) or POVIDONE IODINE 10% solution.

Remove topically applied agents and shave hair where necessary.

◆ Wound care: debride loose dead tissue.

Apply topical antibacterial agents (SILVER SULPHADIAZINE 1% or POVIDONE IODINE 5% cream). Alternatively cover with an occlusive dressing, e.g. sterile gauze and Elastoform, or with a polyurethane dressing (Opsite).

◆ Administer tetanus toxoid 0,5 ml IM. See pages 272-3.

Note

Prophylactic antibiotic is contra-indicated.

Follow-up therapy

◆ Continue with local topical therapy.
◆ Encourage active movement.
◆ Return daily or once a week as needed until healing occurs, which is usually within two or three weeks.

Definitive management of major burns

Admit to hospital and treat as an emergency. The burn wound itself is rarely immediately life-threatening after emergency management at the scene of the accident. Care of other injuries may have to take precedence.

General measures

Establish patency of the airway. Take surface swabs for culture. Pass a nasogastric tube. Keep patient warm.

Specific measures

Fluid resuscitation

Start as soon as possible (the fluid resuscitation schedule given in Table 10.3 gives guidelines). Fluid administration requires constant reassessment to provide haemodynamic stability as measured by the pulse rate, blood pressure and a urine output of at least 1-1,5 ml/kg/hour and urine specific gravity of <1 020. In the presence of clinical shock, ileus, or with burns greater than 20% (BSA), oral intake should be stopped and the stomach decompressed with a nasogastric tube.

Blood

◆ Packed cells if haematocrit <25%.
◆ Transfuse 10 ml/kg.

Catheterize

◆ All burns over 15%.

Monitor

◆ Pulse, blood pressure, respiratory rate, sensorium.
◆ Urine output: aim at 1,0-1,5 ml/kg/hour with SG below 1020.

Relief of pain

Important. Therapy is rarely needed on a regular basis beyond 48 hours. See page 38 for guidelines.

Prevention of peptic ulceration

Antacids or an H_2 receptor blocker should be given to children with burns >50% of the BSA to guard against peptic ulceration.

Table 10.3 Fluid resuscitation schedule

Resuscitation fluid: plasmalyte B or Ringer's lactate (balanced electrolyte solution).
Maintenance fluid: paediatric maintenance fluid.

Burns under 10%

♦ If under one year with burn >5% treat as >10%.
♦ Resuscitation fluid for complicated or full thickness burns.
♦ Maintenance fluid is given orally or by nasogastric tube.

Burns 10 – 20%

♦ Resuscitation fluid 15-25 ml/kg in one or two hours if the patient is shocked, has a full thickness burn and/or haemoglobinuria is present.
♦ Plus stabilized human serum
   first 24 hr: 3,5 ml x mass (kg) x % burn
   second 24 hr: 1,5 ml x mass (kg) x % burn
   Plus maintenance fluid as outlined below.

Burns >20%

♦ Resuscitation fluid 15 to 25 ml/kg in one or two hours (as above)
♦ Plus stabilized human serum 3,5 ml x mass (kg) x % burn as for 10 – 20% burns above.
   0 – two years: calculate at 20% maximum
   three to seven years: calculate at 25% maximum
   seven – 12 years: calculate at 30% maximum
♦ Plus maintenance fluid (+ 10% dextrose) continuously infused
   Infant: 120-150 ml/kg/day.
   two to five years: 100 ml/kg/day.
   five to eight years: 80 ml/kg/day.
   eight – 12 years: 50 ml/kg/day.

Wound management

♦ A gentle but thorough initial cleaning that includes removal of all debris left by combustion and debridement of lost non-viable skin is performed.
♦ Blisters are usually left intact for two or three days and then removed.
♦ Topical therapy (see below) and cover the wound with a sterile dressing. Use an occlusive sterile dressing technique where practical.

◆ Change dressings daily or more frequently.
◆ When dressings are changed, clean the burned surface with an aqueous solution of POVIDONE IODINE 10% (Betadine).

Daily showering of the patient, even with a critical burn, is necessary in order to maintain body hygiene and is an essential part of burn wound management.

Topical therapy

No single agent is totally effective against all burn wound microbes. Treatment should be guided by regular burn wound cultures and *in vitro* results. Recommended agents are:

◆ POVIDONE IODINE (Betadine 5%). Good prophylactic and therapeutic cream. Active for 24 hours with broad spectrum antibacterial, antifungal and antiviral activity. Apply occlusive dressings daily. Good tissue penetration. Minimal side-effects but can cause metabolic acidosis.
◆ SILVER SULPHADIAZINE (Flamazine 1%). Mainly against Gram-negative organisms and effective for 24 hours. A good prophylactic and therapeutic agent. Apply occlusive dressings once daily. Poor tissue penetration. Transient leukopaenia can result. Determine the WBC count twice per week, and discontinue if the WBC count falls below 3 000 cm^3.
◆ MUPIROCIN (Bactroban) is a very effective broad spectrum agent against Gram-positive and Gram-negative organisms. Apply occlusive dressings once daily. Excellent tissue penetration. Unwanted side-effects include metabolic acidosis. Should not be used on a burn with a BSA greater than 20%, unless there are poor results with other agents. In this case, apply MUPIROCIN for only three hours twice daily and remove with saline during the in-between periods.

Prevention and treatment of infection

Topical antibiotics are not recommended. Systemic antibiotics are only administered in the presence of proven clinical burn wound sepsis; septicaemia; thermal injury with respiratory tract infection; β-haemolytic streptococcal infection; a burn wound BSA of more than 40%; if early tangential excision is contemplated; or during skin grafting procedures. Systemic antibiotic therapy should be re-evaluated according to culture results every five days.

Antitetanus prophylaxis is indicated. See pages 272-3.

Surgical management of the burn wound

The single most important principle in burn therapy is to achieve wound closure as expeditiously as possible, thereby reducing the risk of sepsis, decreasing morbidity and restoring function.

Guidelines for surgery

All full thickness fire burns should be excised and grafted as soon as resuscitation has been completed. The depth of hot water burns is more difficult to assess accurately and if not obviously full thickness (Table 10.2) they are best treated expectantly for ten to 14 days. Those wounds not showing evidence of healing should then be excised and grafted.

◆ **Releasing escharotomy** should be done whenever the burn has impeded blood flow to more distal parts, and in full thickness trunk burns which are impairing respiratory movement. The incision must traverse the dead tissue layer and extend beyond the borders of the burn.

◆ **Tangential excision.** Done as soon as the patient is haemodynamically stable. This entails sequential excision of thin layers of eschar until bleeding dermis has been exposed after which there should be immediate grafting. Not more than 15-20% surface area should be excised at any one time.

◆ **Delayed escharectomy.** Surgical removal of dead tissue ten to 14 days after the burn followed by immediate or delayed grafting.

◆ **Spontaneous separation of eschar.** Ideally suited for burns of the perineum. Daily debridement by means of hydrotherapy, and 'thirds solution' (peroxide, saline, acetic acid) or gauze dressings.

◆ **Biological dressings** are used as temporary dressings until grafts are available, e.g. pigskin as a heterograft and cadaver skin as an allograft.

◆ **Skin grafting.** A burn wound is ready for skin grafting when there is a uniform bed of healthy granulation tissue.

   ◇ A split skin graft (Thiersch) is the preferred choice. Topically applied ADRENALINE 1:30 000 may reduce capillary bleeding from donor and recipient areas.
   ◇ Low-grade infection with other organisms does not necessarily preclude skin grafting.

◇ β-haemolytic streptococcal wound infection is a contra-
  indication to skin grafting.
◇ All skin grafting procedures should be covered with a
  cephalosporin for two to five days as antibiotic prophylaxis.

Nutritional support

Caloric and protein demands require attention from the first day.
Most children with small burns can tolerate enteral feeding
within four to eight hours, either orally or via nasogastric or
naso-duodenal tubes. Major burns, due to gastric stasis, require
the placement of a nasoduodenal feeding tube. Tube-feeding
(milk, Ensure) should begin as soon as possible and feeding
volume increased at 1 ml/kg/hour to full feeds. Effective enteral
feeding can replace parenteral nutrition. Parenteral feeding
should provide daily requirements during the initial phase of
intestinal intolerance. Daily needs can be assessed from the
formula:

Protein: 3 g/kg body weight + (1 g/1% burned BSA)
Calories: 250 kJ/kg body weight + (150 kJ x % burned BSA)

The maximum percentage burn area used for the calculation
should not exceed 50%.

Albumin infusions of 1 g/kg/day can be given to maintain
adequate plasma albumin levels (>28 g/dl).

Micronutrients: iron, vitamins, zinc and trace elements should
be given at double RDA dosages until skin cover is completed.
See page 391.

Rehabilitation

The best overall care and preparation for the patient's return to
his or her environment should be provided by a team incorporat-
ing a nurse, physiotherapist, occupational therapist, dietitian,
social worker, teacher, and doctor. Every endeavour should be
made to facilitate the child's return to society.

Basic principles include:
◆ maintenance of function of the affected area;
◆ restoration of physical and functional abilities;
◆ minimization of scarring and contractures, e.g. with pressure
  garments and splints; and
◆ psychological support and encouragement of psychological
  acceptance of self-image.

11 CARDIOVASCULAR DISORDERS

M M A de Moor

The majority of children with symptomatic heart disease will present in the first year of life. They should be considered to be suffering from a congenital heart defect in the first instance and only rarely from other conditions such as myocarditis. Neonates and infants who are cyanosed, who have had hypercyanotic spells, or who are in heart failure require urgent referral. It is important to consult by telephone with a paediatric cardiologist before referral.

Clinical assessment

Clinical assessment for the presence of cyanosis and cardiac failure and of heart sounds, murmurs, peripheral pulses and blood pressure in all four limbs is important. Auscultation for sounds and murmurs other than over the cardiac area, and haemoglobin estimations, help to exclude other causes of cardiac failure such as arteriovenous malformations, anaemia and fluid overload.

An electrocardiogram (ECG) and chest radiograph (CXR) should be obtained.

Innocent murmurs

Innocent (vibratory or non-significant) murmurs are common and occur in about 60% of children. The child is well and not cyanosed nor in heart failure. The heart sounds are normal. The murmur is soft and usually parasternal with no radiation. The murmur is usually systolic only; the soft continuous murmurs of the venous hum and the subclavian bruit are easily distinguished as the murmur disappears when the head is rotated or the position of the child is altered. ECG and CXR are normal.

The hyperoxia test

Cyanosis in the neonate is more likely to be due to a pulmonary or cerebral cause than a cardiac defect. Cold extremities or metabolic disturbances such as hypoglycaemia may cause peripheral cyanosis. The hyperoxia test may resolve the question of whether the patient has a cyanotic congenital heart defect or pulmonary disease.

♦ Give 100% oxygen via an enclosed head box for five to ten minutes.
♦ Obtain a sample of arterial blood from the right radial artery. See page 443.
   PaO_2 >33,3 kPa (250 mmHg) – excludes cyanotic heart disease
   PaO_2 20-33,3 kPa (150-250 mmHg) – unlikely
   PaO_2 <20 kPa (150 mmHg) – cyanotic congenital heart defect or transient fetal circulation (TFC).

A diagnosis of TFC should be considered in a cyanosed neonate during the first 36 hours after birth.

TFC is characterized by persistent pulmonary hypertension with a R-L shunt at atrial level and via the PDA. Underlying conditions such as asphyxia neonatorum, hypothermia, hypoglycaemia and polycythaemia are frequent triggers. Cyanosis is associated with respiratory distress. Treatment includes removal of the underlying causes, treatment of acidosis and hypoxia and possibly mechanical ventilation. The cyanosis may improve rapidly or, if the pulmonary hypertension is severe, it may only resolve slowly after days of mechanical ventilation.

Neonates suffering from TFC are often born outside the hospital.

Blood pressure measurement

Blood pressure determination is an integral part of the routine physical examination of all children.

Technique
Cuff

Use the largest cuff that can comfortably be applied to the upper arm without the lower edge interfering with the stethoscope in the antecubital fossa.

The inflatable bladder must encircle at least two thirds of the upper arm over the artery. Too small a cuff gives erroneously high readings.

Appearance of the Korotkoff sounds on auscultation indicates the systolic blood pressure. Disappearance indicates the diastolic blood pressure.

Flush method

Invariably underestimates the true reading in infants.

Palpation

Palpate pulse distal to cuff. Measures systolic pressure only.

Ultrasound (Doppler) technique

The most accurate method.

Table 11.1 Normal blood pressure levels: upper limit of normal

Age (Years)	Blood pressure (mmHg) Systolic	Diastolic
0-1	100	65
1-3	110	65
3-7	120	70
7-14	130	75

Warning: There is a tendency towards higher blood pressure readings in children with increased height for age and weight for age than in their peers.

Chest X-ray

The exact definition of specific chamber enlargement on the chest X-ray is difficult in paediatric cardiology but should be assessed. See page 100.

The normal cardiothoracic ratio:
in infancy ≤60%. In childhood ≤55%. In adolescence ≤50%. See page 463.

Electrocardiogram

See Table 11.2.

Table 11.2 Normal values in an electrocardiogram

Age	Heart Rate	Mean Frontal Plane QRS Axis	PR Interval
0-1 months	100-180(120)	+75 to 180(+120)	0,08-0,12(0,10)
2-3 months	110-180(120)	+35 to +135(+100)	0,08-0,12(0,10)
4-12 months	100-180(150)	+30 to +135(+60)	0,09-0,13(0,12)
1-3 years	100-180(130)	0 to +110(+60)	0,10-0,14(0,12)
4-5 years	60-150(100)	0 to +110(+60)	0,11-0,15(0,13)
6-8 years	60-130(100)	−15 to +110(+60)	0,12-0,16(0,14)
9-11 years	50-110(80)	−15 to +110(+60)	0,12-0,17(0,14)
12-16 years	50-100(75)	−15 to +110(+60)	0,12-0,17(0,15)
16 years	50-90(70)	−15 to +110(+60)	0,12-0,20(0,15)

Prolongation of the PR interval indicates a first-degree heartblock. DIGOXIN toxicity and rheumatic fever are causes.

Criteria for chamber enlargement ('hypertrophy')

Right ventricular

◆ Incomplete right bundle branch block (IRBBB) with R 'prime' >12 mm in VI
◆ Pure R wave >12 mm in VI
◆ R (with S wave) >20 mm in VI
◆ Upright T wave VI (one week to ten years)
◆ Q wave in VI

Left ventricular

R wave ≥30 mm V6
RV6 + SVl ≥50 mm

Combined ventricular

◆ V3 : R 30 mm + S 30 mm
◆ V4 : R 40 mm + S 20 mm

Right atrial

◆ Lead II peaked P wave, ≥2,5 blocks (upwards)

Left atrial

◆ Lead II widened P wave, ≥2 blocks (across)

Combined atrial

♦ Early portion of P wave peaked, plus
♦ P wave 2 blocks across
♦ Biphasic P wave in VI

QT interval

The syndrome of prolonged QT interval is an important cause of syncope and cardiac arrest in young people. The interval is rate-dependent and should be corrected using Bazett's formula:

$$\text{QT corrected} = \frac{\text{QT interval}}{\sqrt{\text{Preceding RR in seconds}}}$$

Normal ≤0,44 seconds (measured in V5).

ECG changes with electrolyte disturbances

♦ Hypokalaemia: ST depression, flat T-waves, prominent U-waves[1], prolonged P-R interval, arrhythmias.
♦ Hyperkalaemia: peaked tall T-waves, broad QRS, arrhythmia (ventricular fibrillation).
♦ Hypocalcaemia: prolonged QT.
♦ Hypercalcaemia: shortens QT.

Heart disease in the first year of life

Table 11.3 is a guide to the most common conditions seen at different ages in the first year. The groups are not mutually exclusive.

Congestive cardiac failure in infancy
Clinical presentation

The clinical features of congestive cardiac failure result from the pathophysiological changes associated with the failing heart.

♦ **Pulmonary venous congestion:** tachypnoea, dyspnoea, sub-costal recession. Wheeze and basal crepitations.
♦ **Systemic venous congestion:** hepatomegaly and oedema. Distended neck veins are not easily visible but may be prominent on the dorsum of the hands and scalp.

---

[1]Abnormal U-waves have an amplitude of at least 1 mm and are best seen in the middle chest leads in the same direction as T-waves.

Table 11.3 Common heart conditions in babies under 12 months

Lesions	Congestive cardiac failure	Cyanosis	Chest X-ray	ECG
In the first month				
Hypoplastic left heart syndrome	+++ Shock	+	Cardiomegaly	RVH Poor LV forces
Coarctation	+++ Absent femoral pulses	±	Cardiomegaly	RAD, RVH
Transposition	+	++	Cardiomegaly Plethora	RAD, RVH
Obstructed right heart (e.g. pulmonary atresia)	–	+++	Cardiomegaly Oligaemia	RAD, RAH
Arrhythmias	++	±	Normal	Arrhythmia
From one to three months				
Complex VSD (VSD+PDA or VSD+ASD) Intracardiac mixing	++	–	Cardiomegaly Plethora	BVH or RVH
e.g.Atrial(TAPVD)	++	+	Cardiomegaly Plethora	RAH, RVH
Atrioventricular canal	+++	+	Cardiomegaly Plethora	BVH, LAD
Univentricular heart or TGA+VSD	++	+	Cardiomegaly Plethora	BVH, RAD LAD
Truncus arteriosus	++ Ejection click	+	Cardiomegaly Plethora	BVH
From three to 12 months				
Left to right shunts	+	–	Cardiomegaly Plethora	LVH/RVH
Myocarditis/EFE	++	–	Cardiomegaly	ST/T wave changes
			Congestion	LVH

Lesions	Congestive cardiac failure	Cyanosis	Chest X-ray	ECG
Tetralogy of Fallot	–	++ ±Hypoxic spells	No cardiomegaly	RAD, RVH Oligaemia

PDA   = Patent ductus arteriosus
ASD   = Atrial septal defect
VSD   = Ventricular septal defect
TAPVD = Total anomalous pulmonary venous drainage
TGA   = Transposition of the great arteries
EFE   = Endocardial fibro-elastosis
UVH   = Univentricular heart

Note: Remember that heart failure is not always due to a cardiac defect; examples of other causes include severe anaemia, iatrogenic or peripartum fluid overload and peripheral (e.g. cerebral) arteriovenous malformations.

♦ **Low cardiac output**: tachycardia
♦ **Increased sympathetic activity:** pallor, sweating, cold extremities, poor pulses.
♦ **Fluid retention:** abnormal weight gain. Failing urinary output. Evidence of pulmonary and systemic venous congestion.

Treatment of heart failure

♦ **Oxygen:** 40% for acute, severe heart failure
♦ **DIGOXIN (Lanoxin):**

◇ Oral
Initial dose: 0,005 mg/kg/dose, eight-hourly x three doses only
Maintenance dose: 0,005 mg/kg/dose, 12-hourly
◇ Intravenous dose: 0,005 mg/kg/dose, 12-hourly
◇ Availability of DIGOXIN:
Elixir: 0,05 mg/ml
Tabs.: 0,25 mg
Ampoules: 0,25 mg/ml

- ◆ **FUROSEMIDE:** 1-2 mg/kg/day parenteral or oral.
- ◆ **Potassium supplements:** 50 mg/kg/day.
- ◆ **Fluid restriction:** 70 ml/kg/day initially.
- ◆ **Low salt milks:** see pages 50-1.

Failure of above measures

Angiotensin converting enzyme (ACE) inhibitors

Cause afterload reduction for refractory heart failure. Start with a small dose and increase gradually to prevent precipitous drop in blood pressure. See Pharmacopoeia page 606 (Appendix 2) for doses of ENALAPRIL.
Exercise caution when using potassium-sparing diuretics. Stop potassium supplements.
CAPTOPRIL:
   Commence: 0,5 mg/kg/day divided into eight-hourly dosage.
   Increase: 0,5 mg/kg/day.
   Maintenance: 3-5 mg/kg/day.

Maintenance of duct potency

PROSTAGLANDIN E is used to maintain patency of the ductus arteriosus.

Indications

- ◆ Cyanotic congenital heart defect, possibly due to right ventricular outflow tract obstruction.
- ◆ Transposition of the Great Arteries.
- ◆ Suspected Ebstein's malformation (cyanosis and massive radiological cardiomegaly due to severe tricuspid incompetence and a huge right atrium).
- ◆ Severe obstructive lesions of the systemic circulation, e.g. coarctation of the aorta, critical aortic stenosis.

Management

Treatment must be commenced within the first two weeks of life, as soon as the diagnosis has been suspected.

Step 1 Oral PROSTAGLANDIN

PROSTAGLANDIN E2 (Prostin E): 125 µg (one quarter tablet of 500 µg) crushed and suspended in 2-5 ml of water and given hourly via a nasogastric tube.

If the response to 125 µg hourly is unsatisfactory, then 250 µg tab hourly can be given if the baby weighs more than 2,5 kg.

Step 2 Assisted ventilation

If there is no improvement in the degree of cyanosis with oral prostaglandin: commence assisted ventilation prior to the introduction of intravenous PROSTAGLANDIN.

PROSTAGLANDIN E1 (Prostin VR) causes significantly more apnoea than oral PROSTAGLANDIN, particularly at higher infusion rates.

Step 3 Intravenous PROSTAGLANDIN

PROSTAGLANDIN E1 (Prostin VR) 250 µg (0,5 ml solution) is added to 200 ml 5% dextrose water. One ml of this solution contains 1,25 µg PROSTAGLANDIN E1.

Infusion via a microdropper (60 drops per ml) will give 0,02 µg/drop and thus 1 drop/minute gives 0,02 µg/minute.

Recommended infusion rate is 0,005 µg/kg/minute up to 0,05 µg/kg/minute.

Hypercyanotic spells

Hypercyanotic (hypoxic) spells occur in those congenital heart defects where there is right ventricular outflow tract obstruction causing a right to left shunt, e.g. Tetralogy of Fallot, pulmonary atresia with ventricular septal defect, or any complex defect with associated severe pulmonary stenosis.

Clinical presentation

During a spell the patient becomes more cyanosed, tachypnoeic, and acidotic, while previously auscultated murmurs diminish in intensity or disappear.

Management

Prevention

The hypercyanotic spell may be brought on by crying or by any event which provokes systemic vasodilatation, e.g. a hot bath. Explain to the mother both mechanisms responsible for the clinical features of the spell and the prevention of precipitating factors.

♦ Iron deficiency anaemia: common. Diagnose early and treat.

◆ β-adrenergic receptor blockade: PROPRANOLOL 3-5 mg/kg/day orally in three divided doses eight-hourly is effective at preventing spells in children previously noted to have the hypercyanotic spells. PROPRANOLOL is continued until surgery is planned.

Acute management

◆ Oxygen: 100%
  Bend the legs at the hips and knees ('squatting' while supine)
◆ MORPHINE: 0,1 mg/kg IV
◆ IV fluids: 10 ml/kg rapidly
◆ Sodium bicarbonate 8%: 2 ml/kg IV
◆ Blood transfusion: if Hb <10 g/dl.
  β-adrenergic receptor blockade: ESMOLOL (Brevibloc) (rapid onset, short acting) 0,5 mg/kg IV or PROPRANOLOL 3-5 mg/kg/day orally in three divided doses eight-hourly.
◆ Surgery: failure of response to medical treatment. Recurrent hypercyanotic spells occurring despite adequate PROPRANOLOL therapy (5 mg/kg/day orally).

Warning

A hypercyanotic spell is a medical emergency. It always requires urgent action.

Arrhythmias

Bradyarrhythmias vary from a sinus bradycardia to low atrial escape rhythms to various degrees of atrioventricular dissociation.

Complete heart block

In paediatrics it is usually either congenital or follows cardiac surgery.

Clinical presentation

The presentation ranges from being relatively asymptomatic to severe congestive cardiac failure.

Management

Refer to a paediatric cardiologist or cardiac service to consider the placement of a pacemaker.

Indications for pacemaker placement

♦ **Urgent:** complete heart block complicated by heart failure.
♦ **For consideration:** neonate or infant with a heart rate <50/min. Older child with a heart rate <60/min with cardiomegaly and no response with an increasing heart rate to exercise.

Supraventricular tachycardia (SVT)

Relatively common in infancy.

Clinical presentation

SVT may cause heart failure and cardiogenic shock. The ECG indicates a narrow complex QRS tachycardia and frequently the p wave is not visible. Recurrence is common.

Management

The diving reflex

This is the safest and easiest method of terminating a SVT, but is only successful in about 50% of cases.

Method

Hold the baby or older child prone and submerge the face in a basin of ice cold water for one or two seconds (baby will not drown!).

Cardioversion

Cardioversion is a safe method of acute management of any tachyarrhythmia, provided the following steps are taken:

♦ empty stomach: nil per month for six hours or emptied by nasogastric tube;
♦ resuscitation facilities: oxygen, suction, endotracheal tube etc. Drugs, ADRENALINE, calcium, sodium bicarbonate etc. See Chapter 1 and Table 36.4 on page 411;
♦ electrical energy: use synchronized DC electrical cardioversion at 0,5-2 J/kg. Start with the smallest level of electrical cardioversion and increase dose if necessary. Administration of too much electrical energy can result in myocardial damage.

> **Warning**
>
> DIGOXIN: caution should be exercised if the patient is receiving DIGOXIN as cardioversion can lead to ventricular fibrillation. DIGOXIN should preferably be discontinued 48 hours before cardioversion and the serum level checked.

Drugs

Drugs may be used to convert a supraventricular tachycardia although the above measures are undoubtedly safer.

◆ β adrenergic receptor blockade: ESMOLOL (Brevibloc) 0,5 mg/kg IV stat is relatively safe because its half-life is about three minutes.

Maintenance treatment

◆ **To prevent recurrence:** PROPRANOLOL 1 mg/kg/dose eight-hourly for at least one year.
◆ **Failure:** Consult a paediatric cardiologist or cardiac service.

Note

◆ Unifocal ventricular premature beats in the asymptomatic child are not uncommon and are usually benign.
◆ Anti-arrhythmic drugs are toxic and can have dangerous interactions.

Transport of the sick cardiac neonate or infant

The manner and urgency of the transport of the sick cardiac infant will make the difference between life or death. The baby should be warm, nursed in 30% to 50% oxygen, on slow IV 5% dextrose infusion and, if cyanosed, on PROSTAGLANDIN.

> **Warning**
>
> Always consult with a paediatric cardiologist or cardiac service at the tertiary centre before transfer.

Rheumatic fever

This is the most common cause of acquired heart disease in childhood between the ages of five and 15 years in southern

Africa. The condition may first occur at a younger age but is uncommon after adolescence.

The exact pathophysiology is still uncertain but group A β-haemolytic streptococcal infection and socio-economic conditions play a part. Overcrowding leads to a higher incidence. Recurrence is more likely in the young, and especially during the first year after the initial attack.

Clinical presentation and diagnostic criteria

Modified Jones criteria are used. These require evidence of previous streptococcal infection such as a raised ASOT and/or culture of β-haemolytic group A streptococcus and the presence of one major and two minor criteria or two major criteria. Failure to meet the criteria does not exclude rheumatic fever.

Major criteria

◆ Carditis
◆ Migrating polyarthritis
◆ Chorea
◆ Subcutaneous nodules
◆ Erythema marginatum.

Minor criteria

◆ Fever
◆ Arthralgia
◆ Raised ESR
◆ Raised C-reactive protein test
◆ Leucocytosis
◆ History of previous acute rheumatic fever or presence of established rheumatic heart disease
◆ Prolonged PR interval on ECG.

Treatment

◆ Bed rest: until the sleeping pulse is normal and signs of rheumatic activity have resolved.
◆ SALICYLATES (ASPIRIN SOLUBLE): for symptomatic relief of fever and joint pain only – 75 mg/kg/day.
◆ PENICILLIN: therapeutic – PENICILLIN V 250 mg six-hourly for ten days or PROCAINE PENICILLIN 1,2 million units daily for ten days.

◆ Corticosteroids
  Carditis present: PREDNISOLONE 3 mg/kg/day in four divided doses for ten days (maximum 60 mg/day). Tail off over ten days, providing the clinical response is maintained and the ESR remains normal. Should there be a rebound of the ESR then the dosage may need to be increased again.
◆ Prophylaxis against streptococcal infection: BENZATHINE PENICILLIN, long-acting, 1,2 million units IM monthly. This is the preferred method. Primary and secondary prevention also involves the early and aggressive treatment of bacterial sore throats with a ten day course of oral PENICILLIN or
  PENICILLIN V 250 mg twice daily by mouth, ERYTHROMYCIN or SULPHADIAZINE (if allergic to PENICILLIN). Prophylactic therapy should be maintained until the age of 21 years. See Appendix 1.

Chorea

HALOPERIDOL (Serenace) 0,1 mg/kg/day by mouth in three divided doses. Give for as long as symptoms persist. Tail off medication slowly.

Cardiac failure

See page 103.

Surgery

See pages 112-3.
Indications for valve replacement:

◆ low cardiac output state with severe cardiac failure due to severe mitral or aortic regurgitation;
◆ critical mitral stenosis with low cardiac output or pulmonary oedema may require urgent intervention.

Warning

◆ Acute rheumatic fever and infective bacterial endocarditis may be difficult to differentiate at initial presentation. In these instances it is essential to obtain blood cultures (and if possible two-dimensional echocardiography) before commencing specific treatment for acute rheumatic carditis.

♦ Do not start PREDNISOLONE before bacterial endocarditis, TB or other infections have definitely been excluded.
♦ Important: corticosteroids shorten hospital stay for children with acute rheumatic fever but do not affect the eventual outcome of valvular damage.

Infective endocarditis
Clinical presentation

Pyrexia, new murmurs, anaemia, fatigue, splenomegaly, haematuria, splinter haemorrhages, Roth spots.

Warning

Do not commence intravenous antibiotics until at least three blood cultures have been done in a patient with suspected infective endocarditis. Echocardiography will usually confirm the presence of vegetations in the heart. During antibiotic treatment blood samples should be taken regularly to check serum bactericidal activity.

Treatment
Antibiotics

Length and choice of treatment should be discussed with a bacteriologist.

Guidelines

Antibiotic choice depends on the causal organism.

♦ Organism not known: PENICILLIN IV and GENTAMICIN IV and CLOXACILLIN IV for four weeks.
♦ Viridans streptococcus: PENICILLIN IV (four-hourly) and GENTAMICIN IV (1 mg/kg every eight hours) for two weeks followed by oral AMOXYCILLIN and PROBENECID for two weeks.
♦ Enterococci: PENICILLIN IV and GENTAMICIN IV for four weeks.

- Staphylococcus: CLOXACILLIN IV and FUSIDIC ACID IV for four weeks. Change to oral administration once the patient's condition is stable.
- Enteric Bacilli, e.g. Klebsiella: GENTAMICIN IV and CEFTRIAXONE IV for six weeks.

Antibiotic prophylaxis

Children with cardiac lesions should be advised to brush their teeth twice daily with a tooth paste containing fluoride. Before extractions or extensive fillings, children with congenital or rheumatic heart lesions require an antibiotic to prevent infective endocarditis. See Appendix 1.

Without an anaesthetic
Dental extraction or upper respiratory tract surgery

- Adults and child over ten years: AMOXYCILLIN 3 g single oral dose one hour before procedure.
- Child under ten years: AMOXYCILLIN half adult dose.
- Child under five years: AMOXYCILLIN quarter adult dose.

For a patient allergic to PENICILLIN

- Adult and child over ten years: ERYTHROMYCIN 1,5 g orally one to two hours before dental procedure and 0,5 g six hours later.
- Child under ten years: ERYTHROMYCIN half adult dose.
- Child under five years: ERYTHROMYCIN quarter adult dose.

With an anaesthetic

Adult: AMOXYCILLIN 3 g together with PROBENECID 1 g orally four hours before the operation. Modify the dose for children as for previously described drugs. If PROBENECID is not given, then the AMOXYCILLIN dose should be repeated as soon as possible after the operation. For patients allergic to PENICILLIN administer ERYTHROMYCIN accordingly.

Genito-urinary surgery or instrumentation

- GENTAMICIN IM 2 mg/kg stat 15 minutes before surgery given with the AMOXYCILLIN (as above). If the patient is allergic to PENICILLIN: VANCOMYCIN 20 mg/kg IV over 60 minutes and GENTAMICIN IV 2 mg/kg.

Heart valve replacement

Since 1979 all children and adolescents undergoing valve replacement surgery in Cape Town have had a St Jude Medical prosthetic valve inserted. This is a mechanical bileaflet valve which is not normally visible on routine chest X-ray. It is a mechanical prosthesis, and so the important complications are thrombo-embolism from the valve and thrombotic obstruction of the valve.

Management

◆ Anticoagulant therapy: WARFARIN is recommended where this can be adequately supervised, and should be continued for life
   or
◆ Anti-platelet therapy: ASPIRIN SOLUBLE 5 mg/kg/day daily for life.
◆ Prophylactic PENICILLIN.
   ◇ On WARFARIN: PENICILLIN 250 mg twice daily orally.
   ◇ On ASPIRIN SOLUBLE: BENZATHINE PENICILLIN, long-acting, 1,2 million units IM monthly.

12 CENTRAL NERVOUS SYSTEM INFECTIONS

A J G Thomson

Meningitis

The most common causes of meningitis are bacterial and viral. Rarer causes are fungal, cestodal, rickettsial and protozoal. Acute bacterial meningitis is a medical emergency and occurs more frequently in the paediatric age group than in any other.

Acute bacterial meningitis (septic meningitis)

Aetiology

Neonates and infants under three months

Escherichia coli and other enteric bacteria as well as Group B and non-Group B streptococci are the most common organisms in this group. In Cape Town *Listeria monocytogenes* is a rare cause of neonatal meningitis.

Children and infants over three months

The overwhelming majority of cases of acute bacterial meningitis are due to *Haemophilus influenzae*, *Neisseria meningitidis* and *Streptococcus pneumoniae*. Incidence of *H. influenzae* decreases significantly after the ages of three or four years and dwindles by adolescence.

Clinical presentation

A high index of clinical suspicion is required. Early clinical recognition and a diagnostic lumbar puncture are essential.

Neonates

Specific signs and symptoms are often absent and a lumbar puncture is therefore generally indicated. Noteworthy features may be poor sucking, hypothermia, apathy, vomiting and apnoeic attacks.

Infants

Fretfulness, fever, convulsions, vomiting and a tense fontanelle when assessed in the upright position.

Children

Headaches, fever, vomiting, photophobia, stiffness in the neck, Kernig's sign (limitation of knee extension when the thighs are flexed at right angles to the body) and/or Brudzinski's sign (the hips flex when the head is bent forward).

Diagnosis

Lumbar puncture

Lumbar puncture (LP) with thorough examination of the cerebrospinal fluid (CSF), including culture and sensitivity of the organisms, provides a specific diagnosis. Contra-indications to LP in a patient suspected of having meningitis are few. Most patients with acute bacterial meningitis will have some degree of cerebral oedema. However, LP is contra-indicated when a patient develops severe cerebral oedema, with critically raised intracranial pressure (ICP) and a significantly depressed level of consciousness (i.e. will only arouse after noxious stimulation). In such cases, LP should be delayed until the level of consciousness improves. As early deaths may be due to extensive cerebral oedema, which causes brain shifts and **cones**, the critically raised ICP must be reduced by treatment with MANNITOL IV 0,25-0,5 g/kg/dose and DEXAMETHASONE IV 0,25-0,5 mg/kg/day six to eight-hourly. See pages 333-4.

Warning

Antibiotic therapy must not be delayed if raised ICP were to postpone LP and definitive diagnosis. When acute meningitis is clinically suspected, antibiotics should be commenced immediately after blood culture.

Management

All patients with abnormal CSF findings should be carefully monitored for CNS changes for 24 hours after a LP.

Table 12.1 Usual CSF values

	Protein g/l	Glucose[1] mmol/l	Chloride	Cells/mm³
Normal				
Neonate	0,2-1,5	Normal[1]	116-130	0-10 lympho-cytes
Older	0,2-0,4	Normal[1]	116-130	0-5 lympho-cytes
Aseptic Viral	0,2-2,0	Normal[1]	Normal	20 to a few hundred, mainly lymphocytes[2]
Tuberculous	0,5-3,0	Moderately reduced	Very low, 100 or less	20-500, mainly lymphocytes[2]
Pyogenic	0,5-5,0	Reduced, may be absent	Normal, slightly reduced	50 to thousands, nearly all poly-morphs

[1] Normal CSF glucose concentration about two-thirds of the blood glucose concentration.

[2] In early stages polymorphs may predominate.

Antibiotic therapy

Neonates and infants less than three months of age

Initially and prior to availability of culture/sensitivity:

◆ CEFTRIAXONE (Rocephin) 80 mg/kg/day IV or IM once-daily or CEFOTAXIME (Claforan) 200 mg/kg/day IV six-hourly
   AND
◆ AMPICILLIN 200 mg/kg/day IV six-hourly.

Culture results known: treat according to sensitivity. If sensitivity results dictate GENTAMICIN therapy it must be given intra-ventricularly via an Ommya valve as well as IV.

No growth: continue initial therapy if clinically warranted.

Note

The second generation CEPHALOSPORINS (e.g. CEFUROX-IME) should not be used, as there may be delayed sterilization of the CSF.

Children and infants over three months of age

Initially and prior to the availability of culture/sensitivity:

EITHER

♦ PENICILLIN (G or CRYSTALLINE PENICILLIN) 300 000-400 000 U/kg/day six-hourly IV or AMPICILLIN (Penbritin, Pentrex) 200 mg/kg/day six-hourly IV
AND
♦ CHLORAMPHENICOL (Chloromycetin) 100 mg/kg/day IV six-hourly
OR
♦ CEFOTAXIME (Claforan) 200 mg/kg/day IV six-hourly or CEFTRIAXONE (Rocephin) 80 mg/kg/day IV or IM once daily.

Culture results known:

♦ *H. influenzae*: continue CHLORAMPHENICOL. Stop PENICILLIN (alternative: AMPICILLIN, CEFTRIAXONE, CEFOTAXIME). For prophylaxis see page 252.
♦ *N. meningitidis:* continue PENICILLIN. Stop CHLORAMPHENICOL (alternative: CEFOTAXIME or CEFTRIAXONE, see Appendix 1, page 568). For prophylaxis see page 252. For the treatment of shock see pages 7-14.
♦ *S. pneumoniae:* continue PENICILLIN. Stop CHLORAMPHENICOL (alternative: CEFOTAXIME or CEFTRIAXONE, see Appendix 1, page 568).
♦ Other organisms: treat according to sensitivity.
♦ No growth: continue initial therapy if clinically warranted. The combination of PENICILLIN and CHLORAMPHENICOL is a most effective therapy despite the theoretical antagonism of the two antibiotics.

Duration and route of antibiotic therapy at full dosage

Duration

♦ Patients over three months of age: at least ten days.
♦ Patients less than three months: Gram-positive bacterial infection for at least two weeks, Gram-negative bacterial infection for at least three weeks.

Route

IV mandatory for the first 48 hours and preferred route for as long as possible. Change to IM but the oral route may be used with CHLORAMPHENICOL.

Supportive management

Ensure adequate circulatory status (maintain BP and peripheral perfusion) with IV fluids. Monitor weight, serum and urine sodium concentrations. Fluid restriction should be instituted if the syndrome of inappropriate antidiuretic hormone secretion (SIADH) develops. With large doses of PENICILLIN/AMPICILLIN the serum sodium level must be monitored to ensure that sodium overload does not occur.

Indications for repeat LP

Repeat LP is seldom indicated in routine management. It is indicated in neonates and in patients with unusual forms of bacterial meningitis in order to check that the CSF has been sterilized after 72 hours of therapy. It is also indicated if fever and/or encephalopathy persist, or when there are focal signs at the conclusion of therapy.

Indications for computerized tomography (CT)

These include a significantly depressed level of consciousness, focal neurologic deficits, unexplained persistent or recurrent fever, or focal or generalized seizures occurring after three days of therapy (late onset seizures).

Steroid therapy

The increasing evidence that the host's inflammatory response, if unbridled, leads to increased tissue damage has led many authorities to advocate the routine use of steroid therapy in all cases of bacterial meningitis. In the presence of a critically raised ICP, MANNITOL 0,25-0,5 g/kg/dose IV should be added to DEXAMETHASONE IV 0,25-0,5 mg/kg/day six to eight-hourly. See pages 333-4.

Complications

Deteriorating level of consciousness: exclude and treat cerebral oedema, SIADH, mass lesion with cerebral shift and metabolic encephalopathy (hypoglycaemia, hypocalcaemia, hypercapnia etc).

Seizures: exclude a treatable metabolic cause such as hypoglycaemia, hypocalcaemia and hypomagnesaemia. Early onset seizures occurring in the first three days of therapy are usually self-limiting and not of serious prognostic significance. Late onset seizures occurring after three days of therapy are usually more serious and persistent and may require therapy. See page 338.

Persistent fever: lasting for more than a week of therapy. Occurs in about 10% of patients, because of the underlying meningitis. Extrameningeal sources of inflammation such as drug fever and thrombophlebitis should be excluded before CT is undertaken. Repeat LP or tapping of a subdural fluid collection with analysis of the fluid should be performed.

Subdural effusions: usually bilateral. Aspirate (see page 454) only if symptoms are present, e.g. persistent or secondary fever, depressed level of consciousness, seizures and focal signs, and feeding difficulties. Sterile effusions will generally resolve spontaneously.

CT scan may distinguish a subdural effusion from an empyema (i.e. there is no enhancing capsule visible after the IV injection of contrast agents).

Subdural empyema: infected purulent 'effusions' which contain more than 5 000 WBC/cm³. CT scan with IV contrast demonstrates a well-formed enhancing capsule requiring surgical drainage and decompression.

Brain abscess: rare complication in patients with acute bacterial meningitis. Diagnosis difficult.

Sensorineural hearing loss: the most common long-term complication of acute bacterial meningitis. Occurs early in the course of the disease. Test for hearing loss.

Ventriculomegaly: usually due to cerebral atrophy which is more common than communicating or obstructive hydrocephalus as a late sequelae of bacterial meningitis. Patients present with neurodevelopmental disability.

Prognosis

Adverse factors affecting prognosis in meningitis include delay in diagnosis and treatment, inappropriate or inadequate therapy, late onset convulsions during therapy (where the cause is not metabolic), and severe depression of the level of consciousness.

Aseptic meningitis

Aetiology

There are many causes of aseptic meningitis.

Viral

Viral meningitis is by far the most common cause, and usually presents acutely. The presumed diagnosis in the appropriate clinical setting initially depends on the exclusion of bacterial infection (negative Gram stain and negative culture in CSF). The specific diagnosis depends on positive viral culture from CSF or from other sites (throat, faeces, urine) with the demonstration of a rising serum antibody titre to the specific virus cultured. Common pathogens are mumps, enteroviruses, adenoviruses, herpes simplex, measles, rubella, varicella, influenzae and para-influenzae viruses as well as Epstein-Barr virus and cytomegalovirus. AIDS meningitis is of increasing importance.

The differential diagnoses include:

♦ a partially treated bacterial meningitis, tuberculous meningitis, cryptococcal (Torula) meningitis and less common fungal causes;

♦ aseptic CSF reaction due to a parameningeal infection, e.g. mastoiditis, paranasal sinusitis, epidural abscess, dural venous thrombosis, subdural empyema and brain abscess;

♦ secondary syphilis and other spirochaetal meningitides. Cysticeral meningitis needs to be considered in patients from endemic regions; while

♦ less common infective causes in the appropriate clinical setting include infection with *Toxoplasma gondii, Mycoplasma pneumoniae,* Kawasaki disease, leptospirosis, brucellosis and Lyme disease.

Other causes

Allergic and hypersensitivity reactions (including serum sickness and drug reactions), chemical meningitis, leptomeningeal malignancy and vasculitic diseases.

Clinical presentation

♦ Fever, headache and neck stiffness.
♦ Bacteriologically sterile CSF. Classically the CSF is predominantly lymphocytic, although it is initially polymorphic. The

chemistry of the CSF is typically normal. However, in some cases the glucose may be low and the protein may be increased. See Table 12.1

The diagnosis may be perplexing and worrying. A clue to the diagnosis is a dramatic relief of headache after LP.

Management

Symptomatic

Analgesics, bed rest.

Specific

Appropriate treatment of the cause.

Tuberculous meningitis (TBM)

A devastating complication of haematogenous-spread tuberculo-sis resulting from the rupture of a parameningeal caseous focus (Rich focus) with discharge of bacilli and TB antigens into the subarachnoid space.

Clinical presentation

Mortality and long-term disability rates are high and are particu-larly so when there is a delay in diagnosis and treatment. The disease occurs at any age, with the highest incidence in the first five years of life. The illness may start insidiously or may have an acute onset. Clinical manifestations usually progress through three stages:

◆ **Prodromal phase**: apathy, irritability, loss of appetite, nau-sea, vomiting, personality and behavioural changes.
◆ **Meningeal phase**: headache and vomiting. Signs in older children of meningeal irritation with neck stiffness and posi-tive Kernig's and Bradzinski's signs. Fever of varying degree is usually present. Approximately 5% of cases are apyrexial. Cranial nerve palsies (6,3,4,7,2), convulsions, increased ICP, focal motor deficits and dyskinesias (hemi-choreas, hemiballismus) may develop.
◆ **Phase of depressed level of consciousness**: increasing evi-dence of cerebral dysfunction with evolution of stupor to deep coma and decerebrate state. Clinical signs of brain stem dysfunction are usually due to tentorial herniation but may be the result of brainstem infarcts.

Diagnosis

Clinical grounds

TBM should be considered to be a likely diagnosis in a patient with aseptic meningitis when the syndrome of IADH secretion, a clinically consistent illness and a history of TB contact are associated.

Support for the diagnosis includes the presence of pulmonary tuberculosis, fundal choroidal tubercles, and a positive tuberculin skin test (may be initially negative in up to 50% of cases).

CSF findings

The CSF shows a moderate degree of pleocytosis of 50-500 cells per mm^3. Cells are initially predominantly polymorphonuclear but change over days to weeks to an increasingly predominant lymphocyte count. Cell counts over 1 500 cells per mm^3 are rare in TBM. CSF protein levels are elevated between 1,0-5,0 g/l, increasing as the disease worsens. Levels of 10-15 g/l suggest the presence of a spinal block. CSF glucose levels are decreased below 2,2 mmol/l or are less than 50% of a simultaneous blood glucose measurement. In most patients with TBM the combination of hypochloraemia and elevated CSF protein depresses the CSF chloride to less than 110 mmol/l.

Further support for a diagnosis of TBM may be provided by a CSF ADA level of more than 7 units/l and a CSF bromide partition test ratio of below 1,6. Both these tests are helpful in excluding viral meningitis. Computerized tomography may also strongly indicate the diagnosis. See page 459.

Definitive diagnosis of TBM

Microscopic examination of the CSF reveals the presence of bacilli with either Ziehl-Neelsen or fluorescent stains. A positive yield depends on the time devoted to searching and the number of specimens examined. Bacilli are cultured from the CSF. The latter takes four to six weeks.

Management

Treatment

◆ ISONIAZID and RIFAMPICIN for 12 months. PYRAZINAMIDE and ETHIONAMIDE for the first six months of therapy. Liver function must be carefully monitored on this therapy.

◆ Steroid therapy (although controversial) is recommended when a provisional diagnosis of TBM has been made. PREDNISONE 2-4 mg/kg/day for four to six weeks with a subsequent careful clinically monitored reduction of dosage over ten to 14 days.

Surgery

Surgery is directed at the relief of hydrocephalus when this is associated with signs of imminent tentorial herniation despite adequate medical therapy. This is more likely to occur with obstructive than with communicating hydrocephalus. Serial CT scans are useful in the assessment of this situation.

> ### Warning
>
> Bacilli cannot be isolated from the CSF of all TBM patients. It is far safer to commence treatment than to delay while waiting for clarification of a doubtful diagnosis.
>
> Death or poor clinical response to chemotherapy is usually due to delayed diagnosis and treatment.

Cryptococcal meningitis (torulosis)

Organisms are found widely in avian (birds') excreta.

Aetiology

Cryptococcus is a budding yeast. The portal of entry is through the lungs and skin. Infection and dissemination depend on host factors. Great susceptibility exists among patients with an impaired immune response, such as malignant lymphoma, leukaemia, Hodgkins', sarcoid, diabetes mellitus, and AIDS; or who are undergoing corticosteroid therapy.

Clinical presentation

The onset is often insidious with fever, headache and vomiting and signs of raised intracranial pressure and/or of a subacute or chronic meningo-encephalitis. A much less common form is characterized by signs of a focal expanding lesion, possibly simulating a cerebral abscess or a neoplasm. It is usually a gradually progressive disease. Some cases may show remissions and exacerbations with or without therapy.

Diagnosis

LP and CSF examination. The organisms may not be present in the CSF at times during the course of the illness, and Indian ink preparations and cultures may be negative. Ventricular fluid culture is more often positive than that of lumbar fluid. Detection of cryptococcal antigen in the CSF by latex fixation or complement fixation is possible with 95% reliability. It may be the only evidence of infection.

Treatment

◆ AMPHOTERICIN B 0,25 mg/kg/day increasing to 1 mg/kg/ day IV for approximately six weeks (duration depends on response and toxicity; add intrathecal or intraventricular AMPHOTERICIN in the resistant case), and

◆ 5 FLUOROCYTOSINE 150 mg/kg/day for two to six months. Duration of therapy depends on response and toxicity.

◆ MICONAZOLE IV may be used as an alternative therapy in patients with renal insufficiency. Problems include thrombophlebitis from frequent IV injections.

Warning

Following recovery the patient must be followed for two years with periodic LP's.

Acute encephalopathy (including encephalitis)

Diffuse or multifocal involvement of the encephalon. It is a common neurological emergency in childhood. Most patients with encephalitis have meningeal involvement as well.

Aetiology

Important conditions to consider among the many possible aetiologies are metabolic/toxic causes, infectious causes, space-demanding lesions and vascular/anoxic accidents. Amongst the infectious causes, viral illnesses are the most common aetiological agents, and manifest most commonly as acute meningo-encephalitis (most patients have meningeal involvement as well).

Viruses produce acute encephalopathy in four ways:

◆ viral meningo-encephalitis in which inflammation is caused directly by viruses that can be cultured from the CNS, e.g. herpes simplex;
◆ para-infectious inflammatory meningo-encephalitis in which the infecting agent has not yet been recovered from the brain, e.g. infectious mononucleosis, *Mycoplasma pneumoniae* infections and influenza (otherwise clinically and pathologically indistinguishable from viral meningo-encephalitis);
◆ postinfectious meningo-encephalomyelitis in which multifocal inflammatory demyelination due to impaired immune response to neural antigens may follow measles, rubella, varicella and mumps infections; and
◆ para-infectious non-inflammatory acute toxic encephalopathy and Reye's syndrome. These are characterized by a persistent increase in ICP with few or no cells in the CSF. There is diffuse cerebral oedema without inflammation, necrosis, or demyelination of the brain. Presumably the viral illness precipitates cell dysfunction in 'metabolically' predisposed individuals.

Clinical presentation

Severe headache, convulsions, depressed level of consciousness, decerebration and focal neurological deficits associated with pyrexial illness.

Diagnosis in patients with encephalitis

◆ The CSF is abnormal with a lymphocytic pleocytosis, a mild protein elevation and a normal glucose level. In rare cases a CSF sampled early in the course of the illness may be normal.
◆ The EEG, CT scan and technetium brain scan show diffuse or focal abnormalities.

Advice

Suspect herpes simplex infection with fronto-temporal signs or symptoms and with fronto-temporal focal or hemispheric abnormalities on EEG. These are most important clues to the diagnosis and occur early in the disease. An isotope brain scan indicates fronto-temporal changes earlier than does a CT scan.

Management

◆ Admit the patient to high intensive care facility. Maintain airway, fluid balance and general supportive measures.

◆ Control seizures and suppress potential status epilepticus with PHENYTOIN or PHENOBARBITONE. Monitor blood levels to ensure adequate loading, i.e. to high therapeutic range. For control of status epilepticus see pages 338-41.

◆ Treat cerebral oedema with MANNITOL or DEXAMETHASONE as required. See pages 333-4.

◆ For herpes encephalitis ACYCLOVIR 30 mg/kg/day administered three times daily as an IV infusion given over one hour for ten days.

Neurocysticercosis

Neurocysticercosis follows ingestion of tape worm eggs and is caused by infestation of the nervous system with the cysticercal (larval) form of *Taenia soleum* (pork tape worm). The location of the larvae in the CNS may vary from subarachnoid to intraparenchymal to intraventricular, or it may include a combination of these regions. Children from endemic areas, and especially those with pica, are at great risk of developing neurocysticercosis as they may eat contaminated vegetation and soil because of the poor hygiene and lack of sanitation in these areas.

Clinical presentation

The clinical features and CT findings are extremely varied as they are largely determined by the location and the stage of the life cycle of the parasite in the brain as well as by the degree of immune reaction mounted by the host. This varies from immune tolerance to severe meningo-encephalitis.

Diagnosis

Diagnosis depends on a high index of clinical suspicion; typical findings on CT scan or magnetic resonance imaging (MRI) of the brain; and LP (the latter only after control of increased ICP). Examination of CSF shows features of aseptic meningitis with the occasional presence of eosinophils. Blood and CSF immunologic reactions by ELISA and Western blot methods vary widely according to the stage of life cycle, immunoreactivity of the host and localization of the parasite.

Management

General

Determined by clinical features and CT findings.

♦ Viable cysts of the brain (unless very large) are usually asymptomatic, show no pericyst oedema or enhancement on CT scan. Specific therapy is most effective and is indicated in these patients, who are usually adolescents and adults. Note that the cysts are still too small in the brains of children to be visible with present-day neuroradiology.

♦ Dying cysts with varying degrees of pericyst oedema and enhancement on CT scan (radiologic 'granulomas') present with clinical features of focal or multifocal encephalitis or generalized meningo-encephalitis: specific therapy is contro-versial as cysts are already dying but is recommended as different stages of the parasites' life cycle may exist in any one patient and associated small viable cysts will not be visible in scans of those children with encephalitis.

♦ Dead parasites with calcific foci on CT scan or skull X-ray may manifest with epilepsy or other neurologic sequelae, or may be asymptomatic. Specific therapy is not indicated.

♦ Large intraventricular or subarachnoid racemose cysts demonstrated on CT scan (with intraventricular or subarach-noid contrast), or on MRI, manifest with features of space-demanding lesions and/or hydrocephalus: specific therapy is ineffective. Surgical extirpation is required.

Specific treatment

♦ PRAZIQUANTEL 50 mg/kg/day for 14 days or ALBENDA-ZOLE 15 mg/kg/day for five days. These dosages and the length of treatment have been empirically determined.

♦ Patients with numerous viable cysts or multifocal encephalitis should be treated with DEXAMETHASONE 0,25-0,5 mg/kg/day for 24 hours prior to commencing specific therapy and for the duration of such therapy. Steroid therapy is then slowly withdrawn. Watch for signs of rebound cerebral oedema. Patients with few viable cysts or focal encephalitis do not require steroid cover prior to specific therapy. These patients should be observed for raised ICP and focal neurological deficit during the first five days of drug therapy as the inflam-matory response to drug-induced cyst death is maximal during this time.

Supportive treatment

◆ Epilepsy: appropriate anticonvulsants. See page 340.
◆ Raised ICP due to meningo-encephalitis. See pages 124-6.
◆ Raised ICP due to hydrocephalus: ventricular shunt. See page 330.

Acute idiopathic polyneuritis (Guillain-Barré syndrome, acute infectious polyneuritis)

The condition is an acute neurological emergency and is the most common acute neuromuscular disorder. It necessitates intensive care management and possible ventilatory support.

Clinical presentation

Weakness usually evolves over several days up to a few weeks. The evolution may at times be more rapid over some hours. Hypotonia and reduced muscle stretch reflexes followed by absent reflexes are invariable findings. The paresis or paralysis evolves in most patients in a more or less symmetrical fashion from initial distal leg or arm involvement to proximal limb, trunk and respiratory muscle involvement. Occasionally the weakness may begin in the proximal limb girdle muscles. Cranial nerves may be involved in particular bilateral facial paresis or paralysis. Bulbar weakness may be present. Peripheral paraesthesiae with variable objective stocking-glove sensory loss may be features of the syndrome in older children. The latter is not easy to document in younger children. Autonomic dysfunction with cardiac arrhythmias, hypotension or hypertension may be lethal. Urinary retention is uncommon. A syndrome of total ophthalmoplegia, ataxia and areflexia (Fisher's syndrome) is thought to be a variety of acute idiopathic polyneuritis.

Diagnosis

◆ The diagnosis is based on the clinical findings. CSF examination shows cyto-albuminic dissociation. The latter may not manifest during the first week or two of the illness.
◆ Nerve conduction studies show a slowing of conduction velocities in the majority of patients.
◆ It is important to exclude disorders that may mimic acute idiopathic polyneuritis, i.e. hypokalaemia, post-diphtheric

polyneuropathy, tick paralysis, botulism and acute porphyria (in adolescents).

Management

The mainstay of therapy is adequate symptomatic support, i.e. ICU facilities must be available in case of respiratory or autonomic failure.

Specific treatment

Nil. Plasma exchange therapy has a favourable influence on morbidity, length of hospital stay and recovery to independent ambulation in severely affected patients.

Prognosis

Favourable in children with adequate supportive care.

13 CHEMICAL PATHOLOGY

L R Purves and S E Franco

General consideration

♦ Preparation of the patient, method of specimen collection and subsequent handling of the specimen are important variables that all have a bearing on the final result.

♦ Reference ranges are method and laboratory specific. Given reference ranges are for the Chemical Pathology Service of the Red Cross War Memorial Children's Hospital.

♦ Blood for routine chemistry is collected in 3 ml tubes containing LITHIUM HEPARINATE as anticoagulant.

♦ Specialized tubes are available for specific analyses and must be used appropriately. Glucose assays require oxalate and fluoride; pyruvate requires protein precipitation; ammonia requires specially prepared heparinized tubes etc. If in doubt, check with the laboratory. All specimens, whether blood, CSF, or urine etc., should always be transported to the laboratory with minimum delay.

♦ Dark glass containers for 24 hour collections are obtainable from the laboratory. Inform laboratory staff of intended investigation so that the correct preservative can be added.

Inborn errors of metabolism

Screening tests are available for the detection and semi-quantitation of the following substances in urine: mono- and disaccharides, amino acids, mucopolysaccharides, organic acids, long chain fatty acids, carnitine and ketones. Random urine specimens (± 15 ml) are required, accompanied by heparinized blood (2 ml), in the case of suspected amino acid disorders. A list of current medication as well as essential clinical information should accompany each request.

Definitive tests are only done after consultation with the laboratory.

Table 13.1 Clinical chemistry reference (normal) range

* Tests done by outside laboratories may be sent to the Chemical Pathology Laboratory at the Red Cross War Memorial Children's Hospital. They will then be forwarded to the appropriate laboratories by the Chemical Pathology Laboratory.

** Abbreviations: P = Plasma,S=Serum,B=Whole Blood,U=Urine,F=Faeces,CS=Cerebrospinal Fluid, Fld=Fluid.

Test*	Sample**		Reference range	Comments
Acid phosphatase (ACP)	P	Total acid phosphatase	0-4,2 U/l	Unstable. Arrange with laboratory beforehand. Blood into heparin tube on ice and send immediately for analysis.
Adenosine deaminase (ADA)	CS		0-7 U/l	ADA is synthesized by T-lymphocytes in response to infection. Elevated levels while not diagnostic, are more in keeping with TB than other causes of transudates and exudates.
	Fld		0-35 U/l	
Alanine aminotransferase (ALT)	P	0-2 yrs	7-41 U/l (37°C)	Very specific marker of hepatocellular damage. Cytosolic enzyme.
		> 2 yrs	7-35 U/l	
Albumin	P	<2 months	30-45 g/l	Method: BCG (Astra 8). The BCG dye binding method is non-specific, measuring $\alpha 1$ and $\alpha 2$ globulins in addition to albumin. In the nephrotic syndrome and related disorders, the non-specificity is marked and nephelometry or another immuno-chemical assay should be requested.
		2 months-3 yrs	35-47 g/l	
		3-5 yrs	38-50 g/l	
		5-8 yrs	40-56 g/l	
		8-13 yrs	30-55 g/l	
		> 13 yrs	35-49 g/l	

Test*	Sample**	Reference range	Comments
Alcohol*	P	Legal intoxication >17 mmol/l (800 mg/l) Comatosed >64 mmol/l (3000 mg/l)	Doctors should be aware that some paediatric preparations have alcohol as the vehicle. Consult the label.
Alkaline phosphatase	P	0-3 yrs 100-300 U/l (37°C) 3-12 yrs 75-250 U/l (37°C) 12-18 yrs 75-300 U/l (37°C)	Values in pubertal boys higher than in girls but peak at about 15 yrs compared to 11 yrs in girls. Transient normal increases above the reference limits may occur during growth spurt. Major isoenzyme in children derived from bone. 5'Nucleotidase activity reflects the liver isoenzyme.
α1-antitrypsin (A1AT)	P	Birth-3 days 1,43-4,4 g/l 4 days-3 yrs 1,47-2,44 g/l 4-9 yrs 1,6-2,45 g/l 10-13 yrs 1,62-2,59 g/l	Anti-elastase isoproteins: normal: MM Significant variants SS, SZ, ZZ Of the α1-antitrypsin variants, only the ZZ homozygote and null phenotypes are associated with liver and lung disease.
α1-antitrypsin stool clearance	P&F	0,8-5,4 ml/day	Measures enteric protein loss. Requires at least 24 hour stool collection, preferably 72 hours. Submit a plasma specimen for each 24 hour period. Preweighed stool container available from laboratory.

Test*	Sample**	Reference range	Comments
α-fetoprotein* (AFP)	P	µg/l (or ng/ml)	Level should decrease after birth with half-time five to seven days.
		Birth <170 000	
		2 days-1 wk 20 000-60 000	
		>35 days <10	
Amino acids	P&U	Normal values supplied on request	Arrange with laboratory.
Ammonia	P	Neonates 64-107 µmol/l	By arrangement with laboratory only.
		0-2 wks 56-92 µmol/l	
		Children 21-50 µmol/l	
	U	Infants 40-207 mmol/day	
Amylase	P	0-60 U/l (30°C)	Salivary and pancreatic isoenzymes available on request. Should collect urine for at least two hours. Record times on container.
	U	0-16 U/l (30°C)	
Anion Gap Na−(Cl + HCO₃)		8-16 mmol/l	
Ascorbate	P	Normal 28-85 µmol/l	Ascorbate saturation test preferable.
Ascorbate saturation test	P	Rise of >14,2 µmol/l	By arrangement with laboratory. Draw baseline specimen. Administer 15 mg/kg ascorbate orally, and draw three-hour specimen.

Test*	Sample**	Reference range	Comments
Aspartate transferase (AST, SGOT)*	P	0-56 U/l (37 °C)	Mitochondrial and cytosolic isoenzyme. Less specific for liver damage than ALT.
Astrup and PaO₂			See Appendix 4, Table 1, page 661
Phenobarbitone	P	Toxic level (approx): short-acting >13 μmol/l long-acting >130 μmol/l Therapeutic levels (approx): PHENOBARBITONE 45-130 μmol/l	Levels depend on time of sampling after ingestion.
Bilirubin	P	Total 3-17 μmol/l Conjugated 0-4 μmol/l Neonates (total): Age Preterm Term <24 hr 17-103 μmol/l 34-103 μmol/l <48 hr 103-137 μmol/l 103-120 μmol/l 3-5 days 171-205 μmol/l 68-103 μmol/l Adult values achieved at one month.	Levels must be assessed in relation to risk factors such as immaturity, hypoxia, acidosis, infections and increased plasma levels of certain drugs, free fatty acids or low albumin levels. See page 359.
Caeruloplasmin*	S	>1 yr 0,2-0,6 g/l	

Test*	Sample**		Reference range	Comments
Calcium (Total)	P	Preterm Fullterm (1st week) Children	1.50-2.50 mmol/l 1.75-3.00 mmol/l 2.2-2.7 mmol/l	Always correct level for albumin by adding 0,02 x (42-Albumin).
	U		0,005-0,2 mmol/kg/day	
Calcium (ionized)	P	Heparinized syringe on ice	1,12-1,23 mmol/l	Determines physiologically active Ca level in altered acid base and protein states.
Carotenes	P		50-300 µg/dl	Wrap specimen in metal foil and send to laboratory on ice. 3 ml blood required.
Catecholamines* **(Total)**	U	<1 yr 1-5 yrs 6-15 yrs >15 yrs	0.08-0.18 µmol/day 0,18-0,36 µmol/day 0,22-0,57 µmol/day <1,3 µmol/day	Phaeochromocytoma in adults: 1,75 µmol/day. Normal plasma ranges for children have yet to be established but are likely to be similar. Consult laboratory for collection details.
	P	Adrenaline (adult) Noradrenaline (adult)	30-80 pg/ml 200-400 pg/ml	
Chloride	P	<1 year >1 year	96-110 mmol/l 98-106 mmol/l	For diagnosis of cystic fibrosis the following criteria should be met: (a) sweat sodium + chloride >140 mmol/l (b) sweat chloride > sodium Arrange with laboratory, following delta-F-508.
	CS		120-130 mmol/l	
	Sweat		<40 mmol/l	

Test*	Sample**		Reference range	Comments
Cholesterol	P	Neonates (cord blood)	1,17-2,60 mmol/l	For cholesterol in HDL + LDL, contact laboratory for collection details.
		<1 yr	1,81-4,53 mmol/l	
		1-13 yrs	3,10-5,20 mmol/l	
Cholinesterase	P,B	Children	3500-8500 U/l (30°C)	Red cell enzyme not regenerated in ORGANOPHOSPHATE poisoning.
Copper*	S	Infants	<11 μmol/l	2 ml blood required. Avoid contamination. Use disposable plastic syringe and new needle. Collect in trace metal free tubes obtainable from the laboratory.
		Children	13-30 μmol/l	
Cortisol*	P	Three months-adult		Marked circadian rhythm. Note time of collection. Use heparinized chemistry tubes.
	09h00		140-700 nmol/l	
	24h00		0-280 nmol/l	
Creatinine	P	Neonates	27-88 μmol/l	Affected by haemolysis and raised levels of bilirubin and ketones.
		<1 year	18-35 μmol/l	
		>1 year	27-62 μmol/l	

Test*	Sample**	Reference range	Comments
Creatinine clearance	P&U	Neonates 26-68 ml/min/1,73m² <6 months 41-103 ml/min/1,73m² 6 months-1 yr 49-157 ml/min/1,73m² 1-2 yrs 63-191 ml/min/1,73m² 2-12 yrs 89-165 ml/min/1,73m²	Always supply height and weight. 24 hr urine specimen with a blood sample taken during the 24 hours.
Creatinine kinase (CK)	P	23-203 U/l (37°C)	Iso-enzymes done when indicated.
Delta-F-508 gene probe		Reported as normal, heterozygous or homozygous	Preferably arrange buccal scrape with laboratory; or send 0,5 ml blood in EDTA. Detects approx. 70% of cystic fibroses.
Faecal fat	F	1-6 yrs <1 g/day Adults <7 g/day	Patient on appropriate daily fat intake probe to commencement. Arrange with laboratory for collection details. Pre-weighed container used for a three-day collection.
Ferritin*	P	20-210 µg/l	<12 µg/l in iron deficiency.
Free fatty acids	P	0,3-1,1 mmol/l	Collected on ice, unstable. Patient must be fasting.

Test*	Sample**		Reference range	Comments
Gamma glutamyl transferase	P	0-1 month	12-244 U/l (37°C)	
		1-2 months	9-160 U/l (37°C)	
		2 months-2 yrs	3-30 U/l (37°C)	
		2-15 yrs	5-28 U/l (37°C)	
Glucose				NB. Clinically significant hypoglycaemia defined as <2.2 mmol/l. In neonates <1,1 mmol/l. Glucose in neonatal blood extremely labile in vitro: transport rapidly to laboratory on ice and request urgent separation.
		Neonates		
		Preterm	1,1-3,3 mmol/l	
		Fullterm	1,7-3,3 mmol/l	
		Children	3,3-5,6 mmol/l	
Glutamine	CS		0,5-1,2 mmol/l	Patients with grade I hepatic encephalopathy may have values within the reference range.
Homovanillic acid 24 hr (HVA)	U	0-1 yr	2,0-27,0 nmol/μmol Creat	Contact laboratory for collection details.
		1-2 yrs	3,0-26,0 nmol/μmol Creat	
		2-5 yrs	2,0-18,0 nmol/μmol Creat	
		>5 yrs	0-12,0 nmol/μmol Creat	
Immunoglobulins	S or P		See page 681	

Test*	Sample**	Reference range	Comments
Iron	P	17,9-44,7 µmol/l Decreases gradually 17,9 to 7,1 µmol/l 21,4 to 8,9 µmol/l 28,6 to 8,9 µmol/l	Avoid contamination when collecting. Send at least 3 ml blood in heparinized chemistry tube. Use disposable needle and plastic syringe.
	Neonates 1 month-3 yrs 3-10 yrs Adults		
Ketone bodies: aceto-acetate β-hydroxybutyrate	P P	<300 µmol/l <300 µmol/l	Arrange with laboratory beforehand.
Lactate	B	0,5-2,2 mmol/l	Contact laboratory to arrange collection.
Lactate dehydrogenase (LD)	P Fld	153-263 U/l (37°C) >200 U/l	Iso-enzymes done when indicated. Indicates exudate.
Lactose tolerance test	P	Increase in P-glucose of >1,1 mmol/l	Contact laboratory for collection details.
Lead*	B	<30 µg/dl (1,45 µmol/l)	Specimen must be submitted in metal-free containers available from laboratory.

Test*	Sample**		Reference range	Comments
Magnesium	P	Neonates	0,5-0,9 mmol/l	
		Children	0,7-0,9 mmol/l	
		Adults	0,7-1,0 mmol/l	
5'-Nucleotidase (NTD)	P		2-17 U/l (30°C)	Not raised if alkaline phosphatase is of bone origin. Lower values reported in children.
Osmolality	P		275-295 mmol/kg water	Calculation:2[Na] + glucose + urea expressed as mmol/l. The difference between measured and calculated plasma osmolality may indicate additional osmotically active substances, eg. MANNITOL, polyethylene glycol, alcohol etc.
	U	Infants	50-600 mmol/kg water	
		Children & adults: severe dehydration	800-1400 mmol/kg water	
		Water diuresis	40-80 mmol/kg water	
PARACETAMOL	P	4 hrs after ingestion: clinically insignificant:	<0,8 mmol/l	Values apply to adults. If blood values are above the toxic level, liver function tests should be timeously performed
		Toxic:	>2,00 mmol/l	
		12 hrs after ingestion:	to detect hepatic injury.	
		Toxic:	>0,33 mmol/l	

Test*	Sample**	Reference range	Comments
Phosphate	P	Birth 1,78-3,07 mmol/l <1 yr 1,45-2,10 mmol/l 1-3 yrs 1,45-1,78 mmol/l >3 yrs 0,87-1,45 mmol/l	24 hr urine in 10 ml HCl. Blood taken during collection period.
TRP		82-95%	Tubular reabsorption of phosphate. $TRP = 1 - \dfrac{U\text{-phosphate} \times P\text{-creatinine}}{P\text{-phosphate} \times U\text{-creatinine}} \times 100$
Potassium	P	3,4-4,5 mmol/l	Haemolysis raises level.
Protein Total	P	<6 months 40-76 g/l 6 months-2 yrs 51-73 g/l >2 years 60-80 g/l	Serum protein is approximately 2g/l less than plasma protein.
Protein fractions (electrophoresis)	S	Albumin (g/l) 38-58 Globulins (g/l): Alpha 1 Alpha 2 Beta Gamma 1,1-3,2 5,3-11,2 4,2-8,7 5,3-13,7	

Test*	Sample**		Reference range	Comments
Protein selectivity index	P & U	Low selectivity	>30%	May be determined on random urine and plasma sample collected at the same time.
		Medium selectivity	16-30%	Formula:(U-IgG x P-albumin)(U-albumin x P-IgG) x 100
		High selectivity	<16%	
			Above 20%: 85% steroid resistant	
			Below 10%: 85% steroid responsive	
Pyruvate	B		30-100 µmol/l	Contact laboratory for collection details.
SALICYLATE	P	Normally therapeutic	<0,14 mmol/l (blank value) 0,72-1,45 mmol/l	Note overlap between therapeutic and potentially toxic levels. However, toxicity is rare if level <2,17 mmol/l. Falsely elevated if ketones raised.
Sodium	P	Neonates Children	134-146 mmol/l 138-145 mmol/l	
	Sweat		<40 mmol/l	See also chloride and delta-F-508.

Test*	Sample**	Reference range	Comments
THEOPHYLLINE	Therapeutic	8-20 µg/ml	
Thyroxine (free T4)*	P		
<1 yr		variable	
>1 yr		6,3-22,8 pmol/l	
Thyrotropin (TSH)*			Different laboratories give different normal values; these are a guide. Hypothyroidism in the newborn leads to damage of the neonatal brain. Early detection of hypothyroidism and appropriate therapy prevents this outcome.
Cord blood		1,5-20,0 µIU/ml	
Newborn-48 hrs		Very variable	
3-7 days		<25 µIU/ml	
7-14 days		<10 µIU/ml	
14 days-adults		<4 µIU/ml	
Titratable acidity	U		24hr urine collection at 4 °C. Under layer of toluene + liquid paraffin. Contact laboratory for details.
Outside limits		20-30 mmol/24 hr	
		15-40 mmol/24 hr	
Total iron binding capacity (TIBC)	P		Reflects transferrin level.
<1 yr		17,9-71,6 µmol/l	
>1 yr		44,7-71,6 µmol/l	
Transferrin	P	2,2-4,0 g/l	
Triglyceride	P		Patient must be fasted.
<6 yrs		0,11-1,12 mmol/l	
6-12 yrs		0,35-1,22 mmol/l	
>12 yrs		0,41-1,56 mmol/l	

Test*	Sample**		Reference range	Comments
Tryptic activity (stool)	F	<1 yr	1/80 dilution or higher	Decreased activity in cystic fibrosis.
		>1 yr	1/20-1/40 dilution	See also chloride and delta-F-508.
		Adults	Unreliable	
Urea	P	Neonates	1,4-4,3 mmol/l	
		Children	1,8-6,4 mmol/l	
Urate	P	Children	0,12-0,32 mmol/l	
Vanillylmandelic acid (VMA)	U (24 hrs)	0-1 yr	0-20 nmol/μmol creatinine	Contact laboratory for collection details.
		1-2 yrs	0-17 nmol/μmol creatinine	
		2-5 yrs	0-9 nmol/μmol creatinine	
		5-10 yrs	0-8 nmol/μmol creatinine	
		10-15 yrs	0-6 nmol/μmol creatinine	
VIT A*	S	Neonates	1,22-2,62 μmol/l	Wrap specimen in metal foil and send to laboratory on ice.
		Children	1,05-2,79 μmol/l	
		Adults	1,05-2,27 μmol/l	

Test*	Sample**	Reference range	Comments
VIT C	See Ascorbate		
Xylose absorption test (five-hour excretion)	U	<6 months 11-30% of ingested load 6-12 months 20-35% of ingested load 1-10 yrs 20-45% of ingested load >10 yrs 28-51% of ingested load	Must fast overnight. Baseline blood plus urine obtained. 0,5 g of xylose/kg (max 5g) dissolved in 100-500 ml of water given; draw blood one hour post dose. Collect urine for five hours. Notify laboratory beforehand.
Xylose-one-hour blood test	B	>1,3 mmol/l after 5 g dose	

* Tests done by outside laboratories may be sent to the Chemical Pathology Laboratory at the Red Cross War Memorial Children's Hospital. They will then be forwarded to the appropriate laboratories.
** Abbreviations: P = Plasma, S=Serum, B=Whole blood, U=Urine, F=Faeces, CS=Cerebrospinal fluid, Fld=Fluid.

14 CHILD ABUSE AND NEGLECT

A C Argent, D H Bass and P I Lachman

Child abuse and neglect are common problems encountered by all health professionals who work with children. Failure to consider a diagnosis of child abuse may have catastrophic implications for the affected child and the family.

Definitions

Abuse and neglect can be defined in different ways.

Physical abuse

Physical injury to a child where there is reasonable evidence that the injury was inflicted deliberately, or was wilfully not prevented.

Sexual abuse

The use of a child for sexual gratification.

Neglect

The intentional neglect to provide for the child's care and developmental needs.

Approach

The diagnosis, assessment and management of child abuse and neglect are complex. Wherever possible, teams should be established which consist of at least social workers and doctors.

The goals of management of child abuse

♦ Investigate child abuse where appropriate with minimum trauma to the child.
♦ Each investigation should be done once only by a competent person.
♦ Ensure the safety of the child.
♦ Collect all relevant information for medico-legal procedures.

Within this framework the responsibility of the doctor is to consider the possibility of child abuse when appropriate, treat any injuries, and to diagnose and treat any medical complications, such as sexually transmitted diseases.

Assessment

There are at least three questions that need to be addressed during the assessment of possible abuse:

◆ What is the nature of the abuse that has taken place?
◆ With what degree of certainty can the diagnosis of abuse be made?
◆ What is the risk that further abuse will take place?

History

Abuse has occurred until proven otherwise when:

◆ the child describes the abuse;
◆ injuries occur without explanation, or there is a change of explanation for the injury on repeated questioning;
◆ the presentation of any sexually transmitted disease in a child;
◆ the child presents with sexualized behaviour inappropriate to his or her developmental stage; or
◆ any person suspects abuse.

Abuse should be considered in the differential diagnosis of a child who presents with complaints such as repeated urogenital symptoms, enuresis, encopresis, recurrent abdominal pain and a wide range of vague symptoms. If there is concern about abuse, the subject must be broached with the child and the childminder. This must be done in a non-accusatory manner, and ideally together with personnel skilled in interviewing.

Physical findings

No single physical sign alone is diagnostic of child abuse. At least 50% of abused children may have no physical evidence of abuse.

A general physical examination should be done on every child. Measures of growth and development are important, particularly in cases where neglect may be suspected. This examination should be done in a 'child-friendly environment', and must not be painful.

Equipment such as otoscopes which may be used in the later examination of the genitalia can be introduced to the child during this examination.

Unless abuse is thought to have occurred within the previous 48-72 hours, genital examination can be delayed until the child is prepared for the examination, and a suitably experienced person can be present.

Examination of the genitalia of a small child is best done with the child on his or her mother's lap. An older child can be examined when sitting on a chair or lying on a bed. An otoscope can be used to illuminate and magnify the genitalia. This is particularly useful in smaller children. If there is evidence of trauma, and the examination is likely to be inadequate without hurting the child, the examination should be done under anaesthesia.

All physical findings (including growth parameters) should be documented meticulously. If any uncertainty exists regarding the significance of signs it is advisable to describe details rather than to record interpretations of findings.

Results of the physical examination should be carefully explained to the older child and his or her caretaker. Reassurance regarding normal findings is often extremely comforting to parents.

Special investigations

Children and their parents should be informed as to the reason for any special investigation being done before that test is done.

Forensic

Blood- or secretion-stained clothing, vaginal swabs for semen or buccal mucosal swabs (smear on glass slide) should be collected. If sexual abuse within the previous 48-72 hours is suspected, 5 ml of clotted blood, clothing, glass slides and saliva must be submitted to police forensic laboratories. Document collection of specimens on the appropriate form (J88).

Radiology

X-ray appropriately if there is obvious injury. A skeletal survey or bone scan (the latter is preferable) is indicated for multiple injury or suspected chronic abuse.

Blood

Multiple bruising is an indication for obtaining a clotting profile and platelet count. If sexual abuse is suspected or confirmed, do a VDRL. In a high-risk area, HIV serology should be done.

Microbiology

Vaginal swabs should be collected for exclusion or diagnosis of sexually transmitted diseases. In cases of rectal or oral sexual abuse, collect swabs from these areas.

Swabs used for genital specimen collection should be pre-moistened with bacterial transport medium. Collect intravaginal or urethral swabs with thin wire-mounted swabs. As many of the sexually transmitted organisms are fastidious, swabs should be put in a transport medium.

Management

All cases of child abuse and neglect must be reported to the Regional Director of Health and Welfare in terms of the Child Care Act No. 74 of 1983. See page 321.

Emergency

◆ Ensure the safety of the child.
◆ Treat any injuries or medical problems.
◆ Collect and collate all relevant information.
◆ Complete Form J88 with medical evidence to support the diagnosis of abuse.
◆ Meet together with involved personnel to make a decision regarding the reliability of the diagnosis and plan appropriate management.

Long-term

◆ Medical follow-up of all cases is particularly important when there is a possibility of neglect or sexually transmitted diseases.
◆ Social work follow-up to support the child and the family and to identify long-term problems as early as possible.
◆ Support of the child and the family during legal proceedings.
◆ Psychological intervention when indicated.
◆ Communication between all personnel involved in the care of the child is essential.

15 DATA GATHERING

D J Power

These suggestions are aimed at paediatric departments in regional or district hospitals that have links to community services. They cover the minimum data set that would be satisfactory for monitoring the health of a community and for the provision of information necessary for service management and planning.

Data may be collected, stored and analysed by hand, but the use of microcomputers will assist this process. Several units have produced software to gather and analyse essential information and may be able to help others in the setting up of systems.

Much of the data can be captured as part of routine clinical work, especially if the information system offers the inputting staff member a tangible benefit in daily work, such as the printing of discharge summaries or midnight count lists.

Data required

The community

♦ **Population**. Total numbers of people in the community served. Figures can be obtained from census data, informal estimates by aerial surveys of house counts, etc.

♦ **Age structure**. The percentage of the total population in each of a number of age categories. These allow estimation of the numbers of children in each age category in the community. If not known, assumptions can produce reasonable approximations. See Table 15.1, page 153.

♦ **Births**. The number of births (live and still) in the community over a period of time can be reliably obtained if most births take place in the health service or if the registration of births is fairly complete. Otherwise the number of births can be crudely estimated from the population figure by using the real or an assumed birth rate. See page 153 for typical birth rates.

♦ **Birth data**. Information should be gathered about each birth as part of birth notification and registration. These include the date of birth, whether live or stillborn (macerated or fresh), the place of birth, i.e. home or institution (hospital or clinic), and the birthweight.

◆ **Death data**. Information about each death registration should include the date of birth, sex, the normal residential address, the cause and date of death. Neonatal deaths should also include birthweight and the neonatal diagnostic category. See page 153.

◆ **Community service data** should include immunizations given, collected by type and age group.

Hospital admissions

◆ **Newborn nursery admissions**. The following data should be collected on each infant admitted to the newborn nursery: mother's age, address, gravida, parity, obstetric complications, the source of referral, the infant's date of birth, the place of birth, the method of delivery, the Apgar score at five minutes, the birthweight, the estimated gestational age at birth, the admission weight, the discharge weight, the discharge diagnosis, the neonatal diagnostic category, the causes of death, any procedures carried out, and the duration of stay.

◆ **Paediatric admissions**. The following data should be collected on each infant admitted to paediatric wards: address (text and coded; see page 153), date of birth, sex, weight, nutritional category, clinic area, discharge diagnoses or causes of death (ICD9 coded) and duration of stay.

Registers of certain categories of patient

These are kept to facilitate continuing care, and to produce data essential for the motivation for new services or for the evaluation of existing services. Registers that have proved useful include:

◆ **Cardiac**: recording diagnoses, date of birth, sex, address, plan of management.

◆ **Disabled**: recording type of disability, severity, date of birth, sex, address, community facility needed (if the facility is not available the register facilitates planning of services).

◆ **TB treatment**: TB patient register with monthly feedback from treatment point as to doses taken. Allows close monitoring of treatment.

Analyses required

◆ **Infant mortality rate**[1]: this important indicator of child health depends on very complete birth registration and death certification. If these are not available use the Brass survey method (Brass W., 'Indirect techniques for demographic estimation', in: *United Nations Manual X.* New York: Department of Economic and Social Affairs Population Studies No. 81.).

◆ **Perinatal mortality rate**[1]: this should be produced separately for births in hospital, clinic and in the whole community. Each rate relates to a picture of a different part of health and health services.

◆ **Ratio of stillbirths to early neonatal deaths**[1] for hospital deliveries.

◆ **Neonatal birthweight and diagnostic category analysis:** the categories for this are set out on page 154. Such an analysis provides a useful reflection of neonatal health and health services.

◆ **Annual rates per 1 000 total births**: for the 'sentinel' conditions of neonatal tetanus, congenital syphilis, hypoxic ischaemic encephalopathy (birth asphyxia), and low and very low birthweight. Prevalence rates of teenage pregnancy should be recorded.

These conditions reflect the preventable component of perinatal morbidity. Improving trends over time are desirable.

◆ **Admissions for 'sentinel' conditions**. Monthly numbers of measles, gastroenteritis, respiratory infections and severe malnutrition i.e. underweight-for-age, marasmus, kwashiorkor and marasmic-kwashiorkor cases.

◆ **Annual incidence rates** for conditions such as tuberculous meningitis, acute nephritis, gastroenteritis, measles and malnutrition. These reflect child health in the general community, and improving trends with time are desirable.

Note: It is essential to communicate analyses to the hospital and community service staff who provide data. Regular reports should be provided to each clinic of patients discharged from hospital to their area with name, age, address, diagnosis and

---

[1] See Chapter 16 page 156 for definitions

date of discharge. This feedback leads to service development and ensures cooperation with data handling.

Codes, formats and rates

◆ **Age structures for three population types:**

Table 15.1 Percentage of total population in each age category

Age groups in years										
	<5	–10	–15	–20	–30	–40	–50	–60	–70	>70	Total
Pop. A	9	9	9	9	18	12,5	11,7	9,2	8	4,6	100
(Economically prosperous such as found in Europe or North America)											
Pop. B	12	11,5	11	10,5	17	13	10	8	5	2	100
(Transitional)											
Pop. C	13	13	13	11,5	17,5	13,5	9	6	2	1,5	100
(Economically disadvantaged in the developing world)											

◆ **Birth rates**
These are typical figures for the above three types of population: Pop. A = 11, Pop. B = 22, Pop. C = 37 births per annum per 1 000 total population.
◆ **Address coding**. For analysis of conditions by geographic area, some form of coding of addresses is essential. There is no uniformity around the country but examples in current use are (a) census enumerator districts which are coded subdivisions of magisterial districts, (b) allocation of a six-digit code to every village and suburb for use in all government departments; the codes allow aggregation into regions and (c) postal codes (use only as a last resort!).
◆ **Diagnostic coding**. The ICD (9th revision, clinical modification) is the most commonly used around the country. The British Paediatric Association has also published a set of 'Codes for classification of paediatric and perinatal disorders compatible with ICD9', which are available from the British Paediatric Association, 5 St Andrew's Place, Regents Park, London, NW1 N 4LB.
◆ **Nutritional categories**. Those commonly used are: normal, underweight for age, kwashiorkor, marasmus, marasmic kwashiorkor. See Chapter 34, page 376.

◆ **Neonatal diagnostic categories**. Neonatal outcomes are cat-
egorized according to the areas of major clinical concern.
Births and deaths are recorded in each of the following categories: 'prematurity', 'asphyxia', 'infection', 'other' and
'total'. These categories should then be divided into the
following birthweight categories : <1000g, –1249g, –1499g,
–1999g , –2499g, –2999g, –3999g, 4000+ g, totals.

Getting started

The following notes will be useful to anyone starting up a
computerized clinical hospital paediatric information system.

Hardware. The ideal is to have several personal computers
(PC's) linked to form a network so that data can be entered or
extracted at a terminal close to where the patient is being seen in
the outpatient department, the nursery or a ward. In a small paediatric unit, one could start with a single stand-alone PC in the
children's ward. It is ideal to have a printer for each PC so that
reports can be produced locally. Printers can be shared on a
network.

Software. A paediatric hospital information package is
required to handle your data and finding a suitable one is crucial
to success. There are a number of commercially produced packages available but these tend to be expensive. A good start can
be made with a package produced in-house or by drawing on the
experience of other units.

In evaluating a software programme it is best to start by
deciding what 'outputs', such as notes, reports and letters, you
will need for your purposes both now and in the future.

◆ Draw up the format of the discharge summary, letters and
   any other forms that you would like to send out.
◆ Draw up examples of the sort of enquiries about patients currently in the hospital that you might need, such as a listing of
   all patients in a ward, the matron's midnight report and a
   table of ward occupancy.
◆ Draw up examples of data analyses that you will need on a
   regular basis, such as a table of common preventable diseases by month, or a listing of discharges for a period of time
   broken down by clinic area.
◆ Set out examples of the sort of enquiries that you might want
   to make of the system on an occasional basis – such as a
   listing of cases of neurocysticercosis – by residential area.

♦ Decide on the coding format you want to use for diagnoses. The most commonly used is the ICD9.

♦ Assess the input side of the system by listing the items of data that will be needed to produce the required outputs.

Note that packages should make provision for the special data requirements of new-borns if neonatal information is to be processed.

You will now be in a position to judge whether any of the available software packages are capable of meeting your needs. If they are not, then you will need to develop your own software.

It is possible to start with a simple system that meets only basic needs and then with time to add modules that build up to a more comprehensive system. It is essential to set out on paper as much of your ideal system as possible so that each additional module will be compatible with the final product.

It should be unnecessary to use forms at the input stages as direct entry into the computer is best. There is a science to the layout of output forms and help can be obtained in their design from Medical Informatics Departments of the universities.

A list of all residential areas in the region served by the hospital is required, together with a code assigned to each. A list of the names and postal addresses of all referring agencies is also needed so that letters can be automatically addressed by the system.

Personnel. For a successful system one needs one or two enthusiasts who are determined to make the system work and who are computer-literate enough to deal with minor technical problems. However, one does not need to be a computer expert or programmer to run a successful paediatric information system.

H de V Heese and H M Power

Definitions of medico-legal terms are given in Chapter 30, page 305.

Age periods of childhood

Several different ways of describing time periods for the neonatal period are to be found in the literature. The differences reflect different ways of counting time, for example (i) the first week of life, (ii) the period from day 1 to day 7, or (iii) the period from day 0 to day 6. For epidemiological purposes the day of birth is taken as day 0 and time periods as in (iii) above.

Adolescence

The period during which all the dimensions of growth, development and maturation are completed. Most cultures relate the beginning of adolescence to the onset of puberty, but they differ widely in what constitutes its end. As societies become more complex, this point occurs later and later, yet there is at the same time a secular trend towards earlier puberty. The World Health Organization defines adolescence as the period of life between ten and 19 years, a definition used for statistical convenience rather than for biological accuracy.

Early infancy

One to six completed months, excluding the neonatal period.

Early neonatal period

The first week of life, i.e. 0-6 days old.

Infancy

First year of life, including the neonatal period.

Late infancy

Seven to 12 completed months.

Late neonatal period

The second, third and fourth weeks of life, i.e. 7-27 days old.

Neonatal period

The first four weeks of life, i.e. 0-27 days old.

Perinatal period

From the start of the 28th week of gestation to the end of the early neonatal period.

Post-neonatal period

From the start of the fifth week to the end of the first year.

Preschool child

Two to five years.

Puberty

The sequence of events by which the individual is transformed into a young adult by a series of biological changes. During this period the secondary sex characteristics develop. Ratings of pubertal development for clinical use have been devised by Tanner. Genital development in boys, pubic hair in boys and girls and breast development in girls have each been graded into five stages, ranging from pre-adolescence to maturity.

School child

Six years to school leaving. The school child period is divided into pre-adolescence and adolescence. Puberty takes place during this time.

Secular trend

A trend occurring over an 'age' or very long period.

Toddler

12-24 completed months.

Terms used in growth and development

Adaptive behaviour

Adaptive behaviour occurs when a child places fine motor skills in the context of the environment. This includes the ability to initiate new experience and profit from past experience.

Bone age

This is determined by comparing X-rays of the long bones, hand and wrist to age-related standards. It provides a measurement of osseus maturation.

Catch-up growth

A return towards the size that would have been attained if the growth lag had not occurred.

Chronological age

A record in terms of years and months, calculated from the birth date of the individual. The term 'chronological' is used to distinguish the ordinary meaning of age from other 'age' measures of development. It is commonly used and suffices in most circumstances.

Communication

Transmission of information.

Decimal age, decimal date

Age and date measured with a scale calibrated in tenths of a year, rather than months. Decimal dates simplify the calculation of age. Decimal ages facilitate calculations that involve age (such as the computation of growth velocity). A decimal calendar is used to look up decimal age. The calendar is a table in which the year is divided into thousandths and each date has a decimal number. Thus 1 May 1988 is 88,329 and a child born on 12 June 1987 is (88,329 − 87,444) = 0,885 years old on 1 May 1988. A decimal calendar appears on page 666.

Development

The increase in the complexity of structures and of their functions which take place in the same age period and often in a parallel fashion. It has been defined by Burlock as a 'progressive series of orderly, coherent changes'. It is the product of the interaction between the processes of maturation and learning.

Disability
Direct behaviour manifestation of the illness.

Disease
An objectively determined condition of ill health. It is a biological phenomenon, an array of symptoms, signs and pathological processes.

Fine motor development (manipulation)
Fine motor development refers to a series of skills which develop through visually guided prehension, thumb-finger opposition and the transition from unilateral and bimanual manipulation.

Gross motor development
Progression of abilities which ultimately enables the child to assume an upright posture and perform skilled activities while maintaining posture and equilibrium.

Growth
Increase in physical size. It involves changes in the composition and distribution of tissues, and is associated with changes in proportions, shape and functions.

Growth is measured in terms of 'distance' travelled, e.g. the weight, height or head circumference at a particular age. Measures of growth reflect the sum of physiological processes over the child's entire life span. Changes in growth are measured by growth velocity and growth acceleration.

Reference standards for weight, height and head circumference have been published by the National Center for Health Statistics (NCHS) in America and in Britain by Tanner and Whitehouse. These are available as tables and also appear on the familiar 'Road to Health' chart; see also Figures 4-9 in Appendix 4, pages 669-74.

Growth acceleration
The rate of change in growth velocity is expressed in units of growth velocity per year. The unit of height acceleration is cm/cm/year.

Growth spurt

The swift increase in growth rate that occurs at puberty or in response to treatment of impaired growth as, for example, in coeliac disease.

Growth velocity

The rate at which a child grows is expressed as the change per year. Growth velocity reflects physiological processes over periods of months, i.e. it is more sensitive to recent events than are measures of growth. The unit of height velocity is cm/year.

Handicap

Socially determined limitation of performance in specific activities.

Health

Denotes a state of well-being and effective function satisfactory to both the child and his or her social milieu and environment.

Height, stature

Height or stature is measured standing and recorded to the nearest millimetre. The child stands without shoes, the heels and back in contact with an upright surface. The head is held so that the child looks straight forward with the lower borders of the eye sockets in the same horizontal plane as the external auditory meati. A block is moved down until it touches the child's head. During the measurement the child should be told to take a breath, relax the shoulders and stretch up as tall as possible. The examiner helps by applying gentle upward pressure under the mastoid processes. The stretching minimizes the variation in height which occurs from morning to evening, which can otherwise be as much as 2 cm.

Height age

The chronological age at which the individual's height (stature) or length falls on the 50th percentile. This serves as an indicator of skeletal growth.

Illness

The subjective experience of ill health, i.e. the psychological and social ordeal of a human being.

Language

The primary medium of communication which involves the formalization of thought.

Learning

Refers to enduring changes in behaviour that result from contact with the environment.

Length

Length is measured supine and recorded to the nearest millimetre. Up to the age of two years the child is measured supine. One examiner holds the child's head in contact with a fixed board while a second person stretches him or her out to his maximum length and then brings a moving board into contact with the heels. Turning the infant's head sideways makes it easier to straighten the legs. Length averages about 1 cm more than height even when the best techniques are used for measuring height.

Maturation

The process of achieving full growth and development. In the latter it refers to changes in developmental status that occur without practice. The term is used for different systems in distinct yet related ways. It is the process that affects the genetically programmed biological inheritance, and, by implication, it is governed by an inherent regulating and controlling mechanism. Maturation is accompanied by structural and functional changes in the central nervous system and is initially related to myelination. However, maturation can be influenced by external factors, e.g. brain damage may retard the process, as does poor nutrition.

Mental age

This is difficult to define in precise terms, but in essence it is what one child can do when carrying out a large number of tests in comparison with the average achievements of a large number of children.

Milestone

The 'age' at which a specific measurement is achieved. It varies considerably between children. The 'age' may be expressed in terms of the chronological age, decimal age, height age, bone age or mental age.

Personal development

Is assessed on culturally modified skills of daily living.

Social development, socialization

The development of behaviour which is in accordance with social expectations.

Indicators of maternal and child health

Appropriate for gestational age (AGA)

Birthweight between the tenth and 90th centiles for gestational age.

Birth order

The succession number of the birth. Success of family planning and population development programmes is indicated by higher proportions of births that are first order or second order.

Elderly pregnancy

Pregnancy in a woman over 40 years.

Gestational Age

By convention, gestational age is calculated from the first day of the last menstrual period and is usually expressed as the nearest number of completed weeks. True gestational age is shorter and depends on the interval between the onset of menstruation and ovulation, fertilization and implantation.

Low birthweight (LBW)

Birthweight <2 500 g. Low birthweight is associated with a number of measures of poor maternal health and health practices such as lower socio-economic status, lesser use of health services, increased smoking rates etc. The outcome for the newborn is increased morbidity and mortality.

Overweight for gestational age (OGA)

Birthweight above the 90th centile for gestational age.

Post-term

Infant delivered after 293 days, i.e. >42 weeks gestational age.

Preterm

Having a gestational age less than 259 days, i.e. <37 weeks.

Symmetrical UGA infant

An UGA infant with crown-heel length and head circumference on the same centile as weight. This indicates a prolonged period of slow intra-uterine growth.

Teenage pregnancy

Pregnancy in a woman under 16 years.

Term

Having a gestational age of 259 to 293 days, i.e. from the start of the 37th week to the end of the 42nd week.

UGA infant with wasting

Weight below the tenth centile for gestational age, but length and head circumference normal for gestational age. This suggests soft tissue wasting from recent intra-uterine undernutrition.

Underweight for gestational age (UGA)

Birthweight below the tenth centile for gestational age.

Very low birthweight (VLBW)

Birthweight <1 500 g. Reflects similar risk factors and prognosis as low birthweight.

Overall indicators of child health

The term 'crude' is applied to a rate which has not been adjusted or refined for specific subgroups. For example, contrast crude birth rate with fertility rate which is an age- and sex-specific birth rate.

Age-specific death rate

Death rate calculated as the number of deaths in the age group per 1 000 population in that age group.

Attack rate

The proportion of people exposed to infection who develop the disease.

Case fatality rate

The proportion of cases that result in death.

Crude birth rate

Number of births (live or still) per 1 000 population per year. The number of births is counted during the year and the population at mid-year is estimated from census data, registered births and deaths, immigration and emigration. In some communities the number of actual births may significantly exceed the number of registered births. This caveat should be borne in mind when drawing conclusions from statistics derived from registered births.

Crude mortality rate

Total deaths per 1 000 population. This varies with factors such as social background and environment which are not directly under medical or nursing control.

Early neonatal mortality rate

Number of deaths in the period 0-6 days of life per 1 000 live births.

General fertility rate

Number of live births per year per 1 000 women of child-bearing age. 'Child-bearing age' by convention refers to 15-44 years. Age-specific rates, e.g. number of births to women aged 20-39, are also often employed.

Incidence rate

Number of new cases of a disease over a period of time divided by the population at risk. It measures the probability that healthy people will develop a disease during a specified period of time.

Infant and child mortality rate

Annual number of deaths of children under five years of age per 1 000 live births. More specifically, this is the probability of dying between birth and exactly five years of life.

Infant mortality rate (IMR)

Number of deaths of infants in the first 12 months of life per 1 000 live births in the same year. The IMR is widely used as it is regarded as a sensitive indicator of the health status of the population and is derived from data that are readily available in most countries. However, it includes deaths in both the neonatal period and the post-neonatal period. Since the causes of deaths in these two periods are very different, the perinatal mortality rate and postnatal mortality rate are becoming more popular terms of reference.

In some communities a higher proportion of infant deaths is registered than births. Since this will produce a spuriously high IMR, statistics from such communities should be interpreted with due caution.

Late neonatal mortality

Number of deaths in the period 7-27 days of life per 1 000 live births.

Neonatal mortality rate

Number of deaths in the period 0-27 days of life per 1 000 live births. Deaths and births are taken over the same period of time.

Perinatal mortality rate

Number of registered stillbirths plus number of deaths in the period 0-6 days of life per 1 000 total births. It is a measure of the success or failure of the promotion of perinatal health. Rates are affected by maternal age, parity, height and birthweight. Social services and use of antenatal services also have an effect. It is a commonly used indicator of the health status of the population.

Post-neonatal mortality rate (PNMR)

Number of deaths in the period 28 days to 12 completed months of life per 1 000 live births.

Prevalence rate

Total number of existing cases of a disease at a given time divided by the total population. It measures the number of people in a population who have the disease at a given time.

Stillbirth rate, late fetal mortality rate

Number of stillbirths per 1 000 total births. Sometimes, e.g. in United Nations statistics, this is expressed per 1 000 live births.

Terms used in the assessment of nutritional status

Indicator

The term relates to the use or application of indices. The indicator is usually constructed from the indices. As an example the proportion of children below a certain level of weight-for-age is used as an indicator of the nutritional status of children in a community.

Note: At times, an index and an indicator may be the same. For example 'rate' indices are also overall indicators of child health. See page 164.

Indices

Indices are combinations of anthropometric measurements such as age, weight, length (<two years) and height (>two years). Examples are weight for age, height for age and the ratio of the weight of a child to the median weight of the reference group of the same height. Indices are necessary for the interpretation of the measurements in an individual child or for grouping them in a number of children.

Reference

A reference is a device for grouping and analysing data. It is constructed from analysis of measurements, e.g. the median of the weights of children at a given age in a reference population.

Standard

A standard may be defined as a set of values which carries scientific authority and which can be used as a norm against which measured values or observations may be compared. In the field of nutrition the term also embodies the concept of a target which would be reached by interventions such as increased dietary intake, social upliftment or eradication of infection.

Note: An authorative reference may also be used as a standard. In South Africa, anthropometric measurements in a reference population as defined by the US National Center for Health Statistics (NCHS) are used both as references and as standards.

Stunting

Stunting signifies slowing in skeletal growth. The growth rate may be reduced from birth, but may not be evident for some years. Stunting represents the accumulated consequences of retarded growth over a prolonged period. The end result of the process of stunting is termed 'stunted'.

Wasting

Wasting indicates a deficit in tissue and fat mass compared with the amount expected in a child of the same length or height. It may result from failure to gain weight or from actual weight loss. The end result of the process of wasting is termed 'wasted'. The index used to quantify wasting is weight-for-height age.

17 DEVELOPMENT

C M Adnams and P I Lachman

The promotion of normal development is holistic and concerns the physical, emotional and social well-being of the child. A developmental examination forms part of the standard examination of every child and all visits to the health professional afford the opportunity to screen for deviations in development. The purpose of this screening is the early detection of abnormalities, referral for in-depth assessment, and the development of an intervention programme for the child in order to prevent further complications. Children at high risk of developmental delay as a result of problems such as prematurity, perinatal insults, meningitis and head trauma should be followed with particular care.

Screening

The routine screening of development involves taking a pertinent history of pregnancy, birth, and milestones, as well as medical and family histories. This is followed by observation of the child's motor activities, communication and social interaction, and a physical examination. Developmental assessment will entail a number of tests, a more in-depth appraisal of the psychological maturity of the child, and occasional laboratory or radiological tests.

Parents are partners in the assessment process and are the primary screeners of development. Children differ in their rates of development and a range of normality is used. Table 17.1 details the normal stages of development. Warning signs are provided as a guide for referral of potential problems at each age level.

Developmental problems

The WHO defines a disability as a defect that results in some malfunctioning, but does not necessarily affect normal life, whereas a handicap is a disability that has a substantial or permanent affect on normal growth or mental development. Delays need not develop into handicaps, particularly if detected early. As a result of screening and subsequent assessment the following problems may be detected:

Specific developmental delays

The most common delays in development are:

Motor: walking – exclude cerebral palsy, mental handicap, orthopaedic problems such as congenital dislocation of the hip, and muscle disorders.

Communication: exclude mental handicap, hearing loss, oral problems such as cleft palate, emotional deprivation, bilingualism, isolated speech delay and autism.

Coordination: exclude cerebral palsy, fine motor integration problems and mental handicap.

Mental handicap/intellectual disability

A mentally handicapped child has a global delay in development and catch-up to the normal is not possible. Understanding the causes of mental handicap are important in its prevention and management. The causes can be classified as follows:

Prenatal, e.g. intra-uterine insult, infection, structural brain disorder, chromosomal abnormality, or genetic disorders.

Perinatal, e.g. prematurity and ischaemia.

Postnatal, e.g. infections such as meningitis, anoxia, trauma, severe dehydration and shock;

Idiopathic, i.e. despite investigation and history, the cause cannot be determined.

There are four categories of mental handicap which determine placement. Intelligence quotients (IQ) are a guide and are used in determining placement. However, it is the functioning of the child that is more important. Children on the borderline are often difficult to place appropriately.

Mild (IQ 50-74)

These children are educable but have difficulty in formal schooling. They require a small class and individualized tuition. Entry to a special adaptation class in a normal school is the ideal.

Moderate (IQ 35 - 49)

These children are trainable and require specialized schooling where they are taught life skills and simple repeatable tasks. The special training schools admit children in the IQ range 30-50.

Severe (IQ 20-34) and profound (IQ 0-19)

These children require constant supervision and are eligible for care in special care centres. A child in this category can receive a care dependency grant from the State, dependent on regulations that may change in the near future. Referral to a social worker with a detailed medical report that states the diagnosis, severity, aetiology and permanence of the condition is necessary.

Cerebral Palsy

Cerebral palsy is defined as a disorder of movement resulting from a non-progressive lesion of the immature brain. This results in neurological dysfunction that may alter with time. Classification of causes is similar to that for mental handicap. The child usually presents with gross motor delay, but all areas of development can be affected. The clinical types are:

Spasticity (75%)

Spasticity is the result of an upper motor neuron lesion. It may present as hemiplegia (one sided), diplegia (lower limbs more than upper limbs, usually due to prematurity), triplegia (one upper limb spared), or quadriplegia (all limbs, usually due to asphyxia or cerebral infection).

Dyskinesia (7,5%)

This is the result of basal ganglia involvement and presents as athetosis, chorio-athetosis or dystonia.

Ataxia (5%)

This is the result of cerebellar involvement. Other causes of ataxia must be excluded.

Hypotonia (5%)

This is often the early presenting feature, and it develops into one of the above types.

Mixed (7,5%)

This involves a combination of the other types. The common causes are head injury due to motor vehicle accidents and tuberculous meningitis.

The child with cerebral palsy may have associated problems such as mental handicap, seizures, visual and communication problems, learning disabilities or poor fine motor coordination. Common problems include dislocation of the hips, dental caries, constipation and sleep disorders. Physiotherapy, occupational therapy, communication therapy and orthopaedic interventions are part of the overall management.

Many children with developmental disorders have behavioural problems. Behavioural problems associated with developmental difficulties, such as learning disorders, speech and fine motor difficulties and hyperactivity, may be presenting features of a pervasive developmental disorder.

Referral

Early detection and referral for intervention is important. A 'wait and see' attitude can have negative long-term effects on the child. A child should be referred to a specialist in the field for assessment if there is a persistent warning sign present according to the developmental chart, or if there is a history of any of the possible causes of developmental delays. Persistent increased or decreased tone, delays in any of the major milestones — sitting, walking and talking and disproportionately small head size are markers for referral. Children with conditions known to be associated with developmental delay (e.g. Down's Syndrome, Fetal Alcohol Syndrome) should also be referred for appropriate intervention. Parental anxiety should not be ignored.

Management

The management of a child with a handicap consists of a partnership between the child, the parent, the multi-disciplinary team and the community. The health team should consist of doctors, social workers, psychologists, teachers, physiotherapists, occupational therapists and communication therapists. Community rehabilitation workers can play a vital role. While diagnosis may be at the secondary or tertiary level, the management should be at the community level and should aim at attaining the prevention of the secondary complications of the handicap, and at the mental, physical and social well-being of the child.

Management includes:

A **Awareness** of normal development and promotion of prevention of the causes of handicap.

E **Early detection** of any disability or handicap by means of regular child surveillance at every visit to a health professional, and monitoring of all children at risk of developing a handicap.

I **Intervention** by means of appropriate breaking of the news to parents (see page 79), and planning an individual intervention strategy with the parents and the team.

O **Ongoing support** and assessment of the child and the family.

U **Understanding** the effect a disabled child has on the family, and the effects that lack of resources and understanding have on the child.

In summary the disabled child must be treated like all other children — with love, respect and with particular attention given to his or her special needs.

Table 17.1 Milestones and warning signs

AGE	GROSS MOTOR	FINE MOTOR/VISION	HEARING AND SPEECH	PERSONAL/SOCIAL	WARNING SIGNS
Newborn	Almost complete head-lag. Ventral suspension: head droops, hips flexed, limbs hang downwards. Moro reflex present. Palmar and plantar grasp reflexes.	Hands closed. Closes eyes to sudden bright light.	Stills to sound. Startles to sudden loud sounds.	Alternates between drowsiness and alert wakefulness – findings during examination are dependent on these states.	Hyper-/hypotonia. Asymmetrical reflexes. Left and right hand different. Excessive head lag – can be normal. Poor sucking.
6 Weeks	Some head control. Prone: head to side, buttocks moderately high. Moro reflex present. Ventral suspension: head is in line with body and hips semi-extended.	Stares, eyes fixated on objects. Follows horizontally to 90°. Places hand in mouth.	Startle response. Coos responsively to mother's talk from about five to six weeks. Turns to look at sound source.	Smiles at mother.	No visual fixation or following. Asymmetry of tone or movement. Floppy. Excessive head lag. Failure to smile. No response to sound.

AGE	GROSS MOTOR	FINE MOTOR/VISION	HEARING AND SPEECH	PERSONAL/SOCIAL	WARNING SIGNS
3 Months	Pull to sit: little/no head lag. Prone: support on forearms, lifts head, buttocks flat. Beginning to develop reflex standing when held i.e. primary extension phase. Rolls over. Moro begins to disappear.	Follows through 180°. Hands loosely open. Holds rattle when placed in hand. Watches own hand. Pulls at clothes.	Coos and chuckles. Quieting with familiar sounds. Turns head to sound.	Excited when fed. Reacts to familiar situations.	As for previous weeks. Excessive startling to visual stimuli – does not hear well. Absent vocalization.
6 Months	Pull to sit: braces shoulders and pulls to sit. Sits with support. Prone: lifts head and chest wall up. Support on extended arms and hands. Reaches out with one hand supporting on the other. Supine: lifts leg and plays with feet; feet to mouth.	Reaches for objects with the centre of palm and grasps with all fingers. Transfers toy from one hand to the other. Radial approach to toy. Shadow reaction in opposite arm.	Babbling begins at about four months. Repetitive and vowel-like (sing-song). Turns to mother's voice across the room. Laughs aloud.	Takes everything to mouth. Responds to mirror image. Starts holding bottle. Shows likes and dislikes.	Floppiness; failure to use both hands (or symmetry). Squint. Failure to turn to sound. Poor response to people. Little vocalization.

AGE	GROSS MOTOR	FINE MOTOR/VISION	HEARING AND SPEECH	PERSONAL/SOCIAL	WARNING SIGNS
9 Months	Sits without support and can move body without losing balance. Rolls. Crawls – forwards or backwards. Rocks on all fours. Pulls to stand.	Immediately reaches out. Holds a cube in each hand, with flexible finger approach picks up small toy in ends of fingers. Removes peg man or object from hole; cannot return it. Can point.	Vocalizes deliberately: Babbles. Imitates sounds. Understands 'bye-bye' or 'no'.	Stranger anxiety. Holds bottle, drinks from cup.	Unable to sit. Hand preference present. Fisting. Squint. Persistence of primitive reflexes. Monotonous vocalization.
10 Months	Pulls to stand. Lifts one foot. Walks with both hands held. May cruise around furniture. Sitting: beginning protective extension of arms backwards.	Picks up small object between thumb and index finger. Voluntary release begins.	Shakes head for no. Waves bye-bye. One word with meaning.	Plays peek-a-boo / hide and seek.	As for previous months.

AGE	GROSS MOTOR	FINE MOTOR/VISION	HEARING AND SPEECH	PERSONAL/SOCIAL	WARNING SIGNS
12 Months	Bear walks. Walks around furniture lifting one foot and stepping sideways. May walk alone with feet wide and arms in highguard.	Pincer grasp. Releases object on request. Begins to throw objects to floor. Mouthing virtually stopped. Looks for toys when out of sight.	Knows own name. Jargons. Two to three words with meaning. Understands simple instruction.	Finger feeds. Pushes arm into sleeve. Plays games.	Unable to sit or bear weight. Abnormal grasp. Failure to respond to sound. No spontaneous vocalization.
15 Months	Walks alone with uneven steps. Steps with arms out for balance. Collapses backward. Creeps upstairs, goes downstairs backwards.	Two cube tower. Holds two cubes in one hand.	Jabbers with expression. Two to six words spoken. Points at objects on request.	Picks up, drinks from, and puts down cup. Attempts feeding with spoon and spills most. Indicates wet nappy.	As for previous months.
18 Months	Walks well with arms down, and can stop and start. Cannot turn unless still. Throws a ball. Pulls a toy. Climbs onto chair. Seats self on chair.	Three cube tower. Scribbles. May start showing hand preference.	Uses six to 20+ recognizable words. Begins to put two words together.	Handles spoon and cup. Enjoys picture books. Takes off shoes, socks. Domestic mimicry.	Failure to walk. No pincer grip. Inability to understand simple commands. No speech. Mouthing. Drooling.

AGE	GROSS MOTOR	FINE MOTOR/VISION	HEARING AND SPEECH	PERSONAL/SOCIAL	WARNING SIGNS
24 Months	Runs. Up and down steps with two feet per step. Can kick a ball. Squats and rises without hands. Can plan movement (under/over).	Six cube tower. Train with cubes. Imitates vertical line. Hand preference usually obvious.	Short phrases. Uses 50+ words. Puts two or three words together. Asks for drink, toilet, food.	Spoon feeds without spilling. Clean and dry by day. Pretend play.	Unable to understand simple commands. Tremor. Incoordination. Severe clumsiness.
36 Months	Rides a tricycle. Up steps one foot per step. Down steps two feet per step. Climbs. Walks on tiptoe. Throws and kicks ball.	Nine cube tower. Builds bridge with cubes. Copies circle. Cuts with scissors. Three piece formboard; threads large beads.	Knows name and sex. Uses pronouns. Talks incessantly. Large vocabulary, intelligible to strangers.	Toilet trained. Dresses with supervision. Eats with fork. Washes and dries hands.	Ataxia. Using single words only.
48 Months	Up and down stairs with one foot per step. Stands on one (preferred) foot for three to five seconds. Hops on preferred foot.	Copies cross. Five cube gate/bridge. Coloured formboard five out of five.	Full name, home address and (usually) age. Recognizes colours. Speech should be grammatically correct and intelligible.	Eats with spoon and fork. Dresses and undresses. Make-believe play. Always asking questions.	Speech difficult to understand because of poor articulation or omission of consonants.

AGE	GROSS MOTOR	FINE MOTOR/VISION	HEARING AND SPEECH	PERSONAL/SOCIAL	WARNING SIGNS
60 Months	Walks easily on narrow line. Can hop on each foot separately.	Six cube steps. Copies square and triangle. Draws a man with all features. Can print a few letters, good control with writing and drawing.	Fluent speech. Full name, age, (usually) birthday, address. Use of conjunctions e.g. 'although'. Knows three opposites.	Uses knife and fork competently. Undresses and dresses alone. Chooses own friends.	Emotional immaturity. Clumsiness and poor fine motor skills.
72 Months	Sits up without help of hands. Walks backwards along straight line (ten paces).	Ten cube steps. Copies diamond but oddly shaped.	Learns irregular forms of nouns and verbs. Learns comparatives.	Cooperative play – leadership and division of labour.	Clumsy. Poor posture. Poor pencil grip.

Acknowledgements: adapted from Kibel and Wagstaff, *Child Health for All*. Oxford University Press 1991, Cape Town. Members of Developmental Clinics in Cape Town and Johannesburg

18 DIABETIC KETOACIDOSIS

F Bonnici and A Philotheou

Before referring the patient

A few important steps should be taken by the referring practitioner before sending a child with diabetic ketoacidosis (DKA) to a main centre.

Diagnosis

Severe hyperglycaemia (on reagent strips), heavy ketonuria and clinical fluid volume depletion support the diagnosis and may be used as a basis for beginning therapy immediately if considerable delay is envisaged before referral.

Emergency management

◆ Treat shock with IV 0,9% saline and, throughout the journey, infuse at a rate of 25 ml/kg/hr.
◆ Give an initial dose of 0,1 units per kg regular INSULIN as an IV bolus.
◆ Record the time of the injection.
◆ Provide for the maintenance of an airway en route.
◆ Look out for signs of hypoglycaemia.
◆ Have a substitute bottle of 5% glucose in saline available to treat hypoglycaemia during the journey.

Note

Consultation and/or early transfer will minimize the risks to the patient.

Urgent management in hospital

◆ Notify pathologists that urgent results will be required and advise appropriate members of the endocrine-diabetes team, or the appropriate specialist, of the arrival of the patient.
◆ Send blood samples to the laboratory for glucose, acid base,

Warning

Children with DKA are in a state of rapid metabolic flux and should be carefully monitored in hospital to prevent a major catastrophe.

electrolytes, urea, phosphate and ketones (by reagent strip method). Results should be available in minutes and therapy initiated immediately if data support a diagnosis of DKA.

◆ Do ECG early, followed by serial tracings looking for arrhythmias and effects of hyper- or hypokalaemia. See page 102.

◆ Record all clinical and laboratory data on a flow sheet, which should include the volume and composition of the fluids administered and the timing and number of units of each INSULIN dose or rate change.

Clinical and laboratory pitfalls

Children may appear deceptively well despite gross metabolic imbalance. Abdominal symptoms may be severe enough to mimic an acute abdomen.

DKA can occur without pronounced hyperglycaemia. The presence of heavy ketonuria may mask the degree of glycosuria on certain test strips. Factitious hyponatraemia may be caused by hyperglycaemia and hyperlipidaemia. The plasma creatinine concentration may be falsely elevated as a result of interference by acetoacetate.

Fluid therapy

The initial rapid correction of the fluid deficit is a priority and the most important step in management. Volume repletion with restoration of tissue perfusion must be individualized according to the age and haemodynamic status of the patient. Central venous pressure monitoring is rarely indicated.

Hypovolaemic shock

Use saline 0,9% as follows:

◆ 15-25 ml/kg in the first hour.
◆ 10-20 ml/kg in the second hour.
◆ 20-30 ml/kg over the next three or four hours.

Change over to saline 0,45% once shock has been corrected or if plasma sodium rises above 150 mmol/l.

Milder decompensation

Use saline 0,45% from the start and lower infusion rates.

Total fluid volume for first 24 hours (including maintenance)

♦ 5% dehydration—use 3 000 ml/m²
♦ 10% dehydration—use 4 000 ml/m²

Do not exceed 4 000 ml/m² per 24 hours unless the patient is in hypovolaemic shock. Adjust the rate according to the patient's clinical response and fluid volume status. After fluid repletion for shock, replace the remaining fluid steadily over 24 hours. The fluids used for shock should be subtracted from the total 24 hour fluid calculation and the remainder administered from the time of conclusion of therapy for shock to the end of the first 24 hours.

Continuous insulin infusion

Use only orange-coded, no dead-space INSULIN syringes to draw up INSULIN. Use only regular clear INSULIN such as Actrapid HM (ge) or Humulin R. Give a loading dose of 0,1 unit/kg of regular clear INSULIN stat by IV bolus into drip tubing if it has not already been given before arrival, or if the last dose was given more than two hours beforehand. Then follow by a continuous IV infusion at a dose of 0,1 units/kg/hr of regular clear INSULIN.

The solution can be made by adding 50 units regular clear INSULIN to a 200 ml bottle of saline 0,9% (one unit INSULIN/4 ml solution) or 125 units of INSULIN for a 500 ml IV bottle. Allow about 20 ml of mixture to run through the set to prime the tubing and saturate INSULIN binding sites. Haemaccel (Hoechst) may have certain advantages as a carrier when compared with saline 0,9%, but this is of little clinical importance.

For optimal safety, the solution should be connected to the main IV rehydration line either by a three-way tap or by 'piggy-back' (watch for leaks!) and run through an adjustable-rate pressure pump.

In the above concentration (i.e. 1 unit INSULIN/4 ml solution) and with a 60 drops/ml minidropper, the following apply:

◆ 1 unit INSULIN/hr is delivered by a drip rate of 4 minidrops/minute
◆ 5 units INSULIN/hr are delivered by a drip rate of 20 minidrops/minute.

If after two hours the patient's response is inadequate (rate of fall of plasma glucose <4 mmol/l per hour, or no improvement in serum pH or standard bicarbonate), the INSULIN infusion rate should be increased and the adequacy of intravascular fluid expansion reviewed.

Intermittent insulin therapy

The main potential hazards of continuous IV INSULIN therapy are the risk of loss of control over the infusion rate, particularly during transport of the patient and leaking into the tissues at the drip site when effective treatment ceases because of the short half-life of IV INSULIN.

The only alternative to continuous infusion is to inject hourly IV INSULIN boluses (0,1 unit/kg/hr) into the rubber stopper of the IV rehydration set, with particular care to ensure the accuracy of the intermittent doses delivered. Since only U-100 INSULINS (100 units/ml) are available, use low-dose INSULIN syringes (0,3 or 0,5 ml) with widely spaced gradations.

Regimes using IM or subcutaneous (SC) INSULINS are unreliable or impractical because INSULIN syringe needles are very short, and the peripheral perfusion of most patients compromised. Under careful supervision, however, intermittent hourly IM INSULIN doses (0,1 unit/kg/hr) may be tried in patients with mild metabolic decompensation.

Further adjustments
Fluid therapy and INSULIN

When plasma glucose decreases to approximately 13-15 mmol/l, change IV fluids to glucose 5% in saline 0,45%. If acidosis (pH ≤7,2) and severe ketonaemia are still present, continue INSULIN infusion at 0,1 unit/kg/hr. Once acidosis has been corrected and only mild ketonaemia persists, reduce the INSULIN infusion to 0,03-0,06 units/kg/hr. If plasma glucose continues to drop below 11 mmol/l, increase the glucose concentration in the IV fluid to 7,5-10% but maintain the INSULIN infusion rate according to criteria that are based on acid base and ketonaemia. Severe ketoacidosis will not improve with an INSULIN rate of less than 0,05-0,1 units/kg/hr.

Warning

Problems frequently arise when the IV INSULIN therapy is prematurely discontinued on the basis of glucose levels, as this may result in recurrence of the ketoacidosis.

Sodium bicarbonate and acid base status

Use with caution and preferably after consultation.

It is advisable to correct acidosis if pH ≤7,10 or standard bicarbonate ≤5 mmol/l and the patient is clinically unstable. Employ the formula:

base excess x 0,3 x body weight (kg) = mmol bicarbonate

(1 ml 8,5% sodium bicarbonate = 1 mmol bicarbonate), and then assess further requirements. Since this is a theoretical requirement, correct the base excess by 25% over four hours. Administer IV sodium bicarbonate 8,5% slowly (never as a bolus but always mixed in IV rehydration fluid) to avoid rapid potassium decreases. Discontinue sodium bicarbonate 8,5% in IV fluids when standard bicarbonate reaches 8-10 mmol/l or pH >7,15.

Potential disadvantages of IV sodium bicarbonate include: development of hypokalaemia, cerebral oedema and increased oxygen affinity resulting in peripheral tissue anoxia.

In patients with a significantly compromised haemodynamic status and severe acidosis, IV sodium bicarbonate may be given more rapidly.

Potassium

Start potassium chloride immediately if serum potassium is normal or low, or if INSULIN and/or sodium bicarbonate have been given before arrival. The average initial requirements are of the order of 20-30 mmol/hour; larger doses may be needed in severely depleted patients. If initial serum potassium is elevated, begin potassium chloride when serum level falls within the normal range.

If oliguria is present, it is safest to provide potassium on the basis of the serum level only (keep potassium >3,5 mmol/l). In practice, potassium supplements are usually started after the first 30-60 minutes of therapy and an ECG is obtained four hours later.

Note

1 ml potassium chloride 15% contains 2 mmol potassium (1 g KCl = 13 mmol potassium).

Phosphate

Potassium supplements can initially be met by using equal parts of potassium chloride and potassium phosphate solution for the first six to eight hours. Phosphate helps correct the phosphorus depletion syndrome present in DKA.

Note

Potassium phosphate IV ampoules (SABAX) contain 2 mmol potassium and 1,4 mmol phosphate (as HPO_4) per ml.

Magnesium

The serum magnesium concentration should be monitored and replacement instituted as levels fall below normal. Empirically, magnesium sulphate (50%) may be given in a concentration of 2 ml/litre for six hours.

Bladder and stomach

The bladder should be catheterized only if the patient is unable to pass urine. Urine output should be regularly checked and recorded.

If the patient is comatose, or vomiting is persistent, the stomach contents should be aspirated and a nasogastric tube left in place.

Antibiotics

If there is **no** obvious non-infectious precipitating factor for the DKA (e.g. omission of INSULIN), obtain urine and blood cultures and a chest radiograph. Intravenous antibiotics may be given on the basis of general prophylaxis or as a specific therapy for sepsis.

Flow-sheet

Record on a diabetic coma flow-sheet all details of the clinical state (pulse rate, respiratory rate and pattern, BP, urine output, hydration, state of consciousness), laboratory results and therapy given (INSULIN, type) and amounts of fluids.

Complications
Metabolic

Metabolic problems such as hypoglycaemia, hypokalaemia and hypernatraemia can usually be avoided by the judicious use of IV fluids, INSULIN and by frequent monitoring.

Cerebral oedema

Cerebral oedema is the single most common cause of death in children with diabetes. It usually develops a few hours after initiation of therapy while clinical and biochemical improvements are taking place. Deepening coma, fever, bradycardia, widened pulse pressure, and papilloedema may occur. The causative factors remain unclear, though osmotic disequilibrium and brain hypoxia have been suggested. It seems prudent to avoid overtreatment with hypotonic fluids, too rapid alkalinization or too rapid correction of hyperglycaemia with rapid changes in plasma osmolality.

Responsible staff should always be on the look-out for cerebral oedema which must be recognized immediately and reversed with IV MANNITOL (0,25-0,5 g/kg x 3). See page 230. Constant vigilance at the bedside will avert iatrogenic disasters.

Further management in hospital
Investigations
Blood

Bedside blood glucose tests hourly for the first six to eight hours (supervise accuracy to avoid management error). Repeat laboratory glucose, acid base, ketones by strip test every two hours and electrolytes every four hours for at least the first 12 hours. Children with mild decompensation require less frequent monitoring.

Urine

Test urine three-hourly for volume, glucose and acetone and record results.

Fluids and food

When nausea has settled, try oral clear fluids, e.g. sips of water or oral cell repair fluid (glucose 50 g and dipotassium hydrogen phosphate 4 g dissolved in one litre water). If these are retained, give milk and then allow the child to eat. If after ten to 12 hours, oral fluid intake is satisfactory, the IV fluid infusion may be adjusted so as to keep the blood glucose at 6-10 mmol/l.

Change to subcutaneous insulin therapy

Following recovery from DKA (patient fully conscious, retaining fluids and food, substantial improvement in acid base status and degree of ketonaemia), plan to discontinue INSULIN infusion and start **intermittent SC INSULIN** therapy. This should be started at least 30 minutes before the cessation of INSULIN infusion, and preferably to coincide with mealtimes.

Calculate the total daily dose (0,6 units/kg/24 hours) and give 20% of dose as regular clear INSULIN before each meal and 40% as intermediate-acting INSULIN (cloudy appearance, Monotard HM(ge), Protaphane HM(ge), or Humulin N) at 21h00 or 22h00.

Less severely affected children may be switched over immediately on a twice daily 2:1 mixture of **intermediate** and **regular INSULINS** (total dose 0,6 units/kg/24 hours given two-thirds before breakfast and one-third before supper) and changes cautiously made according to blood sugar levels.

Dietary guidelines

♦ Give practical advice and arrange an interview with a dietitian.
♦ Decide upon energy requirement:
  ◊ 4 200 kJ (1 000 kcal) at one year of age;
  ◊ add 420 kJ (100 kcal) for each additional year.
♦ The energy intake is controlled to maintain normal weight gain with growth.
♦ Carbohydrate intake should represent at least 50% of the total energy intake emphasizing complex high-fibre carbohydrates and restricting simple sugars. Fats should make up

around 30% of total energy intake and mainly as poly- and mono-unsaturated fatty acids.

♦ The Carbohydrate Exchange Method, i.e. using glycaemic food indices, should be explained to the parents and child. The proportions are distributed through the day according to the type of INSULIN regime.

♦ Snacks are important between meals, before exercise and at bedtime, to prevent hypoglycaemia.

Glucagon

Explain the indications and use of glucagon to the patient and parents.

Injections and monitoring

Ensure proficiency of injection technique and dose accuracy by the parents or child. Urine tests (Ketodiastix, Ketodiabur) and self-monitoring of blood glucose (Glucostix, Haemo-glukotest) should be taught. Order Medic-Alert badge inscribed: 'Diabetes on INSULIN – Give sugar if confused'. See page 692.

Patient aftercare

If possible, the family should be referred to a Diabetes Education Centre and their local branch of the SA Diabetes Association contacted. Details are available from: SA Diabetes Association, National Office, Cape Town. See Appendix 5.

19 EAR, NOSE AND THROAT DISORDERS

C A J Prescott

Disorders of the ear
External ear disorders
Wax

Use of cotton buds predisposes to wax accumulation.

Treatment

Wax dissolves best in water. Syringe the ear with water at exactly body temperature (otherwise giddiness will occur). If the wax remains impacted, then repeat syringing daily until cleared.

Foreign bodies

Children do not tolerate any probing of the ear canal with hooks or forceps without an anaesthetic.

Treatment

Attempt to remove the foreign body by syringing.

Advice

♦ Live insects are best drowned in olive oil ear drops before syringing.
♦ Vegetable seeds will swell if not dislodged by syringing. Require early ENT referral if unsuccessful.

Otitis externa

A bacterial, fungal or rarely viral infection of the skin of the external ear canal.

Clinical presentation

Itching, pain, discharge, deafness. The ear is tender when the pinna is manipulated to try and see into the canal. The infection may be either localized or generalized.

Treatment

Localized: a furuncle is present in the hair-bearing area.

◆ Gently pack cottonwool around the furuncle and soak it in GLYCERINE ICHTHAMMOL ear drops. Add fresh drops twice daily until resolved, then remove cottonwool.
◆ Give antibiotic (ERYTHROMYCIN) if there is associated cellulitis.

Generalized: pus and debris, inflamed and swollen canal wall.

◆ Syringe out all pus and debris.
◆ Instil ear drops (TINCTURE MERTHIOLATE, Sofradex) four times per day.
◆ Give antibiotic (ERYTHROMYCIN) if there is associated cellulitis.

Advice

Cellulitis may be present but if there is post-auricular swelling then mastoiditis must be excluded. (See page 191).

Middle ear disorders

The inter-relations between these are illustrated in Figure 19.1.

Figure 19.1 The inter-relations between middle ear disorders.

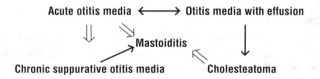

Acute otitis media

A bacterial infection (*H. influenzae, S. pneumoniae, S. pyogenes*) of the mucous membrane of the middle ear with a mucopurulent exudate, that often follows an upper respiratory tract infection. Eustachian tube obstruction results in an empyema with a bulging tympanic membrane that may perforate. The infection may then resolve.

Clinical presentation

Pain, toxicity. Inflamed eardrum, bulging eardrum, fresh perforation with mucopurulent discharge.

Treatment

Antibiotics (PENICILLIN, AMOXYCILLIN) for ten days. (Oral PENICILLIN preparations are poorly absorbed in a toxic child and the first dose should be given IM.) Reassess after 24 hours: persistent pain – see below.

Middle ear effusion may persist after the acute infection has resolved. Treat with a broad spectrum antibiotic e.g. CO-TRIMOXAZOLE orally for ten days.

Advice

Persistent pain is a danger symptom, as it suggests impending mastoiditis. **Urgent ENT referral is required**.

Chronic suppurative otitis media

If the acute infection does not resolve after perforation, it may become chronic when the infecting bacteria change to predominantly coliform organisms. The margins of the perforation become 'sealed' so that even when the infection is subsequently controlled there will remain a persistent perforation. Re-infection is then common.

Clinical presentation

Mucopurulent discharge. Deafness. Central perforation.

Treatment

Broad spectrum antibiotic (CO-TRIMOXAZOLE, AMOXYCILLIN) for ten days, together with dry mopping and antiseptic ear drops (BORIC ACID). If the condition is unresolved, refer to an ENT clinic but continue dry mopping and ear drops. When dry, avoid getting water in the ear.

Advice

Pain is a danger symptom as it suggests impending mastoiditis. **Urgent ENT referral is required**.

Otitis media with effusion

Persistence of a middle ear effusion after resolution of acute or sub-acute infection behind an intact tympanic membrane. There is eustachian tube dysfunction with inadequate aeration of the middle ear.

Clinical presentation

Deafness, delayed speech development. Dull immobile eardrum that may or may not be retracted.

Treatment

Broad spectrum antibiotic: CO-TRIMOXAZOLE, AMOXY-CILLIN for ten days. If the effusion does not resolve after one month then refer to an ENT clinic for possible grommet tube insertion.

Cholesteatoma

Negative middle ear pressure can cause a retraction pocket to form in the tympanic membrane. This is skin-lined and can enlarge within the middle ear where it is both destructive and interferes with drainage of the mastoid. It rapidly becomes infected and breaks down to form a marginal perforation. A complication of infection is mastoiditis.

Clinical presentation

Smelly discharge, deafness. There is marginal perforation with white squamous debris within the middle ear, granulation tissue, and aural polyp.

Treatment

Initiate treatment for infection (as for chronic suppurative otitis media). Refer to ENT for radical mastoidectomy with reconstruction.

Advice

Pain is a danger symptom suggesting impending mastoiditis. **Urgent ENT referral is required**.

Mastoiditis

Mastoiditis occurs when infection is trapped within the mastoid because the drainage channels are obstructed by either swollen mucosa (acute otitis media, chronic suppurative otitis media) or by cholesteatoma. Infection invades the bony walls to cause an osteitis.

Complication: intracranial spread of infection, e.g. meningitis, abscess.

Clinical presentation

Pain, toxicity, post-auricular swelling. Signs of middle ear infection. X-rays show loss of pneumatized mastoid air cells.

Treatment

Initiate treatment with intravenous antibiotics (AMPICILLIN and FLAGYL) and if there will be a delay in referral, then incise and drain the post-auricular abscess. **Refer urgently to ENT for mastoidectomy**.

Childhood deafness

Deafness in childhood will retard speech development. If it is severe it will affect communication, and hence intellectual development. For this reason, if a child is suspected of being deaf it **must** be referred within the first year of life for assessment to an ENT clinic. If deafness is confirmed, intensive rehabilitation is required, including hearing aids, speech therapy, and special schooling.

Clinical presentation

Poor response or no response to sound. Delayed or poor speech development. A history of deafness in the family, maternal rubella, severe neonatal disorders, or meningitis. Abnormal external ears, abnormal facial appearance, signs of middle ear disorder.

Management

Use a Manchester rattle to assess the child's hearing. If there is poor or no response then refer to an ENT clinic.

Advice

Babies with abnormal facial development or abnormal external ears often have hearing disorders and should be referred to an ENT clinic for assessment before six months of age.

Disorders of the nose

Nasal obstruction in the neonate

Facial moulding during birth often causes the nasal septum to buckle and this is associated with swelling of the septal and turbinate mucosa. If the obstruction is significant, use decongestant nasal drops (Drixine, Otrivin, Iliadin) and steroid drops (Sofradex, Betnesol N) for ten days.

Allergic rhinitis

The blocked, mucoid-secreting nose is common in childhood and is frequently due to allergy. The offending allergen can often be identified from the history without the need for further investigation. See page 23 for further comment and management.

Acute sinusitis

Acute sinusitis is usually preceded by a common cold. In younger children the ethmoids are as likely to be affected as the maxillary sinuses.

Clinical presentation

Pain, headache, fever and malaise. Purulent nasal and post-nasal discharge, nasal obstruction with loss of vocal resonance. Some flushing of the overlying tissues may be seen but, in general, cellulitis of the soft tissues of the cheeks results from dental infection. X-rays of sinuses reveal mucosal thickening, fluid levels or opacity of the infected sinuses.

Complication

Orbital cellulitis is a complication of ethmoid infection and vision is at risk in this condition. CT scan will reveal whether or not pus is present within the orbit.

Treatment

- ◆ Antibiotics orally: PENICILLIN, ERYTHROMYCIN, AMOXYCILLIN.
- ◆ Nasal decongestants: (paediatric Otrivin, Drixine, Iliadin)
- ◆ Orbital cellulitis: IV antibiotics. **Urgent ENT** referral.

Purulent rhinitis

Persistent bilateral purulent discharge suggests chronic rhino-sinusitis. This may be associated with adenoid hypertrophy.

Clinical presentation

Purulent (nasal and postnasal) discharge, nasal obstruction, peri-nasal excoriation.

Treatment

♦ Antibiotics: PENICILLIN, ERYTHROMYCIN, AMOXY-CILLIN.
♦ Decongestants: paediatric Otrivin, Drixine, Iliadin.

Advice

♦ Unilateral rhinorrhoea, especially if offensive, is indicative of a foreign body.
♦ Exclude diphtheria if the discharge is sero-sanguineous, mucopurulent and offensive, with excoriation of the nares and upper lip.
♦ If persistent despite treatment – adenoidectory, sinus lavage. In older children minimal sinus surgery may be required. Refer to ENT specialist.
♦ When bilateral purulent rhinorrhoea becomes chronic despite treatment then exclude cystic fibrosis (sweat test), muco-ciliary disorder (mucosal biopsy) and specific immune deficiencies.

Disorders of the throat

Tonsillitis

This is a common infection in childhood.

Clinical presentation

Fever, sore throat, difficulty in swallowing. Inflamed, swollen tonsils, debris and pus in tonsil crypts, cervical adenopathy.

Treatment

♦ When sore throat is associated with a viral upper respiratory tract infection: supportive treatment only.
♦ Acute follicular tonsillitis: antibiotic, i.e. PENICILLIN or ERYTHROMYCIN orally for ten days.
♦ Relapsing tonsillitis or haemolytic streptococcal infection: antibiotic, e.g. PENICILLIN or ERYTHROMYCIN orally for ten days.
♦ Frequent episodes under three years of age: try a course of

long-term antibiotic (PENICILLIN, ERYTHROMYCIN) in half the normal daily dose given once daily for three months.

Indications for Tonsillectomy

♦ Recurrent tonsillitis, i.e. four or more episodes of tonsillitis per year for the preceding two years.
♦ Persistent throat infection with or without cervical lymphadenitis. (Send tonsils for histology).
♦ Peritonsillar abscess (quinsy).

Advice

Acute membraneous tonsillitis is uncommon and the differential diagnosis should include diphtheria, reticulo-endothelial disease and glandular fever.

Adenoid hypertrophy

Often associated with chronic rhinosinusitis (see pages 193-4). It can be a predisposing cause for middle ear disease and deafness in childhood. See page 526 for comment on snoring.

Clinical presentation

Mouth breathing, difficulty with sucking in the young child, snoring, obstructed breathing when sleeping, sleep apnoea, restless sleep, enuresis, symptoms of sleep deprivation, e.g. irritability, lethargy, poor appetite.

Indications for adenoidectomy

♦ The severity of symptoms is the most reliable way of determining the need for adenoidectomy. A lateral X-ray of the nasopharynx is unreliable in determining the degree of obstruction.
♦ Chronic upper airway obstruction, especially if episodes of obstructive sleep apnoea occur.
♦ Recurrent or persistent middle ear problems.

Advice

A late complication of upper airway obstruction can be cor pulmonale and cardiac failure. Chest X-ray and ECG should be obtained before an anaesthetic is given.

Laryngeal stridor

Stridor is indicative of pathology causing airway obstruction. Urgent diagnosis is essential.

Acute stridor

These children require urgent referral to a hospital paediatric service. If the airway obstruction is life-threatening, intubate or perform tracheotomy prior to transfer. See page 513 for comment on croup (laryngotracheobronchitis), page 519 for epiglottitis and page 520 for foreign bodies. Other conditions to be considered are post-intubation laryngeal inflammation, recurrent laryngeal nerve palsy (especially after cardiothoracic and thyroid surgery) and retropharyngeal abscess.

Diagnosis

Anterior-posterior and lateral X-rays can be of assistance prior to viewing the larynx directly, either awake using a flexible fibre-optic endoscope, or under anaesthetic.

Management

Usually includes either endotracheal intubation or tracheostomy to relieve the airway obstruction, in addition to treatment of the specific causes listed above. Drainage of a retro-pharyngeal abscess.

Chronic stridor

Laryngomalacia (see page 521) is the most common cause of stridor in infants and has a characteristic variability of its inspiratory component in both rhythm and intensity. Other causes include recurrent laryngeal nerve palsies, congenital laryngeal cysts and haemangiomas, congenital laryngeal stenosis, tracheal stenosis and vascular rings, recurrent respiratory papillomatosis (associated with hoarseness).

Diagnosis

Detailed clinical examination. Chest and lateral neck X-rays, high kilovoltage airway studies and a barium swallow (vascular ring). Direct examination of the larynx and trachea. This requires experienced management, especially in the severely obstructed patient who may require tracheostomy. Awake flexible fibre-optic endoscopic examination, if available, is useful in that it gives a dynamic view of the airway.

Management

♦ General: maintenance of airway. This may require tracheostomy.
♦ Specific: depends on the cause.

Drooling of saliva

Children who drool usually have a neuro-muscular disorder that impairs control of mouth closure and swallowing. Attention to improving mouth closure may be of benefit and often the removal of tonsils and adenoids will help in this regard. Children still drooling by school-going age will be helped by surgery that relocates the submandibular salivary gland ducts from the front to the back of the mouth. Refer to an ENT specialist.

Corrosive oesophageal burns

Diagnosis

Aims initially at identification of those children who have actually swallowed the corrosive and burned their pharyngeal, oesophageal or gastric mucosa. The history of children is unreliable but indicators of significant injury are a reluctance to swallow and drooling of saliva. Adequate examination of the pharynx is difficult. Endoscopy with either a rigid or a flexible scope is required in order to get this information.

> ### Warning
> Perforation of oesophagus or stomach, inhalation pneumonia and airway embarrassment carry a high mortality if unrecognized.

Management

Emergency treatment in all children

♦ Institute measures recommended by a Poisons Reference Centre in regard to potential poisoning. See Chapter 37, page 414.

In children with minimal burns

Able to swallow, no drooling of saliva: observe for 24 hours. If swallowing remains unimpaired then discharge. Follow up at two weeks to check that swallowing is still normal.

In children with significant burns

Not swallowing, drooling saliva: **refer urgently to a centre with facilities for endoscopy.**

Further management

♦ Passage of a nasogastric tube to maintain a patent lumen in the oesophagus and to provide a channel for nutrition.
♦ Measures to reduce further damage that exacerbates stricture formation as the oesophageal mucosa heals include IV antibiotics and antacids via the NG tube.
♦ The use of steroids has not been shown to be of benefit.

Once saliva can be swallowed, encourage fluids by mouth with the nasogastric tube in place and thereafter introduce solids.

♦ Re-examination of the oesophagus, with dilatation, is done at two-weekly intervals until mucosal healing has taken place. Delay in healing is indicative of deep burns and stricture formation can be expected. These children will require long-term hospitalization and repeated dilatation.
♦ Oesophageal bypass by colon transposition may eventually become necessary, should stricturing be severe.

20 EYE DISORDERS

A D N Murray

Congenital anomalies

Congenital anomalies of the eyes are often associated with congenital abnormalities elsewhere in the body.

Blepharoptosis (droopy lid)

This may be associated with muscle anomalies of the upper lid affecting Muller's smooth muscle or the levator palpebrae superioris. Space-occupying lesions in the eyelid or paresis of the third cranial nerve or sympathetic nerve (Horner's Syndrome) may also cause blepharoptosis. Surgical correction of the ptosis is usually done at about four years of age.

Refer to an ophthalmologist for non-urgent baseline assessment as soon as the condition is diagnosed.

If the pupil is obscured, early surgery is necessary to prevent amblyopia. **Refer on an urgent basis.**

Lacrimal drainage apparatus

A watery eye **without** a runny nose may be caused by blockage of the lacrimal drainage system. Repeated expression of the contents of the lacrimal sac, followed by the instillation of antibiotic eye drops, will help to prevent infection. The majority of blocked ducts open spontaneously. In the absence of infection, probing by an ophthalmologist should be deferred until at least nine months of age.

A watery eye with a runny nose may result from irritation, e.g. a subtarsal foreign body, eyelashes growing inward or from corneal oedema due to congenital glaucoma. **Refer on an urgent basis.**

Congenital glaucoma
Clinical presentation

Infants with this condition present with a watery eye, photophobia, enlargement of the globe and a cloudy cornea. The condition may be bilateral. It commonly results from incomplete development of the angle of the anterior chamber which causes obstruction to the outflow of aqueous humour from the eye. **Refer immediately for urgent surgery.**

Cataract

Clinical presentation

Absent red reflex, poor fundal view, 'white pupil'.

The condition may be present at birth or it may develop subsequently. It may affect one or both eyes, be idiopathic, heredofamilial or result from intra-uterine insults, e.g. maternal rubella or galactosaemia. Surgery, where indicated, should be undertaken within the first few weeks of life. The infant requires some form of optical correction (spectacles, contact lenses or an intraocular lens implant) post-operatively. **Refer immediately for surgery.**

Retinopathy of prematurity (retrolental fibroplasia)

Clinical presentation

May have a normal red reflex or a white reflex behind the crystalline lens. May be mistaken for retinoblastoma. Always bilateral.

Seen in premature infants following nursing in an oxygen-enriched environment during the neonatal period. The lower the birthweight and the greater the exposure to oxygen, the greater the risk.

Refer all infants with a birthweight under 1 500 grams for assessment at 32 weeks conceptional age (gestational age plus weeks of life).

Infections

Lid

Acute infections occur in the eyelash follicles (styes) or Meibomian glands (tarsal cyst or chalazion).

Styes are treated by heat, e.g. 'hot spooning'; local, and if severe, systemic antibiotics. The offending eyelash should be removed.

Meibomian cysts require incision and curettage from the

inside of the eyelid by an ophthalmologist. **Refer on an urgent** basis.

Chronic infections of the eyelids, e.g. due to dandruff, chronic sepsis or lack of personal hygiene, are treated with topical antibiotics and by the elimination of associated factors, such as dirty finger nails. In all lid infections, proper hygiene is important in prophylaxis.

Conjunctivitis

Clinical presentation

Both eyes are red with purulent discharge. Swollen lids.

Acute conjunctivitis in the newborn is commonly due to staphylococcal, chlamydial or gonococcal infection. Identify the organism, if possible, by Gram's stain and culture.

Gonococcal conjunctivitis is particularly dangerous and can lead to corneal perforation in 12-24 hours. **Admit the patient and request urgent ophthalmological opinion.** For management see page 353.

Trachoma

This is endemic in certain areas of southern Africa, and is transmitted by direct eye-to-eye contact in over-crowded communities. Fingers, clothes and flies, attracted to discharging eyes, all serve to inoculate the causative agent. Presents as acute conjunctivitis, later becoming chronic, and results in scarring of the lids and cornea. Treatment is with topical TETRACYCLINE ointment four times daily for six weeks, accompanied by ERYTHROMYCIN by mouth, and instructions to the patient to improve personal hygiene.

Phlyctenular keratoconjunctivitis

This is an ocular sensitivity reaction (a positive ocular Mantoux reaction) which occurs when an allergic individual is exposed to the tubercle bacillus or occasionally to staphylococcal infection. Investigate for tuberculosis. See chapter 46, page 562.

Refer to an ophthalmologist for treatment with topical steroid.

Dendritic ulcers

The commonest cause is the herpes simplex virus. Unilateral painful red eye. The typical dendritic pattern can be demonstrated with fluorescein. **Never use topical corticosteroids.**

Refer for specialist assessment and management with topical ACYCLOVIR ointment.

Strabismus (squint)

Refer all children with suspected esotropia or exotropia immediately for full ophthalmological assessment. There is a familial tendency to strabismus.

Refer siblings and offspring of involved individuals at two or three months of age, whether strabismus or amblyopia is detected or not.

Normal binocularity will occur if:

◆ there is one clear acceptable image presented by each eye;
◆ the images are close together and can be superimposed; or
◆ the brain is sufficiently developed to be able to appreciate and fuse the two images.

If not, squint will occur.

A newborn baby's eyes may wander but should be 'straight' and working together by six weeks of age. If by then the eyes are still crossed, the infant will not outgrow the squint. If one eye is constantly deviated, suppression amblyopia will develop. Treatment can rectify amblyopia, but the chances of success worsen progressively, the longer the squint is allowed to persist, and the older the child becomes. After the age of approximately six years, little or no improvement can generally be expected.

Treatment is aimed at attaining the best possible vision in each eye, e.g. by occlusion or spectacles, improving binocular function by orthoptic exercises and surgical alignment of visual axes.

Early treatment makes a functional result a realistic goal.

Important

Every child with a squint requires a dilated fundal examination to exclude intra-ocular pathology.

Retinoblastoma

A malignant retinal neoplasm, occurring in hereditary (autosomal dominant) and non-hereditary forms. About 20% of new cases have a family history. In about 25% of cases it is bilateral. Occurs in 1:20 000 live births.

Clinical presentation

◆ Squint.
◆ A yellow or white pupillary reflex-amaurotic cat's eye.
◆ Intra-ocular inflammation.
◆ Blood or pus in the anterior chamber.
◆ Loss of vision in one or both eyes.

Early treatment may save the child's sight and life. Treatment comprises surgery, cytotoxics and radiotherapy, as well as life-long follow up and genetic counselling.
    Refer immediately.

Trauma
Lids

Lacerations involving the lid margin require careful apposition of the free edges of the wound to avoid notching of the margin. **Refer for closure of the lid in layers by an ophthalmologist or plastic surgeon.**

Conjunctiva

Small tears need not be sutured, but one should bear in mind the possibility of deeper damage.
    Refer for assessment.

Corneal abrasions

Instil an antibiotic ointment and pad the eye.

Corneal foreign bodies

These may require general anaesthesia for removal. Local anaesthesia will suffice if the child is cooperative. Remove the foreign body with a sterile cotton-bud. Instil an antibiotic ointment after removal and pad the eye.
    Refer if the child is apprehensive, or if the foreign body is deeply embedded. Do not risk corneal penetration with a sharp instrument.

Haemorrhage into the anterior chamber (hyphaema)
Clinical presentation

Diffuse haemorrhage or fluid level of blood in anterior chamber.

This usually results from blunt trauma, e.g. fist or catapult injuries.

Management

◆ Occlusion of the involved eye.
◆ Sedation to restrict activity, if necessary. No ASPIRIN. See page 38.
◆ ATROPINE 1% drops three times per day.
◆ DEXAMETHASONE drops four times per day.
◆ TRANEXAMIC ACID (Cyklokapron) 25 mg/kg orally every eight hours for five days. (Maximum 1 500 mg per day.)
◆ Bed rest until the haemorrhage has been absorbed.
◆ Hyphaema may be complicated by a secondary haemorrhage with glaucoma. **Refer for specialist treatment**.

Vitreous haemorrhage

Clinical presentation

Poor fundal view.

This may take months to disperse. As with any obstruction to vision, a squint may be precipitated. There may be retinal damage, including detachment, concealed behind the haemorrhage. Ultrasound is often of diagnostic value. Strict bed rest for three days may allow a view of the fundus.

Refer suspected vitreous haemorrhage for urgent assessment.

Orbit

Trauma may produce a fracture, commonly through the floor of the orbit (blow-out fracture) with herniation of orbital contents into the maxillary sinus. Ocular movements become restricted, especially elevation, and diplopia results. Management may be conservative or surgical, depending on the amount of tissue entrapment.

Refer for urgent baseline assessment and treatment.

Perforation of the globe

Refer immediately for urgent microsurgical repair.

Protect the eye with an eye pad and eye shield. Starve the patient in preparation for anaesthesia. See page 29. Prognosis must be guarded, especially when the lens has been damaged.

Untreated perforation with incarceration of uveal tissue may result in sympathetic ophthalmitis which is characterized by severe uveitis in both the injured and uninjured eyes.

Burns of the eye

Emergency treatment of chemical burns consists of immediate and adequate irrigation with water (wash basin, hose-pipe, shower). Also see page 424. The irrigation should be prolonged and copious and particulate matter should be removed from under the lids. Further management is aimed at preventing scarring, and adhesions between the lid and the globe. For thermal burns see pages 89-96.

Refer on an urgent basis.

Blindness

May be ocular, or central due to visual tract, occipital cortex or frontal cortex involvement.

Refer for assessment and **refer on an urgent basis if blindness is of recent onset.**

21 FLUID THERAPY

M D Bowie

Fluid therapy is aimed at restoring and maintaining normal water and electrolyte equilibrium in the individual. It is of particular importance in paediatric practice, as infants and children have a high water and electrolyte turnover and abnormalities of homeostasis can occur rapidly and frequently. Requirements vary, depending on the age and size of the child, and on the disease state which affects the source of fluid loss. The recommendations given are but guidelines to safe practice and may require frequent modification in response to changes in patient status. Constant reassessment is the key to fluid therapy. Methods of assessment include clinical examination, body weight and input/output measurement, augmented if necessary by serum electrolyte, acid base and urine flow studies.

Fluid therapy may be administered by bolus oral feeds, continuous intragastric drip or by intravenous infusion. The same general principles apply to every route. Intravenous therapy is commonly and extensively used in:

♦ acute states, i.e. treatment of shock or severe dehydration;
♦ subacute states, i.e. where oral feeding is inadvisable or impracticable, such as with severe respiratory disease, peri-operative management or protracted vomiting; and
♦ chronic states, i.e. where maintenance of hydration and electrolyte homeostasis is impossible by the enteral route, e.g. post-intestinal surgery, intractable diarrhoea. The nutritional status of the child is not maintained by conventional intravenous therapy, and total parenteral nutrition must be considered in such a situation.

Assessment of hydration

The best and most objective method of assessing dehydration is on short-term weight changes. Previous weights are not always initially available and the amount of replacement fluid has to be assessed on clinical signs of dehydration (see page 222) and shock. The clinical signs only appear after there has been significant water loss.

Signs of dehydration

Loss of tissue turgor, sunken eyes, dry mouth and tongue, depression of the fontanelle and diminished urine volume.

Degree of dehydration

See page 222.

♦ 5% – symptoms and signs appear
♦ 10% – signs marked

Shock

Occurs mostly when there is an inadequate circulating blood volume (hypovolaemic). Clinical evidence includes:

♦ tachycardia
♦ poor peripheral circulation – prolonged capillary filling time (more than four seconds)
♦ diminished level of consciousness
♦ hypotension – a late and ominous sign.

Fluid and electrolyte requirements

This can be divided into:

♦ maintenance: necessary for maintaining hydration and replacing normal ongoing losses;
♦ replacement: necessary for restoring hydration to normal, replacing losses that have already occurred, and abnormal ongoing losses; and
♦ resuscitation: necessary for restoring an effective circulating blood volume.

In reality there is considerable overlap of requirements, but these divisions are useful when approaching fluid therapy.

Maintenance fluid

Normal ongoing losses are from three main sources and are usually replaced by dietary water and electrolytes.

Insensible water loss

This occurs mainly from the skin and lungs. It is the volume of fluid leaving the body as a result of the difference in vapour pressure between the skin and lung surface and the surrounding atmosphere. Preterm infants have a high insensible water loss. A rise in body temperature of 1°C will increase insensible loss by 10%.

Renal loss

The water component of renal loss is primarily a vehicle of excretion of various substances, i.e. the urinary solutes. The volume depends on the amount of solute requiring excretion and the ability of the kidney to concentrate the urine. The catabolic products derived from protein represent the major excretory solutes, i.e. urea, creatinine and electrolytes. Protein metabolism is proportional to the metabolic rate and so, therefore, are renal water losses. The concentrating power of the kidney also plays an important role. It is diminished in small infants and in dehydrated and ill children.

Gastrointestinal loss

Under normal circumstances, loss of water from the gastrointestinal tract is small and may be as low as 5 ml/kg/day. When there is diarrhoea these losses may be very large.

Maintenance requirements

Amount

Fluids lost are mainly insensible water and renal losses. The amounts lost are proportional to the metabolic rate and this is proportional to the surface area. The maintenance amounts required for infants and adults are identical when expressed per surface area, i.e. $1\,800$ ml/m^2. Dehydration and replacement fluid are directly related to weight. Surface areas are cumbersome to use in practice and it is preferable to have a common denominator for both maintenance and replacement fluids. Maintenance requirements are therefore expressed per kilogram of body weight. However, the smaller the infant and its weight, the relatively greater the surface areas. A sliding scale should be used that is related to weight, or less accurately, to age. See Table 21.1, page 209.

Composition

Insensible and renal losses are mainly water, and the composition

Table 21.1 Maintenance requirements ml/kg/day related to age or to weight

	Age	Volume	Weight	Volume
Neonate	1 day	60 ml		
	2 days	90 ml		
	3 days	120 ml		
	4 days and over	150-180 ml		
Infants	<1 year	120 ml*	<10kg	100-120 ml
	1-2 years	100 ml	10-20 kg	1 000 ml + 50 ml/kg >10 kg
	2-4 years	85 ml		
	4-10 years	70 ml	>20 kg	1 500 ml + 20 ml/kg >20 kg
	10 years and over	2-3 l		

*Preterm: 4 days 150 ml/kg, 5 days 150-180 ml/kg, 6 days and over 150-200 ml/kg.

Note: Under one year of age, 120 ml/kg/day is advised for intravenous administration. Larger amounts are required for oral maintenance, i.e. 150 ml/kg/day.

of maintenance fluid should be the same. Carbohydrate is essential for its protein-sparing effect in reducing protein breakdown, renal solute load and consequent renal water loss. Carbohydrate requirements for this purpose are at least 3 g/kg/day and in practice most children should receive 5-10 g/kg/day. In addition there are relatively small electrolyte losses in sweat, urine and stool, and the composition of maintenance fluid should replace these. Maintenance fluids are mainly water with added carbohydrate (dextrose) and low concentrations of electrolytes.

Replacement fluids

The symptoms of dehydration are directly proportional to the percentage diminution of extra-cellular fluid and body weight. They are the same at all ages, as the body water proportion of an individual changes only slightly over a lifetime. Furthermore, the initial effects of dehydration are haemodynamic rather than metabolic. The rate of fluid loss is a function of metabolic rate and since this is greater on a weight basis in an infant than in an

wt x deficit x 100
5 x 10 x 100   1 ℓ

Table 21.2 Fluid therapy

	Type	Amount	Rate
Resuscitation	Plasma volume expander Plasma DEXTRAN Plasmolyte Blood[1] Sod. bicarb 8,4%	20 ml/kg Inadequate response: further 10 ml/kg[2] 2 ml/kg	Rapid
Replacement source loss			
Gastroent. Diarrhoea	½ Darrow's and 5% dextrose water	Dehydration 5% - 50 ml/kg 10% - 100 ml/kg	Fast 6-12 hrs Slow 24 hrs Malnutrition[3] Hypernatraemia[4]
Vomiting Gastric Ileostomy Bile	½ N saline and K+ 20 mmol/l Plasmolyte	Ongoing losses measured or estimated	Volume replacement as occurs
Respiratory	Maintelyte or ⅕ N saline		
Maintenance			
General Neonate	Maintelyte Neonatalyte	See Table 21.1	Total volume constant rate
Gastroent.	½ Darrow's[5]		24 hours
Respiratory disease	Maintelyte ⅕ N saline	Reduce volume[6]	
Renal disease	5% dextrose water	Insensible loss 10-30 ml/kg	

See Chapter 42.

Explanatory notes:

1. Blood should only be given if there has been blood loss.
2. Assuming hypovolaemic shock: if response is still inadequate, further management requires monitoring with CVP line. See page 10.

3. Slow rehydration is safer in malnourished (see page 382), small or chronically ill children.

4. Hypernatraemic dehydration. Hypernatraemia serum Na >150 mmol/l. Electrolyte transfer is much slower than water transfer – giving a hypotonic electrolyte solution rapidly may result in water intoxication (i.e. excess intracellular water), causing brain swelling and convulsions. Rehydration should be gradual over 24 hours or longer.

   The degree of hydration is almost invariably underestimated in hypernatraemia. This can be used to the patient's advantage. Aim to correct the apparent clinical degree of dehydration in 24 hours. No modification of the standard therapy regimen with half-strength Darrow's is then necessary in hypernatraemic dehydration as actual dehydration will be corrected slowly. Shock and circulatory collapse must be treated and the metabolic acidosis corrected.

5. Half-strength Darrow's is used as maintenance fluids in gastroenteritis as it makes a further allowance for ongoing electrolyte losses. It should not be used as maintenance fluid where there are no small bowel losses.

6. Overhydration is a problem as water will leak into inflamed pulmonary tissues readily. Oral milk feeds can be given in conventional amounts. Children on maintenance intravenous fluids only should be restricted to 50-60 ml/kg, and hydration carefully monitored (weight, urine output, urine S.G. 1010-1015).

   Give solutions containing bicarbonate or lactate only if specifically indicated. Concomitant gastrointestinal losses, i.e. diarrhoea, if present, will require additional fluid and electrolyte replacement.

---

adult, an infant will suffer a 10% loss more rapidly than an adult. See Table 21.2, page 210.

Replacement requirements

Amounts

Following, if necessary, resuscitation and the restoration of circulation, the correction of dehydration and replacement of losses should be unhurried. Aim at complete correction in the well-nourished child within six to 12 hours, and in the malnourished, small or chronically ill child, within 24 hours. In the latter, replacement fluids together with calculated maintenance fluids are given at a steady rate over 24 hours. Rather err on the side of correcting too slowly but also remember that constant reassessment is necessary to keep ahead of continuing losses.

Replacement amounts are calculated on estimated dehydration and body weight (e.g. 10% of 5 kg = 500 ml).

Note

Do not calculate replacement fluid on more than 10% dehydration. Replace as 10% dehydrated and re-assess – further replacement requirements can then be estimated.

Composition

This will depend to a large extent on the source of the fluid lost. As replacement occurs in the extracellular compartment the fluid used should resemble the lost fluid in composition and contain the major electrolytes (sodium, chloride and potassium) that are found in that space.

◆ Gastrointestinal loss (gastroenteritis) is the most common cause of dehydration, and electrolytes, which are lost in significant amounts, should be replaced.
◆ Dehydration arising in association with pneumonia (fever and increased respiratory rate) would be mainly water, and electrolyte losses are minimal. Replacement fluid in this case should resemble maintenance fluids with lower electrolyte concentrations.

Resuscitation

This is the treatment of shock and a medical emergency. The circulating blood volume must be re-established as rapidly as possible. See page 7.

Other factors in fluid therapy

Acid base status

Three variables are required to interpret the acid base status by the Astrup microtechnique, i.e. base excess (mmol/l), the metabolic component; $PaCO_2$ (kPa), the respiratory component; and pH, the combined metabolic and respiratory component.

Metabolic acidosis is most commonly encountered. Correction of hydration and improved renal function will correct mild to moderate acidosis. If severe, sodium bicarbonate 8,5% is used for more rapid correction.

◆ Base excess x 0,3 x body wt/kg = mmol bicarbonate (1 ml 8,5% $NaHCO_3$ = 1 mmol bicarbonate).
◆ Correct fully in infants. Half-correct and then reassess in older children. Give slowly in neonates.

♦ Metabolic alkalosis most commonly occurs in gastric losses and is usually accompanied by potassium loss.
♦ Respiratory acidosis and alkalosis may require attention to ventilation.

Electrolytes

The aim of maintenance electrolyte therapy is to provide quantities that will cover renal and extra-renal losses without overtaxing the abilities of the mechanisms of conservation and excretion. The recommended fluid schedules cover the daily requirements of sodium, chloride and potassium (each 1-3 mmol/kg/day).

Correction of mild abnormalities is usually not indicated as the restoration of fluid balance achieves this in most instances. If necessary, supplements may be used (see Table 21.3).

Table 21.3 Electrolyte supplements

Electrolyte	Availability	mmol/ml
Potassium	15% Potassium chloride	2
Sodium	0,9% Sodium chloride	0,15
Calcium	10% Calcium gluconate	0,225
Magnesium	50% Magnesium sulphate	3

Warning: do not add bicarbonate or phosphate to solutions containing calcium.

Potassium

Anuria must be excluded before potassium is given.

Hyperkalaemia may produce cardiac arrhythmia or arrest and solutions should not contain a concentration of potassium of more than 35 mmol/l.

In the presence of a serum potassium greater than 6 mmol/l the following steps should be taken:

♦ stop all potassium administration, both intravenous and oral;
♦ check acid-base status and correct acidosis;
♦ do an ECG to establish baseline pattern and serially thereafter to monitor changes in the potassium levels. See page 102; and

◆ if no response to the above then treat as for hyperkalaemia as found in renal disease (see page 500).

Normally the maximum amount of potassium given per 24 hours should not exceed 3 mmol/kg/day. In severe depletion or excessive loss, amounts of up to 9 mmol/kg/day can be given, but constant monitoring and extreme caution should be exercised when exceeding 3 mmol/kg/day.

Sodium

Hyponatraemia need only be corrected if severe, and after the acid base status and hypokalaemia have been treated. Note that hyponatraemia occurs in some sodium retaining states, e.g. malnutrition and hepatic disease. An additional sodium load may precipitate oedema.

The sodium deficit can be calculated as follows:

sodium deficit (mmol) = (normal serum sodium less the observed serum sodium) x 0,6 x body weight (kg)

Replace half the deficit initially and reassess the electrolyte status.

Hypernatraemia – see explanatory note 4, Table 21.2.

Calcium and magnesium

Daily intravenous requirements (IV) have not been defined. If fluid therapy continues for more than a few days, magnesium can be given in a concentration of 1-3 mmol/l and calcium 1-2 mmol/l. In deficiency states dosage is empirical, e.g. calcium gluconate 10%, 2-10 ml/day IV and magnesium sulphate 50%, 2 ml/day IV.

Nutrition

If the child is on conventional IV therapy, it must be remembered that he or she is being starved. There is no protein intake and energy requirements are not being met. Intravenous therapy should therefore be kept as brief as possible.

Protein

Plasma 10 ml/kg/day will help in maintaining plasma proteins, but this does not meet daily protein requirements.

Carbohydrate

A 10% dextrose solution may be used to supply additional kilo-joules and prevent hypoglycaemia (particularly in the first few days after birth) but does not cover energy expenditure.

Vitamins and trace elements

It is necessary to add vitamins only if intravenous therapy is prolonged for more than a few days, in which case the normal requirements are met. See page 378. Trace element require-ments can be met by giving plasma at weekly visits. See page 378.

Blood transfusion

Never exceed 20 ml of blood/kg body weight unless the patient is actively bleeding or has a history of recent blood loss. Anaemia *per se* is not an indication for blood transfusion and the cause should be investigated before planning treatment.

Warning

If IV therapy has to be prolonged, total intravenous nutrition using amino-acid solutions, intravenous fat and carbohydrate becomes necessary. This technique is best left to experienced units.

Advice

There are no short cuts in fluid therapy. Consideration of the whole problem in each individual patient is essential. Constant reassessment of the child, particularly by clinical examination augmented by serum electrolyte and acid-base studies, is the key to successful fluid therapy.

The contents of commonly available solutions for infusion are given in Table 21.4, page 216.

Table 21.4 Solutions for infusion

Solution	Na	K	Mg	Ca	PO₄	Cl	Lactate	HCO₃	Other
				Content (mmol/l)					
Half-strength Darrow's solution with 5% dextrose	61	17				52	27		50 g Dextrose/l
Dextrose 5% in water									50 g Dextrose/l
Haemaccel*	145	5,1		6,25		145			Degraded polypeptides
Maintelyte	35	25	2,5			65			
Neonatalyte (SABAX)	20	15	0,5	2,5	3,75	21	20		100 g Dextrose/l
Paediatric maintenance solution (SABAX)	35	12				47	—	—	50 g Dextrose/l
Plasmolyte B*	130	4	1,5			110	—	27	
Ringer's Lactate+	131	5	—	1,8		112	29		
Sodium chloride 0,9%* (normal saline)	154					154			
Sodium chloride 0,45% (half-normal saline)	77					77			

* = Isotonic fluids

GASTROINTESTINAL DISORDERS

M D Bowie

Anal fissure

◆ Acute anal fissure and painful defecation are treated using anaesthetic creams (Anethaine, Scheriproct) which are applied to the anal verge.

◆ Chronic anal fissure usually requires anal stretching under general anaesthetic and removal of the underlying faeco-loma. The management programme outlined for faecal loading should also be followed in cases of both acute and chronic anal fissure.

Aphthous ulcers

Aetiology

Unknown. Food hypersensitivity, allergic or toxic drug reactions, infectious agents, endocrine factors, emotional stress etc. have all been implicated.

Clinical presentation

Recurrent painful ulcers of the oral mucous membranes. Solitary or multiple lesions occur on the labial, buccal and lingual mucosa as well as on the gums and palate. Often cyclical in occurrence. Initially an erythematous indurated papule that erodes rapidly to form a sharply circumscribed, necrotic ulcer with a grey fibrinous exudate and an erythematous halo. The lesions heal spontaneously in ten to 14 days.

Note

Aphthous ulcers are not a manifestation of recurrent herpes infection which remains localized to the lips and rarely crosses the mucocutaneous junction; only primary herpes involves the oral mucosa.

Management

Palliative as in primary herpes stomatitis, but Acyclovir is of no value.

Faecal loading

Faecal loading in childhood is characterized by the retention of stools in the colon and rectum and occurs as a result of repeated incomplete evacuation of faeces. The condition is much more common than is generally believed.

Aetiology

The cause of the condition is usually not apparent and may be multifactorial, i.e. low fibre diet, disturbance of toilet routine, and behavioural disturbances. Although not common, an organic cause such as hypothyroidism, anal fissure, anorectal malformation or Hirschsprung's disease should also be considered. The younger the child at presentation the more the likelihood that the cause is organic.

Clinical presentation

Symptoms may include constipation, loose stools, faecal soiling, mild abdominal distension and peri-umbilical pain, either singly or in combination. Presenting patients are often misdiagnosed as having chronic diarrhoea, encopresis or recurrent nonspecific abdominal pain of childhood. Recent onset of constipation and painful defecation are commonly caused by an acute anal fissure.

◆ Under five years: children tend to present most commonly with the complaint of constipation.
◆ Over five years: the most common presenting complaints are faecal soiling and/or abdominal pain.

Note

If only classic constipation (the passage of infrequent hard stools) is considered, many of these children will be missed as some pass apparently normal regular stools. Correct diagnosis is important as symptoms respond to therapy.

Diagnosis

Faecal loading should be suspected when abdominal and rectal examination shows palpable faeces, confirmed by straight abdominal radiographs showing faecal content which may fill the entire colon. Gross distension of the bowel is not commonly seen.

Management

Faecal loading

◆ Initial clearance of the colon using repeated Fleet or Microlax enemas, or by the oral administration of large volumes of a balanced electrolyte polyethylene glycol solution (Golytely).

   The constituents of the balanced electrolyte polyethylene glycol powder are available from the Red Cross War Memorial Children's Hospital pharmacy. To one litre of water add 75,77g of the powder and the resultant solution is given in a dose of 20-25 ml/kg/hour. Smaller children should be encouraged to drink these large volumes and the solution can be made more palatable by the addition of artificial sweeteners or diabetic drinks. Do **not** add any sugar-containing mixture to the solution. After one hour of administration a microlax enema should be given. Administration of the solution is continued until the anal effluent is 'clear'. This usually takes between six and eight hours.

   The efficacy of clearance can be checked clinically (soft, mass-free abdomen), but in particularly troublesome cases a repeat abdominal radiograph is useful.

◆ Adjust the diet to include more fibre and supplement this with bulk laxatives (Fybogel or Metamucil). These should be continued for several months as premature withdrawal almost invariably results in relapse. Should this occur then treatment must begin again with colonic clearance.

◆ In occasional cases the above may not be sufficient to keep the colon and rectum empty. A stool softener (LACTULOSE) or bowel stimulant (Senokot 1-3 tabs at night for three to six weeks) may be useful additional measures.

◆ Regular daily bowel habits must be encouraged and the objectives of treatment (daily complete evacuation of the large bowel) carefully explained to both parents and the child. This tends to prevent premature stopping of treatment.

Warning

Chronic faecal loading which does not respond to the above management programme requires further investigation, as do children with early onset constipation, peri-anal abnormalities or gross abdominal or large bowel distension. Refer these cases to a centre of expertise where appropriate investigations can be undertaken.

Gastroenteritis
Acute infectious diarrhoeal disease

Gastroenteritis is caused by an infective agent that damages the gut mucosa and disturbs the balance between the mechanisms controlling secretion and absorption within the bowel. The excessive net loss of electrolytes and water into the gut lumen results in diarrhoea characterized by the passing of frequent unformed stools.

In the well-nourished child acute diarrhoeal disease tends to be self-limiting with minimal mortality. Prolonged diarrhoea is more common among malnourished or very young infants and is associated with an increase in mortality and morbidity.

Aetiology

The infective agents responsible for infantile gastroenteritis may be viral, bacterial or parasitic. Aetiology varies from area to area and depends on environmental and social conditions as well as on the age of the patient. In developed societies, viral pathogens are the major cause and the disease tends to occur in winter. In developing societies diarrhoea occurs mainly in the summer months and bacterial pathogens are more common. Parasites are relatively uncommon in the young infant, but increase in aetiological significance in the second year of life.

Intestinal pathogens causing diarrhoea and/or vomiting

Viruses

Rotavirus, adenovirus, others.

Bacteria

Escherichia coli, shigella, salmonella, *Campylobacter jejuni*, *Yersinia enterocolitica*, aeromonas, others.

Parasites

Entamoeba histolytica, Giardia lamblia, Cryptosporidium.

Note

The term 'parenteral diarrhoea' refers to a clinical state in many children who present with diarrhoea where the primary disease may be outside the gastrointestinal tract, e.g. otitis media, respiratory or urinary tract infection.

Clinical presentation

Diarrhoea

It is wise to ask specifically about the number and character of the stools as the interpretation of what constitutes 'diarrhoea' varies widely. Severity is often underestimated because of initial pooling of secretion in the gut or because watery diarrhoea is easily mistaken for urine. Blood in the stools suggest an invasive organism (shigella, amoebae or necrotizing enterocolitis) or a haemorrhagic colitis induced by enema therapy with toxic substances. Blood-stained stools may also occur in *Campylobacter* infection. Frothy stools suggest carbohydrate intolerance. Pale malodorous stools suggest steatorrhoea and infection with *Giardia lamblia*.

Vomiting

Usually present but its severity is variable. May precede diarrhoea by hours or even a day, particularly in those of viral aetiology. If bile-stained or persistent, surgical conditions must be excluded.

Constitutional signs

Fever and toxicity are uncommon and their presence suggests parenteral or viral aetiology. An abrupt onset of diarrhoea with high fever and no vomiting is characteristic of shigella enteritis.

Dehydration

Occurs in a minority of cases but is the most common complication of gastroenteritis. If untreated, dehydration accounts for 60-70% of deaths. Accurate and immediate assessment is critical to management. Weight changes are the most accurate

Table 22.1 Clinical signs of dehydration

Body weight loss %	Clinical state	Signs
<5	Not unwell	Thirst
		Dry mucous membranes
5-10	Apathetic	Sunken eyes or fontanelle
	Unwell	Reduced tissue turgor
		Tachypnoea
		Oliguria
>10	Shocked	Peripheral circulatory failure
		Small pulse volume
		Tachycardia
		Diminished consciousness
		Hypotension

Notes:
1. In hypernatraemia the above signs underestimate the degree of dehydration. Signs of cerebral irritation occur early.
2. Shock may precede other evidence of dehydration when losses are rapid and severe.

method of assessment but are usually not initially available and clinical assessment is necessary.

Acidosis

Invariably present if there are signs of dehydration. Characterized by deep sighing respiration and an anxious appearance. Persistence of acidosis suggests that dehydration has not been corrected. Metabolic alkalosis virtually excludes the diagnosis of gastroenteritis. The most common cause is protracted vomiting of pyloric stenosis or other surgical conditions.

Ileus

A distended, relatively silent abdomen suggests this diagnosis. This acute 'toxic' dilatation of the gut may be caused by infection, toxaemia or hypokalaemia. Potassium supplementation reduces the incidence of this complication. Necrotizing enterocolitis can occur in young malnourished infants who have had an episode of shock. It presents with the signs of ileus and blood in the stools.

Seizures

These are quite common but their cause is often obscure. Causes to be excluded are: fever, hypoglycaemia, electrolyte disturbances (e.g. sodium, calcium, magnesium), cerebral vein thrombosis and meningitis. Seizures with fever at the onset of illness suggest shigella enteritis. Seizures and other disturbances of central nervous function such as coma, drowsiness, irritability and hyper-reflexia are more common in hypernatraemic dehydration.

Hyper- and hypoglycaemia

Hyperglycaemia may present in both hypernatraemic and normonatraemic dehydration. It is easily confused with diabetic ketoacidosis but in the latter, urine output is maintained or excessive, whereas in dehydration due to diarrhoea there is oliguria or anuria. Insulin treatment is contra-indicated and rehydration and correction of acidosis will return the blood glucose level to normal. Hypoglycaemia may occur, particularly in malnourished, septicaemic and hypothermic infants.

Protein-losing enteropathy

May complicate gastroenteritis in young infants. Clinically evident as generalized oedema and is often confused with kwashiorkor occurring at an unusually early age (two to three months).

Electrolyte disturbances

See page 213.

Diagnosis

Clinical examination is necessary to exclude parenteral disease and system infections such as meningitis. Consider the possibility of surgical conditions, particularly if there is persistent or bile-stained vomiting, gross abdominal distension or redness and oedema of the abdominal wall.

   Dehydration is the most common complication and must initially be assessed clinically (see Table 22.1). Regular weighing thereafter allows an objective measure of the process of rehydration. Many complications follow on dehydration.

Investigation

If there is no more than mild dehydration, most cases of

gastroenteritis can be managed without further investigation. In severe cases it may be useful to measure the plasma electrolytes, urea, glucose and to determine the acid base status.

Correction of dehydration and treatment of shock should never be delayed because of the difficulty in obtaining these parameters. See page 9.

Microbiology of stools (microscopy and culture) is necessary if a definite aetiological diagnosis is required. The clinical characteristics of the illness may be helpful in identifying the probable infective agent, but in most cases symptoms and signs are so similar as to make this impossible. Urine examination, blood culture and CSF examination may be indicated.

Management

The prevention of gastroenteritis involves socio-economic development and betterment of the environmental conditions of the community. Preventing and correcting electrolyte and fluid loss is most important in the management of gastroenteritis.

Fluid and electrolyte treatment

The early use of oral fluids by the lay public, local health centre or general practitioner before clinical dehydration occurs is the ideal. It will reduce the morbidity and mortality associated with gastroenteritis.

Early or mild fluid loss (not dehydrated, and vomiting not a problem)

Continue breast or cow milk formula feeds with additional oral fluids (electrolyte carbohydrate solution) interspersed (10-20 ml/kg) per stool passed, or more as required.

Moderate (5% dehydration, and vomiting not severe)

It is important to restore and maintain normal hydration. Frequent reassessment is advisable. Vomiting is usually transient. Small frequent feeds or nasogastric drip of oral rehydration fluid are usually retained.

Breast-feeding should be continued but cow milk feeds should be withheld for six to 12 hours (while rehydration is being achieved) and an electrolyte and sugar solution given by mouth or by nasogastric tube. Prolonged periods (>24 hours) of `clear fluids' or diluted milk feeds must be avoided, especially in malnourished children. Once rehydrated, milk feeds are restarted and can be given as full strength feeds in amounts that are smaller than usual. Oral electrolyte and sugar solution is continued, but by 24 hours full volume (i.e. 150 ml/kg) full-strength milk feeds should begin.

Severe (5-10% dehydrated and/or serious vomiting)

Requires intragastric drip of electrolyte/sugar solution but intravenous fluids are necessary if the patient suffers from shock, ileus or severe vomiting. Refer the child to a hospital for treatment.

Note

The child **must** be sent with an intravenous line running or an intragastric drip. An intragastric drip may be life-saving until IV therapy can be commenced (see Fluid therapy, pages 206 and 451).

Electrolyte solutions containing carbohydrate

♦ Half-strength Darrow's in 5% or 2,5% dextrose water.
♦ Sorol or other commercially available packaged electrolyte carbohydrate powders.
♦ Where no commercially prepared electrolyte solutions are available, give the following by mouth in appropriate amounts:

Boiled water — 1 litre
Salt   — half a level teaspoonful
Sugar   — 8 level teaspoons

Specific treatment

Potassium: in moderate or severe dehydration potassium-containing ORS or intravenous fluids is adequate for normal requirements. They do not supply sufficient for the correction of deficits, and potassium chloride 3-6 mmol/kg/day should be given in addition.

Antibiotics or chemotherapeutic agents are of no value in the majority of cases. Indications for antimicrobial administration include: shigella infection, salmonellosis (systemic infection), prolonged *Campylobacter* infection, *Yersinia enterocolitica* infection, amoebiasis, giardiasis and clinical septicaemia.

In the very malnourished (see page 385) or very young (under one month of age, see page 355), there is always diagnostic doubt between gastroenteritis and septicaemia. The prescribed antibiotic should provide Gram-positive and negative cover, e.g. CO-TRIMOXAZOLE or PENICILLIN and GENTAMICIN.

Note

Anti-diarrhoeal agents such as opium preparations, pectin, kaolin, CODEINE PHOSPHATE are not recommended. LOPERAMIDE is of some value in much older children and adults but the potential complications in infants and young children far outweigh this. Its use is not recommended.

Prolonged acute diarrhoea

In a small percentage of children, particularly the very young and/or malnourished infant, severe dehydrating diarrhoea may persist for more than seven days.

Management

Children with prolonged acute diarrhoea remain at risk from the complications of dehydration and continued nutrient loss. Treat with oral NEOMYCIN 100 mg/kg/24 hours/four-hourly for three days and oral CHOLESTYRAMINE 1 g/six-hourly for five days.

Note

A mild metabolic acidosis often occurs while on CHOLESTYRAMINE.

Hepatitis

Many viruses can cause acute hepatitis (Table 22.2) but hepatitis is the dominant feature of the illness in only a few. These are hepatitis A, B and the non-A non-B group. The term viral hepatitis is usually used to include only the foregoing. Clinical severity varies widely and in most the infection is asymptomatic or subclinical with anicteric hepatitis. In some an acute illness results with malaise and jaundice, while fulminant hepatitis may occur in a few.

Hepatitis A (HAV)

The most common cause of jaundice in children, spread predominantly by the faecal oral route. Incubation 15-50 days.

Table 22.2 Infective hepatitis — virus aetiology

Hepatitis A	
Hepatitis B	
Hepatitis non-A, non-B	
EB virus	} Clinical picture of
Cytomegalovirus	'glandular fever'
Exotic haemorrhagic fevers	E.g. yellow fever
Herpes simplex	} Usually only in neonates
Coxsackie B	or immunocompromised
Varicella zoster	subjects.

Clinical presentation

♦ Prodrome: nausea, anorexia and malaise.
♦ Clinical: dark urine, jaundice, tender palpable liver.

Diagnosis

Hyperbilirubinaemia is present if jaundiced. A rise in plasma transaminases precedes jaundice. No evidence of chronic liver disease such as low serum albumin or increased prothrombin ratio (high international normalized ratio). Diagnosis is confirmed by finding raised specific IgM antibodies denoting recent infection. Raised IgG antibodies denote previous infection.

Management

Prevention
Post-exposure (within one or two weeks) or pre-exposure prophylaxis: a single dose of human immunoglobulin of 0,04 ml/kg IM is recommended (minimum 1 ml).

Acute infection

♦ **Isolation** is not required as virus shedding ceases at onset of jaundice.
♦ **High energy diet**. Fat is seldom tolerated.
♦ **Bed rest** may be needed but does not alter the course of the disease.

Prognosis

In children jaundice usually abates in two or three weeks and a prolonged cholestatic phase is not common. There is no progression to chronic active hepatitis or cirrhosis. Fulminant hepatitis is rare and danger signals include protracted vomiting, continuing fever, hypoglycaemia, confusion and increased prothrombin ratio which does not respond to Vitamin K.

Hepatitis B (HBV)

This is a common cause of jaundice in South Africa, and has an incubation period of two to six months. Transmission is mainly by the parenteral route (infected blood or blood products), but may occur via the oral route.

Clinical presentation

The clinical presentation may be indistinguishable from hepatitis A but may be more insidious with a longer prodrome of non-specific ill health.

Diagnosis

Acute infection

A diagnosis of HBV is the same as for all viral hepatitis except that HBV presents with serological markers, i.e. HBsAg, HBeAg.

Chronic infection

Occurs commonly in children. About 90% of neonates and 30-40% of children with acute HBV infection become chronic carriers. Typically they are male and initially have asymptomatic disease. Some chronic carriers develop chronic active hepatitis and cirrhosis.

Management

Prevention

Hepatitis B immunoglobulin can be used in non-immune individuals exposed to HBV. A dose of 2 ml in children (3 ml in the adult) is recommended and should be given as soon as possible between one and seven days after exposure. In proven high risk exposure a second injection should be given one month later.

Hepatitis B vaccine — see Immunization, page 252.

Treatment

Same principles as for other types of hepatitis.

Hepatitis non-A and non-B (NANB)

Until recently these have been a diagnosis of exclusion. Hepatitis C, D and E, and more exist. Hepatitis C is considered to be the major cause of transfusion-associated hepatitis. It runs a mild, often asymptomatic course but has a tendency to progress to chronic liver disease in 50% of patients. Hepatitis D is a defective virus only associated with hepatitis B infections and is very rare in South Africa. Hepatitis E is an epidemic disease resembling HAV.

Hepatic failure

Acute liver failure

Acute liver failure (ALF) or fulminant hepatic failure refers to the development of liver failure in children without pre-existing liver disease. It appears within a few weeks of the onset of the illness. There are similarities and differences to those with chronic liver disease who thereafter decompensate.

Aetiology

Viral hepatitis (particularly A and B), Reye's syndrome, drugs (PARACETAMOL, anti-TB) and toxins (including traditional medicines).

Clinical presentation

Protracted vomiting, jaundice (not in Reye's syndrome), disturbed mental function, coma, bleeding diathesis, various metabolic and renal disturbances, and infection.

Investigations

Liver function tests, plasma proteins and prothrombin ratio, blood ammonia and glucose, serum electrolytes and acid base studies.

Management

Hepatotoxic drugs must be withdrawn and sedation avoided.

Encephalopathy

◆ Protein and salt restriction.

◆ LACTULOSE in a dose sufficient to produce loose stools.
◆ NEOMYCIN 100 mg/kg/day in four divided doses for three days. This may be omitted. It is of doubtful value and possibly nephrotoxic.

Cerebral oedema

◆ Ultrasound or CT scanning essential to prove the diagnosis of this common complication.
◆ IV fluids only given at 2/3 normal maintenance requirements.
◆ MANNITOL 0,5 g/kg bodyweight by rapid IV bolus infusion. May be repeated in the same dose once or twice within the next few hours if the clinical response is inadequate. Do not repeat if there is no clinical response. Beware of causing hypovolaemia and oliguria (urine volume <1 ml/kg/hour).
◆ **Note:** Signs of fluid overload may occur in oliguric patients.
◆ Treat by dialysis.
◆ Steroids and PHENOBARBITONE are of no proven value.

Bleeding diathesis

◆ Vitamin K 5 mg IV or IM and repeated.
◆ Fresh frozen plasma daily if necessary.
◆ Cryoprecipitate and platelets can be given to cover invasive procedures.

Metabolic disturbances

◆ Hypoglycaemia is common. Monitor routinely with dextrostix.
◆ High carbohydrate feeds or IV 10% dextrose infusion.
◆ Hypo- and hypernatraemia, hypokalaemia, hypocalcaemia and hypomagnesaemia may occur.
◆ Correct acid base status if necessary. Respiratory alkalosis and metabolic acidosis may occur.

Renal

◆ Pre-renal uraemia secondary to hypovolaemia.
◆ Acute tubular necrosis secondary to hypotension, septicaemia or drugs (aminoglycocides etc.).

Infections

◆ Broad spectrum antibiotic cover. Prescribe AMOXYCILLIN or third generation cephalosporins.

Prognosis

Poor. Even in the best hands, the mortality rate is high (30%).

Decompensated chronic hepatic disease

There are similarities to ALF but the major differences are: cerebral oedema is rare; the hepatorenal syndrome, portal hypertension and ascites are common. This requires a different approach, particularly to fluid balance, and paracentesis of ascites with intravenous colloid replacement is recommended.

Herpes simplex

Herpes simplex is a common viral infection. Two strains of the virus exist (HSV1 and HSV2). HSV1 commonly infects the skin and mucous membranes, eyes and central nervous system, and HSV2 the genitalia. Generalized systemic disease may occur, particularly in newborns and severely malnourished children.

Clinical presentation

Primary infection

The host's first experience of the virus is either subclinical or results in local superficial lesions and an accompanying systemic reaction. Herpes stomatitis is the most common clinical presentation and the primary infection involves the mucosa of the gums, buccal mucosa and tongue. The lesions are shallow ulcers covered with a yellow-grey membrane. Pain, fever, and increased salivation accompany the lesions, and the child generally refuses to eat. The acute phase lasts from four to nine days and is self-limiting.

Recurrent infection

Reactivation of a latent infection in an immune host following non-specific stimuli such as environmental changes or other infections. Lesions are localized and are not associated with a systemic reaction. Fever blisters on the mucocutaneous junction of the mouth are an example.

Management

Primary infection: in mild cases symptomatic treatment by attending to oral hygiene (GLYCO-THYMOL mouth wash) and the application of an analgesic gel (Teegel or TANNIC ACID GEL with 0,5% LIGNOCAINE).

In more severe cases the use of ACYCLOVIR (Zovirax) cream will shorten the attack and lessen the chance that it will spread. Apply five times daily. In the malnourished child, consider intravenous ACYCLOVIR because of the danger of generalized systemic disease.

Infantile colic (three month colic)

A loosely defined disturbance of infancy which is common, occurring in about one in ten infants.

Aetiology

Unknown but occurs in families, and most frequently in first-born babies.

Clinical presentation

◆ Practically always starts within three weeks of birth.
◆ Periods of irritability and crying with apparent abdominal pain associated with drawing up of the legs.
◆ Episodes are often related to feeding – midway through a feed.
◆ Characteristically worse in the afternoon and evening.
◆ Commonly remits by three months but not always.
◆ Occurs in bottle-fed or breast-fed infants.
◆ Association with anxious mothers probably secondary rather than causative.

Management

Reassurance once other possible causes of intermittent pain have been excluded (i.e. pyelonephritis, otitis media, anal fissure, intestinal obstruction). A few may respond to withdrawal of cow milk from their diet or their mothers' diet if they are breast-fed. Treatment with DICYCLOMINE (Merbentyl) is no longer recommended as respiratory collapse, coma and death in infants under six months have been reported with this drug.

Recurrent abdominal pain (RAP)

Aetiology

There are numerous causes of recurrent abdominal pain (RAP) and it is one of the commonest complaints of children. A few cases are due to recognizable organic disease so all require a careful clinical evaluation. The dilemma is which children should be investigated further and to what degree investigation should be pursued.

Functional abdominal pain (irritable bowel syndrome or chronic non-specific abdominal pain of childhood) is claimed to be the commonest cause of RAP, accounting for 95% of cases.

Clinical presentation

♦ Typically affects children aged between five and 14 years.
♦ Commonly sensitive, thoughtful, introverted children.
♦ Rarely major psycho-social stress or problems.
♦ Pain.
  ◇ Characteristically periumbilical but not always.
  ◇ Often severe but short-lived (less than one hour).
  ◇ Pain periods occur in clusters lasting days to weeks.
  ◇ Episodes of pain may occur several times a day or as seldom as once a week.
  ◇ Pain-free periods varying from weeks to months. Accompanying symptoms may include: headache, pallor, nausea, dizziness, fatigue and low grade fever.

Management

Investigation: kept to a minimum but should include FBC, ESR, urine analysis and microscopy, stool examination for parasites and occult blood.

Warning

Features suggesting organic disease in RAP

♦ Age of onset <5 or >14 years.
♦ Pain localized away from umbilicus.
♦ Epigastric tenderness.
♦ Nocturnal pain awakening patient.
♦ Food aggravating or relieving pain.
♦ Signs of gastrointestinal bleeding – overt, occult or anaemia.
♦ Abdominal distension, mass visceromegaly.
♦ Weight loss.

A straight X-ray abdomen should always be performed to exclude faecal loading (see pages 218-20) which presents in a very similar fashion in the over-five year old.

Treat the cause. If none apparent give explanation and reassurance.

Teething

Teething (the eruption of teeth) may cause inflammatory changes in the gums with swelling of the gums, general malaise, irritability and loss of appetite. Symptomatic treatment of pain with PARACETAMOL in more severe cases may be indicated. It is unwise to attribute any other symptoms or signs to teething.

Dental caries

This is due to the progressive decay of teeth by organic acids produced locally by bacteria that ferment dietary carbohydrate, particularly sucrose. Fluoride reduces the incidence and severity of caries by converting the enamel mineral to the more acid resistant fluorapatite and by promoting remineralization. Dental caries can be reduced by avoiding food between meals (sweets or sweet drinks in nursing bottles), by regular cleaning of teeth and an adequate intake of fluoride. This last is particularly important in South Africa where most water supplies are deficient in fluoride. See page 377.

Thrush

Infection with the fungus *Candida albicans*.

Clinical presentation

Common in the newborn. Later in life it is relatively uncommon except in debilitated infants and children or those receiving antibiotics or who are immunosuppressed (e.g. AIDS). The oral lesions are white adherent flaky plaques covering all or part of the tongue, lips, gums and buccal mucous membranes. A brightly inflamed base is seen when the plaques are removed. Discomfort may interfere with food ingestion. Nystatin solution 1 ml (100 000 units) four times a day. The solution should be slowly and gently instilled to allow for wide distribution before it is swallowed.

23 HAEMATOLOGY

C D Karabus and P S Hartley

The anaemic child

Anaemia is the most common blood abnormality in childhood. It occurs when the concentration of haemoglobin (Hb) or number of red cells is below the normal range for the age (and gender after puberty) of a child. Like fever, anaemia is not a diagnosis *per se,* but should be regarded as an indication of an underlying nutritional problem or disease.

Anaemia should be qualified by morphological type (microcytic, normocytic, macrocytic), mechanism (decreased marrow production, haemolysis, blood loss) and aetiology (undernutrition, infection, Meckel's diverticulum, leukaemia, chronic disease etc.). A complete diagnosis can be made in most children with anaemia after a thorough history and examination and with relatively little in the way of laboratory equipment.

Approach to diagnosis

Detection

Pallor is a common feature of anaemia but is not always obvious, especially in milder cases. Clinical assessment of anaemia is therefore best made from the conjunctival mucosa rather than the skin. The diagnosis is confirmed by measuring the Hb or haematocrit. It is good practice to screen infants and children routinely at periods when anaemia is most likely, i.e. at 12 months of age, a preschool check and again during early adolescence. Preterm infants should in addition be checked at six months of age. As a child grows, major changes occur in the range of normal reference blood values, and during the first few months of infancy there is striking variation in the normal Hb concentration. At birth infants have higher Hb levels and larger red cells than adults but this situation reverses by two months of age. Knowledge of the normal blood values at a particular age is a prerequisite to interpreting blood parameters. For example, a

Hb of 9,5 g/dl is acceptable for a two month old infant, indicates moderate anaemia in a child of five years and severe, life-threatening anaemia in a newborn infant. For normal red cell values for infants and children, see page 680.

Evaluation of the anaemic child

History

Most anaemias develop insidiously and provoke few symptoms until an advanced stage is reached. Irritability, anorexia, lethargy and early fatigue are non-specific features of any anaemia resulting from decreased oxygen delivery. Pointers of diagnostic importance in the history which should be specifically asked about are given in Table 23.1.

Table 23.1 Anaemia — features of importance in history

History	Consider
Low birthweight	Iron deficiency
Diet (inadequate, excessive milk)	Iron deficiency
Pica	Iron deficiency
Chronic diarrhoea	Folate, iron lack
Genetic factors (e.g. coloured, Asian, Mediterranean)	Thalassaemia, G6PD deficiency
Jaundice (neonatal, recurrent)	Haemolysis
Sudden onset, no overt bleeding	Haemolysis
Drug exposure	
CHLORAMPHENICOL	Aplastic
Oxidant	Haemolysis
Systemic illness (tuberculosis, rheumatoid arthritis, renal disease)	Marrow production defect
Purpura, bruising	Bleeding disorder, marrow infiltration

Examination

♦ Mucosal pallor, an increased heart rate and a palpable spleen are common to many different types of anaemia and do not suggest a specific aetiology.

♦ Koilonychia is uncommon in children but is specific to iron deficiency.

◆ Other findings of diagnostic importance include jaundice, suggesting haemolysis, bruising associated with a bleeding disorder or leukaemia, and enlarged lymph nodes or abdominal organs which may indicate a systemic disease as the cause of anaemia.

Investigation of the anaemic child

Many of the necessary investigations may be performed cheaply and reasonably accurately with a microcentrifuge, capillary tubes, slides, staining fluid and a microscope. Determination of Hb or haematocrit, mean cell volume (MCV) and reticulocyte count are necessary for the assessment of anaemia. Another simple but important procedure is examination of a peripheral blood film. With very little practice, abnormalities in the shape or size of red blood cells can be assessed as can platelet and white cell counts. If clumps of platelets are easily seen the patient does not have significant thrombocytopaenia. Abnormalities in the number of white cells and the presence of primitive cells can also be readily identified. An important screening investigation in patients with anaemia is examination of the stool for occult blood or parasites. A chest X-ray and other specific investigations are indicated if systemic disease is suspected.

Morphologic classification of anaemia

The MCV (the second most important investigation after Hb) provides an effective way of grouping and starting the diagnostic workup of anaemia (see Table 23.2). Normal developmental changes in RBC size especially during infancy and early childhood must be taken into account. (See page 680.) Microcytic anaemia is the most common morphological type followed by normocytic anaemia, while macrocytic anaemia is relatively uncommon. The ethnic origin of the patient may be relevant. While iron deficiency is the most frequent cause in all population groups, inherited Hb disorders are an important cause of anaemia among coloured and Asian South African children. Haemoglobinopathies are extremely rare among blacks in South Africa.

Mechanism of anaemia

There are three main pathogenic mechanisms of anaemia, i.e. decreased red cell production, excessive haemolysis and blood

Table 23.2 Morphological classification of anaemia

Microcytic	Iron deficiency. Thalassaemia. Chronic systemic disease or lead poisoning.
Normocytic	Mixed deficiency, e.g. iron and folate. Recent blood loss. Infection. Chronic systemic disease. Haemolytic anaemias. Massive splenomegaly.
Macrocytic	Folate (rarely vitamin B_{12}) deficiency. Marrow failure, e.g. aplastic anaemia. Liver disease. Hypothyroidism. Dyserythropoietic anaemias.

loss. Consideration of the morphologic type and mechanism of anaemia contributes towards a more rational investigative plan as well as therapy of the disorder. A simple diagnostic approach to the anaemic patient, utilizing the results of the Hb, MCV, reticulocyte count and blood smear is outlined below. In only a minority of children (see step 5) will referral for more specialized investigations be indicated.

Diagnostic approach to the child with anaemia

STEP 1   Is the Hb below normal for age?

STEP 2   What is the MCV?

        LOW   Suggests iron deficiency or thalassaemia.
                        Look for cause of deficiency – diet, blood loss.
                        Give trial of oral iron.
                        If no response: serum Fe, TIBC, ferritin, HbF, HbA2.

        HIGH   Suggests folate deficiency or marrow failure.
                        Look for cause of deficiency – diet, malabsorption.
                        Give trial of folate.
                        If no response: RBC folate, serum B_{12}, bone marrow, reticulocyte count.

        NORMAL   See step 3.

STEP 3   What is the reticulocyte count?

        LOW   Suggests production defect – see step 4, WBC/PLATELETS.

        HIGH   Suggests haemolysis or recent blood loss:
                        Haemolysis – see step 4, red cells.
                        Blood loss – look for site of bleeding.

STEP 4   What is cell morphology on BLOOD SMEAR?

WBC/PLATELETS	(and low reticulocytes)
NORMAL	Suggests system disease – infection, renal, liver, cancer, connective tissue or RBC aplasia. Check systems; if RBC aplasia suspected – see step 5a.
ABNORMAL	Suggests marrow disease: leukaemia or aplastic anaemia – see step 5a.
RED CELLS	(and increased reticulocytes)
SPHEROCYTIC	Suggests hereditary sphero-cytosis or auto-immune haemolytic anaemia – see step 5b.i).
NONSPHEROID	Suggests drug-induced or G6PD deficient haemolytic anaemia or haemoglobino-pathy – see step 5b.ii).

STEP 5   REFER TO A TERTIARY CENTRE FOR APPRO-
PRIATE INVESTIGATIONS
a. Bone marrow biopsy.
b. i) Family study, osmotic fragility or Coombs test.
   ii) Drug history, Motulsky test or Hb electro-
       phoresis

Abbreviations:
Fe   – Iron
G6PD – glucose-6-phosphate dehydrogenase
Hb   – haemoglobin
MCV – mean corpuscular volume
RBC   – red blood cell
TIBC – total iron binding capacity
WBC – white blood cell

Principles of management

Once a complete assessment has been made of the degree, type and in particular the underlying cause of anaemia, treatment should be considered. The agents available for correcting the common childhood anaemias are listed in Table 23.3. Emphasis should be on the use of specific haematinics rather than the extremely expensive mixtures of drugs. The most effective treatment of iron-deficient anaemia is an oral ferrous iron salt without supplementary vitamins or minerals. The cause of the iron-deficient anaemia whether nutritional, chronic trichuris infestation or a peptic ulcer must also be established and corrected. Transfusions are seldom indicated in the management of anaemia in children and a decision to transfuse should never be based on Hb concentration alone. Children tolerate fairly low levels of Hb before becoming symptomatic and unless there is an acute haemolytic event, immediate transfusion is generally not indicated to correct anaemia. If anaemia is restricting activity or causing cardiac failure, a small transfusion (5-10 ml/kg) may be sufficient to improve symptoms without putting the child at risk of circulatory overload.

Nutritional anaemia

Manifestations are most severe in children where the need for nutrients is increased by growth.

Iron deficiency anaemia

This is the most common anaemia in the world, rife in poorer socio-economic groups. Maximal incidence is from six months to two years when the cause is usually dietary. In older children blood loss is a more common cause. If a suggestive history and typical microcytic anaemia are present, no further investigations (other than for a cause of blood loss) are necessary.

Prophylaxis

Oral iron should be given to all artificially-fed infants from one month of age and breast-fed infants from three months of age.

Methods

◆ Milk powder — iron enriched
  or
◆ Oral elemental iron supplement: term infants 1 mg/kg/day.
  Preterm infants 2 mg/kg/day.

Parenteral iron (see page 614) is indicated for preterm infants only if parental compliance in giving oral iron is expected to be poor.

Management

◆ The cause of iron deficiency such as inadequate diet and blood loss should be investigated and corrected.

◆ FERROUS SULPHATE 3 mg elemental iron/kg/day in two
  or three divided doses. Check the haemoglobin after two to
  three weeks. If there has been no response, consider poor
  patient compliance, continued blood loss, infection which
  interferes with iron utilization or investigate for an alternative diagnosis such as thalassaemia.

◆ Iron-deficient anaemia should be fully corrected by oral iron
  within four to eight weeks but therapy should continue for a
  further eight weeks in order to replenish body iron stores.

Folate deficiency

Deficiency of this B-complex vitamin was common in preterm
infants prior to the prophylactic addition of folic acid to milk
powder and may still occur occasionally in infants fed on whole
cow milk (especially if boiled) or goat milk. Children with
intestinal malabsorption and those receiving anticonvulsant
drugs are also at risk. Folate deficiency is invariable in protein

Table 23.3 Treatment modalities in anaemia

Treatment	Application
Iron	Nutritional deficiency, chronic blood loss, prophylaxis in all preterm infants and term artificially-fed infants.
FOLIC ACID (rarely B₁₂)	Megaloblastic anaemia.
Corticosteroids	Auto-immune haemolytic anaemia, pure RBC aplasia.
Androgens	Aplastic anaemia, especially Fanconi type.
Antithymocyte globulin	Aplastic anaemia.
Marrow transplantation	Aplastic anaemia, thalassaemia major.
Splenectomy	Symptomatic hereditary spherocytosis, massive splenomegaly in thalassaemia or Gaucher's disease.
Transfusion	Severe blood loss, hypoxic symptoms in aplastic anaemia, haemolysis or leukaemia; regular maintenance in thalassaemia major.
DESFERRIOXAMINE	Transfusional iron overload (thalassaemia, aplastic anaemia, pure red cell aplasia).

energy malnutrition but the typical macrocytic red cell picture may be obscured by the concomitant iron deficiency.

In children with macrocytic anaemia, always check the serum vitamin B$_{12}$ level, as well as the serum and RBC folate to exclude the very rare patient with B$_{12}$ deficiency. If folate deficiency is confirmed, the cause should be corrected and folic acid 1 mg daily administered for a few weeks.

Bleeding disorders

Haemostatic defects may result from deficiency of platelets, coagulation factors or of both elements as in disseminated intravascular coagulation. Acquired bleeding disorders are more common than congenital.

Acquired

Disseminated intravascular coagulation (DIC)

Consumption of platelets and clotting factors II, V, VIII and fibrinogen is followed by secondary fibrinolysis with production of fibrin-split products. DIC should be considered in children with suspected Gram-negative infection with severe systemic illness, shock, bleeding, purpura or gangrene. In the neonate, DIC may occur in association with toxaemia, birth asphyxia, acidosis, hypothermia, respiratory distress syndrome and sepsis, while in older children it is chiefly associated with septicaemia, purpura fulminans, severe burns and acute promyelocytic leukaemia.

Vitamin K deficiency

The vitamin K dependent factors II, VII, IX and X are reduced. Occurs in otherwise healthy neonates (especially breast-fed) who have not received vitamin K at birth and in older children with diarrhoea, kwashiorkor or malabsorption. Clotting factors are restored to normal by vitamin K therapy.

Liver disease

Vitamin K-dependent factors are reduced. In severe hepatocellular disease there may be a poor response to vitamin K and factor V and fibrinogen may also be decreased.

Thrombocytopenia

Usually immune in origin (e.g. idiopathic thrombocytopenic

purpura – ITP) but may be caused by drugs, sequestration of platelets in a large spleen, DIC, infections or marrow disorders.

Congenital

The history is the most important part of the diagnosis. The critical point to be determined is whether bleeding is disproportionate to the degree of trauma. In addition the history will suggest the cause of abnormal bleeding and which investigations should be performed.

Haemorrhage into muscles and joints suggests a coagulation disorder, while purpura, superficial bruising, epistaxis, bleeding gums or menorrhagia suggest von Willebrand disease or a platelet problem.

The severity of bleeding and the occurrence of bleeding in other family members should be noted.

Investigations

Hb, platelet count and blood film should be performed in all patients.

Suspected coagulation disorder

Screening tests

♦ Prothrombin time (PT): normal 10-14 seconds. Usually given as the international normalized ratio (INR), normal less than 1,3. Prolonged in deficiency of factors I, II, V, VII and X.
♦ Partial thromboplastin time (PTT): normal 35-45 seconds. Prolonged in deficiency of all factors except VII and XIII.

Specific tests
Coagulation factor assays.

Suspected platelet function disorder

This occurs in children with purpura or superficial bleeding who do not have thrombocytopenia or Henoch-Schonlein purpura.

Screening tests
Bleeding time (BT): normal two to nine minutes. If unavailable do a capillary fragility (Hess) test. Normal = <5 petechiae in an area 2,5 cm x 2,5 cm.

Specific tests
Platelet aggregation studies.

Interpretation of tests

♦ Thrombocytopenia, anaemia with red cell fragments, increased INR, prolonged PTT, fibrin-split products = DIC.
♦ Prolonged INR and PTT = vitamin K deficiency, liver disease.
♦ Isolated thrombocytopenia in a well child = ITP.
♦ Thrombocytopenia, anaemia, neutropenia = marrow aplasia, leukaemia.
♦ Prolonged PTT, normal INR and BT = haemophilia.
♦ Prolonged BT and PTT, normal INR = von Willebrand disease.
♦ Prolonged BT, normal platelet count, INR and PTT = platelet functional disorder.

Treatment

Investigations should be performed before haemostatic agents are given.

Neonatal haemorrhage

1 mg vitamin K1, fresh frozen plasma (FFP) 10 ml/kg. Platelets or fresh blood if necessary.

DIC

Correct underlying cause; FFP 15-20 ml/kg, platelet transfusion.

Thrombocytopenia

Bed rest until platelet count rises above 20 000. Platelet transfusion for bleeding in aplastic anaemia or leukaemia but not for ITP when platelet transfusion is ineffective. If the platelet count needs to be increased urgently in a patient with ITP, intravenous immunoglobulin (0,4 g-2 g/kg) is the most effective therapy.

Haemophilia

Haemophilia A
Factor VIII 15-25 U/kg for the average joint bleed but 40 U/kg for cerebral bleeding or prior to surgery. Repeat every 12-24 hours until bleeding ceases.

Haemophilia B
Factor IX 25-50 U/kg or more for serious bleeding. Repeat every 24 hours.

> ### Warning
> IM injections and aspirin-containing compounds must not be given to patients with haemophilia.

Indications for transfusion of clotting factor in haemophilia
♦ Pain in joint or muscle.
♦ External bleeding not controlled by pressure.
♦ Pre-operative.
♦ Head trauma or headache: urgent.

Other treatment: splint the involved limb, physiotherapy as soon as tolerated.

Blood transfusion

Whole blood should rarely be transfused. The appropriate blood component should be used for specific conditions. The use of plasma components and platelets is discussed under bleeding disorders (see page 242). Vital signs should be carefully monitored during a transfusion and elective transfusions should not be given at night.

> ### Warning
> Over-transfusion is more dangerous than under-transfusion. See page 306 for medico-legal aspects.

Whole blood

Bloodloss with hypovolaemic shock is the only indication for transfusion of whole blood but packed red cells with crystalloid is a satisfactory alternative. The speed of administration and volume required depends on the severity of blood loss. Transfusion of a large volume of blood may affect coagulation and cause dilutional thrombocytopenia. After the rapid administration of 30 ml/kg of whole blood, 5 ml/kg of FFP should be given and after 70 ml/kg, platelets should also be administered.

Packed red blood cells

Some of the plasma has been removed from whole blood. This is the most rational product for the improvement of oxygen-carrying capacity in chronic anaemia with hypoxic symptoms or cardiac failure. The volume given should not ordinarily exceed 10 ml/kg over three to four hours. If severe chronic anaemia is present (Hb <5 g/dl), myocardial function may be severely compromised. A safe volume to transfuse is 2 ml/g of the patient's Hb/kg body weight, i.e. if the Hb is 3 g/dl transfuse 2x3 = 6 ml/kg.

A transfusion of 3 ml packed red cells/kg will increase the Hb concentration by about 1 g/dl. It is rarely necessary to correct anaemia completely by transfusion and an optimal oxygen-carrying capacity is present with a Hb 10 g/dl (HCT 35%).

Filtered or washed red cells

The process removes white cells and it is the product indicated in children with thalassaemia major or pure red cell aplasia who require repeated transfusions and have febrile reactions to the blood.

Transfusion reactions

The most common transfusion reaction is a febrile or allergic reaction to infused leukocytes or plasma proteins. An acute haemolytic reaction may follow an incompatible blood transfusion. This is heralded by heat and pain along the vein used for infusion, facial flushing, backache and constricting pain in the chest. During surgery these features may be masked by anaesthesia, and hypotension and bleeding may be the only signs.

Management

Allergic febrile reactions

PROMETHAZINE IV. Continue the transfusion slowly and observe closely. Washed or filtered red cells should subsequently be given to children who require regular transfusions.

Acute haemolytic reactions

◆ Stop the transfusion immediately and return the blood with the administration set to the laboratory. See page 306.
◆ Infuse 0,5 g/kg of 25% MANNITOL solution over 30 minutes.
◆ Measure urinary output. If this is less than 1 ml/kg/hour give FUROSEMIDE 2 mg/kg.

Should urinary output not improve, treat as for acute renal failure (see page 496).

Disseminated intravascular coagulation may occur and necessitate FFP and platelet transfusion.

Obligatory action

Send post-transfusion anticoagulated and clotted blood specimens with a urine sample to the laboratory for investigations. Keep accurate records.

24 IMMUNIZATION

G D Hussey

Immunization has proven to be the most cost-effective public health intervention against infectious diseases. It is imperative that all children be immunized against tuberculosis, measles, poliomyelitis, tetanus, diphtheria and pertussis. Immunizations to prevent these diseases are provided free of charge as part of the national immunization programme. Immunization to prevent other diseases is encouraged but is not as yet part of the national programme.

Table 24.1 National Immunization Schedule issued in 1995. (This brings the national schedule in line with the WHO Expanded Programme on Immunization)

Age at immunization	Vaccine
Birth	TOPV(0) [Trivalent Oral Polio], BCG [Bacillus Calmette Guerin, i.e. Tuberculosis]
Six weeks	TOPV(1), DPT(1) [Diphtheria, Pertussis and Tetanus], HBV(1) [Hepatitis B Vaccine]
Ten weeks	TOPV(2), DPT(2), HBV(2)
Fourteen weeks	TOPV(3), DPT(3), HBV(3)
Nine months	Measles(1)
Eighteen months	TOPV(4), DPT(4), Measles(2)
Five years	TOPV(5), DT [Diphtheria and Tetanus]

Lapsed immunization

A lapse in the immunization schedule does not necessitate restarting the whole schedule. The remaining dose or doses should be given as if the prolonged period had not occurred.

Immunization of unimmunized older children not immunized in infancy

These children should receive measles vaccine and three primary doses of TOPV and DPT (children over the age of two years must not be given pertussis vaccine – give DT) spaced at least four to six weeks apart. A booster DT, TOPV and measles vaccine must be given about a year after the last primary dose. BCG may be given if the tuberculin test is negative and there is no immunosuppression.

Immunization of children with HIV/AIDS*

These children should be immunized according to the normal schedule. Do not, however, give BCG to HIV-symptomatic infants. Where resources permit they should also be given *Haemophilus,* pneumococcal and *Influenzae* vaccines.

Immunization of pregnant mothers

Live vaccines including rubella should not be administered during pregnancy. Susceptible pregnant mothers, particularly in areas of high risk for neonatal tetanus, must be given tetanus toxoid i.e. two doses of 0,5 ml IM six to eight weeks apart. A third dose is given six months after the first, with two boosters every five years or during subsequent pregnancies.

Cold chain

The cold chain is the means by which vaccines are maintained at a safe temperature from the time of manufacture until they are given to the individuals being immunized. In clinics and hospitals, all vaccines must be kept in a refrigerator at 0-8°C and should not be frozen in the ice compartment. Reconstituted vaccines (particularly measles and BCG) should be used within one working session. Advise parents who may purchase vaccines from other sources that they should be administered immediately and not left lying in the motor vehicle or at home.

---

*HIV=Human Immuno-deficiency Virus
  AIDS=Acquired Immune Deficiency Syndrome

Missed opportunities

Many opportunities to immunize are missed when:

◆ immunizations are not offered at every contact;
◆ they are denied because of false contra-indications (see below); or
◆ only one vaccine is given when the child is eligible for more than one.

Missed opportunities may be reduced by:

◆ checking the immunization status of every child attending a health care facility;
◆ encouraging the immunization of children at centres which are not designated as immunization clinics, e.g. hospitals. All children admitted to hospital or seen at outpatient clinics must be given measles vaccine if there is no documented evidence of prior immunization to prevent nosocomial transmission; and
◆ avoid false contra-indications to immunization.

Contra-indications to immunization
Egg allergy

Children with a history of egg sensitivity (manifested by generalized urticaria, shock, wheezing, upper airway obstruction) should not receive vaccines, such as measles, mumps, yellow fever and influenza vaccines, which are produced in eggs or chick embryos.

Immune suppression

Children with malignant disease, or those who are receiving cytotoxic, high dose prolonged steroid or irradiation therapy should not be given live vaccines such as BCG, measles, MMR (measles, mumps and rubella), TOPV. Vaccination should be deferred for at least three months following cessation of immunosuppressive therapy.

Pertussis vaccine

Do not give DTP if a child has a progressive central nervous system disease or if there was a severe reaction to a previous dose, e.g. shock, collapse or anaphylaxis, persistent screaming for more than three hours, fever above 40,5°C, convulsions within three days, or encephalopathy within seven days.

Polio vaccine

Immunosuppressed children and their household contacts should receive inactivated polio vaccine. The World Health Organization does, however, recommend live TOPV for children with HIV or AIDS.

Administration of plasma or immunoglobulin

Measles, mumps and rubella vaccines should be deferred for three months following such administration. Other vaccines need not be deferred.

False contra-indications to immunization

♦ Minor illness with low grade fever (less than 38,5°C), diarrhoea and respiratory infections.
♦ Malnutrition.
♦ Breast-feeding.
♦ Prematurity – immunization should commence at the same chronological age recommended for term infants.
♦ Family history of convulsions.
♦ History of non-specific allergies, asthma, hayfever or rhinitis.
♦ Dermatoses, eczema or localized skin infections.
♦ Allergy to antibiotics, except anaphylactic reactions to NEOMYCIN or STREPTOMYCIN (they are contained in some vaccines).
♦ Soreness, redness at injection site or mild fever following a previous DPT vaccine.
♦ Treatment with antibiotics.
♦ Children treated with topical, inhaled, short-term (less than two weeks) or low dose maintenance steroid therapy for a condition that is not immunosuppressive.
♦ Chronic diseases of the heart, lung, kidney or liver.
♦ Static neurological disorders such as cerebral palsy and Down's syndrome.

Vaccines not currently part of the routine schedule

Cholera

The current cholera vaccine is not recommended for use as it does not prevent latent or subclinical infection. It is, however, available for travellers if they wish to be immunized.

Haemophilus influenzae type b (Hib)

Hib is a common cause of meningitis, pneumonia and osteitis. Most cases occur in infancy. The conjugate Hib vaccines can be administered in conjunction with DPT. Children aged less than six months require three primary doses, those aged 7-11 months two doses and those aged 12-14 months one dose. A booster dose is given at an age greater than 15 months. Doses should be spaced six to eight weeks apart. Children over the age of 15 months require a single dose only.

Hepatitis B virus (HBV)

The current recommendations are for three primary HBV doses at birth, one and six months with boosters every five years. HBV will soon be part of the routine immunization schedule in South Africa and will be administered together with the primary DPT schedule. Health care workers should also be immunized.

Influenzae

This annually updated vaccine is recommended for children with chronic lung, heart or renal disease, diabetes, HIV infection, immunosuppression and those on long-term SALICY-LATES (ASPIRIN SOLUBLE) therapy. It should be ideally be administered during March to provide adequate protection before the commencement of winter.

Measles, mumps and rubella combined (MMR)

This can be given instead of the monovalent measles vaccine after the age of one year. It is also recommended for non-immune women of childbearing age. Pregnancy must be avoided for three months after vaccination.

Meningococcal vaccine

Vaccines against serogroups A, C, Y and W-135 are available. They have limited efficacy in children aged less than two years and are only recommended in outbreaks or for those individuals travelling to areas outside South Africa where these serogroups are common. They are not, however, recommended in South Africa since serogroup B is currently the major cause of disease.

Pneumococcal vaccine

Polyvalent pneumococcal vaccine is recommended for children over two years of age with asplenia, splenic dysfunction, nephrotic syndrome, chronic lung disease and HIV infection.

Rabies

This human diploid cell vaccine is given to at-risk individuals. The pre-exposure schedule is 1ml IM on days 0, 7 and 28 with boosters every one to three years depending on the level of exposure. Post-exposure the vaccine must be given on days 0, 3, 7, 14, 30 and 90. Human rabies immunoglobulin must also be prescribed (see page 272).

Typhoid vaccine

Heat-phenol-inactivated and oral vaccines are available. They are not as yet recommended for routine use. Vaccination may be required for international travel to endemic areas and may be of benefit during outbreaks.

Yellow fever

Children over the age of six months travelling to or from areas where yellow fever exists (outside South Africa) should be immunized with a single dose. Revaccination is required at ten-yearly intervals for international travel purposes.

Passive immunization

Passive immunization entails the administration of preformed antibody to a susceptible individual to prevent disease. To be effective it should be administered before or soon after exposure. Normal immunoglobulin may be used to prevent measles (page 268) and hepatitis A (page 227, while specific immunoglobulin may be used to prevent tetanus (page 272), rabies (page 272), chicken pox (page 261) and hepatitis B (page 228).

25 RECURRENT INFECTIONS

D W Beatty

Recurrent infections of childhood are a common clinical problem. Normal preschool children may have six to 12 relatively minor and self-limiting infections a year. In some cases this problem is more severe or persistent in which case underlying factors should be considered.

It is important to recognize that many of these factors may co-exist and are additive, e.g. poor hygiene and malnutrition in a young child. Attention must be paid to each component.

Increased exposure to infectious agents

Overcrowding, poor environmental hygiene and poverty contribute to increased exposure. Children attending preschools are exposed to numerous infectious agents, especially when in confined spaces in winter.

Anatomical abnormalities

Obstructed drainage of secretions leads to stagnation which promotes microbial growth and persistence. Examples are middle ear infection due to blocked eustachian tubes, chronic sinusitis, upper respiratory tract infections due to enlarged adenoids and more rarely a foreign body in the bronchus, urinary tract abnormalities and cerebrospinal leaks. The distinctive feature of these is that infections recur at the same anatomical sites.

Allergy

Allergy frequently presents as recurrent infections. Allergic inflammation and swelling of mucosal surfaces leads to anatomical obstruction, and patients with allergy may have associated subtle immune deficiencies.

Delayed maturation of the immune system

Recurrent infections are much less common in the school-age

child as immunological competence is approaching adult levels by this age. The natural immune defences (complement, neutrophils, local barriers) of newborn infants are reduced and T and B lymphocytes have not been stimulated and expanded by antigen exposure. Passive immunity (maternal IgG) provides some protection for the first six months. IgG and IgA levels including IgG2 and IgG4 subclasses are slow to develop and physiological hypogammaglobulinaemia persists for up to two years and in some cases for longer. See page 686 for age-related normal concentrations and ranges of IgG, IgM and IgA.

Secondary immune deficiency

The common causes are severe malnutrition and HIV infection. The nephrotic syndrome, splenectomy, prolonged steroid therapy, malignancy and cytotoxic drug therapy occur less frequently. AIDS leads to a progressive and irreversible immune deficiency and usually presents with recurrent severe infections, including diarrhoea. Other viral and parasitic infections such as measles and malaria often cause a temporary immunosuppression which enhances susceptibility to other infections.

Primary immune deficiencies

Primary immune deficiencies are rare and many are familial. Infections are usually more severe, do not respond well to treatment and the organisms are often atypical.

Antibody deficiency syndromes are more common than all the other primary immune deficiences combined. Because replacement therapy with Ig is relatively easy and effective, early diagnosis is important to prevent irreversible tissue damage, especially in the lungs.

Diagnosis

◆ Establish whether there are environmental, anatomical, allergic, nutritional or infective (e.g. HIV) reasons for recurrent infections.
◆ A family history, e.g. siblings or close relatives with severe or recurrent infections, may indicate an immunodeficiency syndrome.
◆ Measure serum IgG, IgM, IgA. Compare results to age and laboratory-matched normal values. Agammaglobulinaemia is

defined as an IgG of less than 2 g/l, or less than 1 g/l under a year of age. Hypogammaglobulinaemia is defined as an IgG greater than these levels but less than the normal range for age (for reference values, see page 686).

♦ Determine the total and differential white blood cell count. Neutropenia or lymphopenia are suggestive of severe primary or secondary immune deficiency.
♦ A positive Mantoux, Tine or Candida delayed hyper-sensitivity skin test indicates grossly normal cell-mediated immunity.

Management

General

♦ Identify and give attention to underlying factors, e.g. over-crowding, poor hygiene, anatomical abnormalities, allergy, undernutrition and causes of secondary immunodeficiency.
♦ Prescribe antibiotics for infection in full dosage for longer than usual periods, i.e. for two to three weeks in the presence of any of these underlying causes. Most useful antibiotics are AMOXYCILLIN or an antibiotic with equivalent antimicro-bial activity. See page 568.

Hypogammaglobulinaemia

This may be due to prolonged physiological hypogammaglobu-linaemia where specific therapy is not usually required or hered-itary factors. Intramuscular immunoglobulin (IMIg) 0,6 ml/kg every four weeks may be tried for three to six months. Prophy-lactic antibiotics for three to six months (e.g. AMOXYCILLIN) are an alternative treatment. If there is a response to IMIg treat-ment, long-term IVIg replacement therapy may be indicated and full immunological evaluation is required. Note that IMIg is painful and much less effective than IVIg. IVIg is expensive and its administration requires supervision.

IgA absent or low

Most patients with IgA deficiency are asymptomatic. If they do get recurrent infections, concomitant allergy or IgG subclass deficiency may be present. Management of allergy and three to six months of antibiotics (e.g. AMOXYCILLIN) or referral for investigation may be indicated.

Absolute agammaglobulinaemia

The only effective treatment is intravenous immunoglobulin (IVIg) replacement of 200-400 mg/kg/IV every four weeks. The patient should be referred for formal evaluation of immune functions.

Hypergammaglobulinaemia

Suspect chronic infection, especially HIV (see page 258).

Suspected primary immune deficiency

A positive family history of immunodeficiency, severe recurrent infections or persistent unusual infections require referral for full immunological evaluation.

Indications for IVIg therapy

There are three established uses in paediatrics:

◆ Replacement in IgG antibody deficiency disorders (IMIg and IVIg contains only IgG and no IgA or IgM) dosage 200-400 mg/kg/IV every four weeks.
◆ Kawasaki disease – within ten days of development of signs or symptoms to prevent coronary aneurysm formation. Dosage 2g/kg single dose.
◆ Chronic ITP in children. Most cases of childhood ITP resolve spontaneously. Treatment with IVIg may be indicated in the remainder but should be undertaken in a specialized paediatric haematology unit.

Adverse reactions to IVIg

Anaphylactic reactions are extremely rare and have been described in absolute IgA deficient patients with anti-IgA antibodies. Infusions should be given under the same supervision required for blood transfusions. Most side-effects (nausea, chills, headache, etc.) are related to the speed of infusion and the initial infusion rate should be ten drops per minute. If well tolerated this may be increased to 40 drops per minute. IVIg is expensive, but local production (Polygam, Natal Blood Transfusion Service) has reduced the cost. There is no risk of HIV or hepatitis B viruses transmission by IM or IV gammaglobulin preparations.

26 INFECTIOUS DISEASES[1]

G D Hussey

Acquired Immune Deficiency Syndrome (AIDS)

AIDS is a syndrome characterized by opportunistic infections and malignancies as a result of infection by the human immunodeficiency virus (HIV). More than 85% of children who are HIV positive are infected vertically – either antenatally but mainly during delivery. Children born to mothers who are HIV infected have a 20-40% chance of infection. The latter can also be acquired horizontally via infected blood or blood products or sexual practices. Breast milk is a less likely source of infection and thus breast-feeding of her infant by the HIV mother is encouraged in a developing country, depending on circumstances. Infection is not spread via eating utensils, touching, hugging, or kissing.

Clinical presentation

The majority of children with perinatally-acquired AIDS present by three years of age. The incubation period is usually four to six months.

The common presenting syndromes are as follows:

Wasting syndrome

Failure to thrive is usually associated with chronic or recurrent diarrhoeal disease, either as a result of the direct effect of HIV infection on the gastrointestinal tract or as a result of secondary opportunistic infection. The latter includes *cryptosporidium, cytomegalovirus,* other viruses and bacteria. Oropharyngeal or gastrointestinal candidiasis occurs frequently.

---

[1] See Table 26.2 page 275 for the incubation, prodromal and isolation periods of common infectious diseases and pages 276-7 for statutory notifiable diseases.

Persistent generalized lymphadenopathy

With or without hepatosplenomegaly and parotid enlargement.

Recurrent bacterial infections

These are of varying severity and include septicaemia, meningitis, pneumonia, otitis media, tonsillitis, cellulitis and urinary tract infections. The common causative organisms are *S. pneumoniae, H. influenzae* and Salmonella.

Pulmonary syndromes

Pneumocystis carinii pneumonia and lymphoid interstitial pneumonia (a possible result of chronic Epstein-Barr virus infection).

Neurological syndromes

Progressive encephalopathy, developmental delay or loss of motor milestones.

Opportunistic infections

These include *Pneumocystis carinii, Candida, Cytomegalovirus, Cryptosporidium, Toxoplasma gondii, Mycobacterium tuberculosis,* Herpes simplex and *Cryptococcus neoformans.*

Other manifestations

Rarely secondary malignancies (lymphoma and Kaposi's sarcoma), hepatitis, cardiomyopathy, and renal disease.

Diagnosis

World Health Organization criteria: suspect AIDS in a child if two major and two minor criteria are present.

Major criteria

Failure to thrive, persistent fever, chronic diarrhoea.

Minor criteria

Chronic cough, lymphadenopathy, recurrent infections, chronic dermatitis, oral candidiasis and mother HIV antibody positive.

The definitive diagnosis can be a problem. Many of the symptoms and signs of AIDS in children are similar to other common childhood conditions. In addition, a positive antibody

test in the first 15 months may be the result of passively transferred maternal antibodies. In this situation the diagnosis can be
confirmed by viral culture, or if there are clinical and immunological findings such as a decreased CD4 cell count, reversed
CD4:CD8 ratio and hypergammaglobulinaemia.

The ELISA test for antibody detection is most commonly
used for screening. Confirmatory tests include the Western Blot
(detects antibody to specific viral proteins) and Immunofluorescence Antibody test.

Management

The mainstay of therapy is general medical care; ongoing psychological and educational supportive care; counselling for the
child and family, and treatment of opportunistic infections.

Nutritional needs require particular attention.

Isolation

Children with AIDS should not be discriminated against when it
comes to their management in hospitals and in the community.
Isolation of such a patient from other patients, school, or day
care is only advised if the patient has bloody secretions such as
dysentery, severe ulcerative and bleeding oral or skin infections,
or if they exhibit unusually aggressive behaviour such as biting.

Immunizations

Children should be immunized in accordance with the standard
schedule except that BCG is not given to children with AIDS.

Treatment

Bacterial or opportunistic infections

Children with AIDS who present with fever or signs suggestive
of an opportunistic infection should be investigated appropriately and antibiotic therapy prescribed accordingly. Immunoglobulin in high intravenous doses (400 mg/kg monthly)
reduces episodes of infection and improves quality of life. It
should be used if resources permit. Recommended drugs are
prophylactic CO-TRIMOXAZOLE (TRIMETHOPRIM and
SULPHAMETHOXAZOLE) at a dose of 10 mg/kg/day of the
TRIMETHOPRIM component thrice-weekly to prevent *Pneumocystis carinii* pneumonia.

Antiretroviral therapy

Where resources permit, nucleoside analogues such as Zidovudine (AZT) can be used to treat patients with AIDS.

Chicken pox

A mild disease in normal children.

Clinical presentation

Presents with fever and a papular-vesicular eruption which commences on the trunk.

Complications

◆ Common: secondary skin sepsis.
◆ Rare: includes pneumonia, encephalitis and haemorrhagic lesions. These can be lethal in the immunocompromised.

Management

◆ Conservative, supportive and symptomatic.
◆ ACYCLOVIR 15 mg/kg/day IV for seven days is recommended for severe cases and for immunocompromised children with chicken pox.
◆ Human anti-Varicella Zoster (VZIG) 0,15 ml/kg (minimum 1 ml, maximum 5 ml) is recommended for:
  ◇ Susceptible, immunocompromised children within 96 hours after exposure to chicken pox.
  ◇ Newborns of mothers who developed chicken pox within five days before or two days after delivery.
  ◇ Newborns exposed postnatally to chicken pox.

Isolation

Infectious until lesions scab (usually ten to 14 days).

Cholera
Clinical presentation

An acute, usually water-borne, infectious disease caused by *Vibrio cholera*. It is characterized by profuse watery diarrhoea (rice-water stools) which leads to dehydration, shock and even death if not treated. The diagnosis can be confirmed by stool culture.

Management

◆ Vigorous fluid replacement and correction of electrolyte and acid base imbalance are required.
◆ TETRACYCLINE or CO-TRIMOXAZOLE for three days shortens the course of the disease. Killed cholera vaccine is of limited efficacy and is no longer recommended by WHO. New oral vaccines hold much greater promise.
◆ **Notify by telephone.**

Congenital syphilis

Clinical presentation

Usually manifests as a multisystem disease.

Early manifestations in infancy

Erythematous maculopapular rash (may be bullous), involving the palms and soles, hepatosplenomegaly with or without jaundice, mucopurulent nasal discharge (snuffles), fissures and mucous patches, pseudoparalysis of the limbs and rarely nephritis and pancreatitis.

Later manifestations

Interstitial keratitis, chorioretinitis, optic atrophy, deafness, Clutton's joints (effusions into the knee joints) and sabre tibia. Gummas in the nasal septum, palate, long bones and subcutaneous tissue. Neurodevelopmental delay.

Late stigmata

Saddle nose, rhagades, Hutchinson's teeth (upper permanent central incisors are peg-shaped with a central notch), bossing of forehead and rarely neurosyphilis.

Diagnosis

◆ Suspect if the mother has syphilis or a positive serology. A negative test early in pregnancy does not exclude the diagnosis, as the mother may have been infected later in pregnancy.
◆ Neonate (first three days): total IgM or rheumatoid factor raised.

- ◆ Screening tests: WR, VDRL, Kahn.*
- ◆ Specific tests: FTA-ABS, TPHA.*
- ◆ Radiography of long bones. See page 462.

Management

Infants with congenital syphilis may have central nervous system involvement with normal CSF findings. PROCAINE PENICILLIN 50 000 U/kg/day IM for ten days is recommended. BENZATHINE PENICILLIN does not produce sufficiently high concentrations in the CSF to eradicate the organisms.

Diphtheria

The disease is caused by *Corynebacterium diphtheria*.

Clinical presentation

Commonly presents in three stages.

Membrane

Usually oropharyngeal, but may be on conjunctiva or the skin and associated with toxaemia. May present with stridor. Cutaneous diphtheria is rarely associated with toxaemia.

Myocarditis

Beginning after ten days: arrythmias, shock, hypotension, hypertension or failure.

Motor neuropathy

Beginning in the third week. Palatal, ocular, pharyngeal, respiratory muscles and limb involvement occurs in sequence.

Complications

Bronchopneumonia, severe respiratory distress, cardiac failure, nephritis and paralysis.

---

*WR	= Wassermann reaction
VDRL	= Venereal Diseases Research Laboratory
FTA-ABS	= Fluorescent treponema antibody test – absorbed
TPHA	= Treponema pallidium haemagglutination test

Diagnosis

Clinical features. Smear and culture of the membrane or lesions.

Management

PENICILLIN or ERYTHROMYCIN for 14 days. Antitoxin 20 000-100 000 U (depending on severity) must be administered intravenously as soon as the diagnosis is suspected. Great care is required with the administration of antitoxin as it can cause severe reactions in individuals sensitized to horse serum products. Tests for sensitivity include 1:10 antitoxin dilution for conjunctival testing or 1:100 dilution for intradermal testing.

Isolation

Until three consecutive throat swabs are negative.

Advice

Any membrane of the pharynx should be considered as diphtheretic until proven otherwise.

Erythema infectiosum, fifth disease

See Table 26.1.

Gonococcal infections

Neonatal infection

Management

See page 353.

Infections beyond infancy

These are usually due to sexual abuse or they may occur in sexually active adolescents. Vulvovaginitis, urethritis, pelvic inflammatory disease, bacteraemia, arthritis and meningitis may occur.

Treatment

AMOXYCILLIN 50 mg/kg and PROBENECID 25 mg/kg as a single oral dose. For penicillinase-producing *Neisseria gonorrhoea* infections, CEFTRIAXONE 125 mg IM in a single dose (250 mg if older than nine years) or SPECTINOMYCIN 40 mg/kg as a single IM dose are recommended.

Table 26.1 Important childhood erythematous exanthems

Disease	Agent	Exanthem	Other features	Main complications
Erythema infectiosum	Parvovirus B19	'Slapped cheeks', maculopapular rash on the trunk and extremities, becomes lace-like.	Generally well, mild flu-like symptoms.	Rare – arthritis and encephalitis.
Infectious mono-nucleosis	Epstein-Barr virus	Maculopapular rash. Accentuated by AMPICILLIN.	Fever, pharyngitis, adenopathy, splenomegaly.	Purpura, haemolytic anaemia, jaundice myopericarditis, meningo-encephalitis.
Kawasaki syndrome See page 267	Unknown	Polymorphous rash. Morbilliform, urticarial, scarlatiniform.	Fever, cervical adenopathy, conjunctivitis. Skin changes on hands and feet. Oral and lip mucosal changes.	Myopericarditis, urethritis, meningitis, uveitis, arthritis, diarrhoea, hepatitis.
Measles See page 268	Measles virus (Paramyxo-virus)	Diffuse maculopapular rash with coalescence starting on the face; staining and desquamation after five days.	High fever, Koplik's spots, conjunctivitis, photophobia, media, coryza and cough.	Diarrhoea, encephalitis, croup, pneumonia, otitis media, blindness.
Meningococcaemia	*Neisseria meningitidis*	Petechial or purpuric rash. Rarely macular or papular, erythematous.	Fever and irritability.	Meningitis, coma, shock.

Disease	Agent	Exanthem	Other features	Main complications
Roseola infantum	Herpes virus 6	Discrete pink macular rash on the trunk, face and proximal limbs.	Preceding fever for three to four days, which settles when rash appears.	Febrile convulsions.
Rubella	Rubella virus (Togavirus)	Discrete maculopapular rash starting on the face, lasting one to three days.	Mild fever, malaise, sub-occipital and post-auricular adenopathy.	Rare – arthritis, encephalitis, thrombocytopenia.
Scarlet fever	Group A β-haem streptococcus	Punctate erythematous rash. Red sandpapery appearance with flushed cheeks. Circumoral pallor.	Tonsillo-pharyngitis, fever, strawberry tongue.	Myocarditis, nephritis, rheumatic fever.
Toxic shock syndrome	*Staphylococcus aureus* (TSST-1)	Diffuse macular erythroderma. Peripheral desquamation later.	High fever, hypotension and myalgia.	Hepatitis, renal failure, thrombocytopenia, stupor or coma and diarrhoea.
'Viral'	Coxsackie and ECHO viruses	Variable rash: macular, papular, petechial.	Fever headache, myalgia.	Meningitis, encephalitis, pneumonia, diarrhoea.

Bacteraemia, arthritis and meningitis must be treated with CEFTRIAXONE 50 mg/kg/day for seven, 14 and 28 days respectively.

Kawasaki syndrome

Clinical features

An acute, febrile, self-limiting exanthematous multisystem disease of unknown infectious aetiology. It occurs predominantly in children less than five years old.

Complications

Life-threatening cardiac complications are common. These include coronary artery aneurysms, myocarditis, pericarditis and arrythmias. Others include: uveitis, diarrhoea, urethritis, meningitis and arthritis.

Diagnosis

A diagnosis requires that five of the following six criteria are met:

♦ fever lasting for more than four days;
♦ polymorphous exanthemata;
♦ bilateral conjunctival congestion;
♦ changes of extremities such as indurative oedema, red palms and soles or peripheral desquamation;
♦ cervical adenopathy;
♦ changes of oral cavity such as reddening and fissuring of lips, strawberry tongue or injection of oral cavity.

Characteristic peripheral desquamation occurs between days 10 and 20 of the illness.

Laboratory findings include: thrombocytosis, leucocytosis, anaemia, and elevated acute phase reactants, IgE, IgM and C3.

Management

ASPIRIN 100 mg/kg/day in four divided doses for two weeks followed by low dose 5 mg/kg/day for four to six weeks. IV gammaglobulin 400 mg/kg/day for four days.

Warning

Steroids are not recommended.

Measles

Clinical presentation

The prodrome lasts for three to four days and is characterized by high fever, coryza, conjunctivitis, cough and Koplik spots. Maculopapular rash (initially discrete and later confluent) begins at the end of the prodrome. It first appears behind the ears and then spreads to the rest of the body. The rash begins to fade after day 5 and is followed by post-measles staining and desquamation of the skin.

Infectious period

From the start of the prodrome until about five days after the rash has appeared.

Complications

Pneumonia as a sequela is a major cause of death and is usually due to secondary adenovirus, herpes virus or bacterial infections. Croup can be life-threatening and diarrhoeal disease is frequently debilitating. Other complications include otitis media, corneal ulceration and, rarely, acute encephalitis, nephritis, myocarditis, hepatitis and ileocolitis. Recovery following acute measles may be prolonged for many weeks and even months, and is characterized by failure to thrive, recurrent infections and persistent pneumonia and diarrhoea.

Subacute sclerosing panencephalitis (SSPE) is a rare long-term complication of measles. It is characterized by progressive behavioural and intellectual deterioration and bizarre neurological symptom complexes. CSF measles antibody titres are excessively high.

Diagnosis

Essentially clinical. It can be confirmed serologically. A simple bedside diagnostic test is to examine a buccal or conjunctival smear stained with Haemotoxylin and Eosin for the presence of giant cells.

Management

There is no specific therapy for measles. Management is therefore supportive. Vitamin A therapy (200 000 IU orally on two successive days) significantly reduces morbidity and mortality.

ACYCLOVIR is recommended for all children with herpes stomatitis and for children with post-measles croup (which is frequently due to herpes virus infection). Notify the relevant authorities.

Advice

Exposed susceptible children, particularly those who are immunocompromised, may benefit from human anti-measles immunoglobulin 0,25 ml/kg IM and 0,5 ml/kg for immunocompromised children (maximum 15 ml) if given within five days of exposure.

Immunize all children, six months and older, admitted to hospital to prevent nosocomially acquired measles.

Do not refer uncomplicated cases of measles to hospital.

Meningococcal infections

Infection with *Neisseria meningitidis* usually presents as meningitis and/or septicaemia. See page 114 for meningococcal meningitis. Occasionally as arthritis, pneumonia, myocarditis, endophthalmitis, pneumonia or chronic meningococcaemia. **Notify by telephone.**

Clinical presentation

Abrupt onset of fever, chills, malaise, prostration. The former, when associated with a petechial, or less commonly with a urticarial or maculopapular rash, is highly suggestive of meningococcal infection. Neck stiffness may or may not be present. In fulminant cases, purpura, dessiminated intravacular coagulation and shock may be followed by coma and death within hours.

Management

Acute treatment

♦ Meningitis: see page 114. Septicaemia: see page 115. Shock: see pages 115-6.
♦ Give DEXAMETHASONE 0,6 mg/kg/day in four divided doses IV for the first four days of antibiotic treatment or until the patient is stable.
♦ RIFAMPICIN prophylaxis (see below) is recommended prior to the discharge of the patient from hospital.
♦ Notify by telephone.

Exposed contacts

Household members are at increased risk and may be given RIFAMPICIN prophylaxis for two days. Daycare Centre contacts and close contacts in overcrowded hostels should be treated in the same manner. Normal school and work contacts should not be treated. Hospital contacts should only be treated if intensive and intimate exposure has occurred, e.g. giving mouth-to-mouth resuscitation. High-risk contacts of a patient with meningococcal meningitis or septicaemia should show clinically apparent signs and symptoms within five days in 50% of cases.

Prevention

Outbreaks in closed communities (e.g. hostels) are best controlled by administering antimicrobials that reduce meningococcal carriage. Sulphonamides are not useful, because many strains of meningococci are sulphonamide resistant. RIFAMPICIN is the drug of choice.

◆ **Adults:** RIFAMPICIN 600 mg twice a day for two days.
◆ **Children:** one month to 12 years of age. RIFAMPICIN 10 mg/kg twice a day for two days.
◆ **Infants:** under one month of age. RIFAMPICIN 5 mg/kg twice a day for two days.

CEFTRIAXONE 125 mg IM as a single dose (250 mg if over 12 years) may be given in situations where RIFAMPICIN is contra-indicated.

Poliomyelitis

Only about 1% of infected individuals will develop the disease. The disease is being targeted by the WHO for eradication by the year 2000. To this end all suspect cases must be notified.

Clinical presentation

Abortive poliomyelitis

Most common presentation. Presents with minor symptoms including fever, pharyngitis and headache.

Nonparalytic poliomyelitis

Presents as a viral meningitis and resolves within a week.

Paralytic poliomyelitis

The hallmark is an asymmetrical lower motor neurone flaccid paralysis.

Complications

Respiratory failure, mild hypertension, gastric dilatation and malaena.

Diagnosis

The diagnosis is clinical and confirmed by culture of the polio virus from the faeces and the throat, and rarely from the CSF.

Management

Supportive with strict bed rest in the first week following onset of paralysis. Intensive physiotherapy after seven to ten days. Frequent assessment for paralysis of the muscles of respiration and ventilatory support.

Notify all suspect cases of poliomyelitis. The current WHO definition of the disease is 'a suspected case of poliomyelitis is any child under five years of age with acute flaccid paralysis (including Guillian-Barré syndrome) for which no other cause can be identifed or a paralytic illness at any age when polio-myelitis is suspected.' Faecal specimens for polio virus culture must be sent for all cases of suspected poliomyelitis.

Rabies

Infection with rabies virus follows a bite by a rabid domestic or wild animal. Unprovoked attacks by animals in endemic areas are an indication for commencing therapy. Incubation periods can vary from four to 90 days.

Clinical presentation

Patients with furious rabies present with hydrophobia, spasms, convulsions, and periods of alternating excitation and lucidity. Paralytic rabies presents with progressive flaccid paralysis and sensory disturbances.

Diagnosis

Infection in animals can be diagnosed by the demonstration of virus-specific fluorescence in brain tissue.

Management

Treatment

♦ Human rabies immunoglobulin (HRIG) 20 IU/kg body weight – one half is infiltrated into the tissues surrounding the wound, especially in close proximity. The other half is given by deep IM injection away from the lesion. Any immunoglobulin left over after administering the calculated dose may be run into the wound after cleansing.

♦ Human diploid cell strain virus (HDCSV) IM in the deltoid region on days 0, 3, 7, 14, 28 and 90.

♦ Treatment can be stopped if the animal remains healthy for ten days or more or if the immunofluorescence test of the animal brain is negative.

♦ Prescribe PROCAINE PENICILLIN 50 000 U/kg/day for ten days.

Prevention

See page 253.

Roseola infantum

See Table 26.1.

Rubella

See Table 26.1.

Scarlet fever

See Table 26.1.

Tetanus

A disease caused by tetanospasmin, a neurotoxin produced by *Clostridium tetani*.

Clinical presentation

Characterized by muscular rigidity and spasms. Tetanus of the neonate results from infection of the umbilical stump. It presents within the first week with inability to suck, trismus, rigidity, spasms and convulsions. Susceptible older children usually acquire infection following contamination of wounds and may present with tetanus or rarely with local or cephalic tetanus.

Management

◆ Admit the patient to an Intensive Care Unit.
◆ Neutralize unbound toxin. Administer human anti-tetanus immunoglobulin (HTIG): newborn 500 U IM and children 2 000 U IM.
◆ Remove the source of tetanospasmin: wound debridement and PENICILLIN.
◆ Control of spasms and rigidity: DIAZEPAM and PHENO-BARBITONE or CHLORPROMAZINE. Adjust dosages according to the clinical response.
◆ Tracheostomy and IPPV: severe cases with respiratory failure or compromise.
◆ Control of fluid and electrolyte balance. Provide adequate nutritional support. Nurse in quiet environment.

Prevention

◆ Immunize susceptible pregnant mother with tetanus vaccine: two doses of 0,5 ml IM six to eight weeks apart. A third dose is given six months after the first, with two boosters every five years or during subsequent pregnancies.
◆ Prophylactic HTIG for incompletely immunized children with severe wounds: 75 U if under five years, 125 U for five to ten years and 250 U for over ten year-olds.
◆ Incompletely immunized children with clean, minor wounds should be given tetanus toxoid.
◆ After recovery from tetanus, children should be immunized, as the disease does not confer immunity.

Typhoid fever

Caused by *Salmonella typhi*.

Clinical presentation

Protean manifestations include diarrhoea, pneumonia, unexplained fever, acute abdomen, meningitis, jaundice and splenomegaly. Constipation and rose spots are rare findings in children.

Management

◆ CHLORAMPHENICOL or AMOXYCILLIN for 21 days.
◆ Patients should be isolated until three negative consecutive stools have been passed following therapy.
◆ **Notify by telephone.**

Whooping cough

This is caused by *Bordetella pertussis* and on occasions also by *B. parapertussis.*

Clinical presentation

Patients present with a catarrhal stage followed by paroxysmal cough, whoop, cyanosis and apnoea. Young infants and older children and adults may not present with the classical symptoms.

Complications

Include persistent cough (100-day cough), convulsions due to hypoxaemia or encephalopathy, pneumonia and atelectasis.

Diagnosis

Clinical. Absolute lymphocytosis supports the clinical diagnosis. Lymphocytosis may be absent in infants, in partially immunized infants and in those with an atypical illness.

The differential diagnosis includes paroxysmal cough due to *Chlamydia trachomatis,* tuberculous lymphadenopathy and viral infections.

Management

Young infants and those with severe disease should be hospitalized. ERYTHROMYCIN 50 mg/kg/day in four divided doses for 14 days is necessary to eradicate the infection and to prevent relapse. Unless given during the catarrhal stage, it has no ameliorating effect on the course of the disease. In cases with severe cough SALBUTAMOL 0,6 mg/kg/day in four divided doses to counteract the β_2 blockade effect of pertussis toxin and steroids may be helpful. CHLORPROMAZINE may also be tried in inpatients.

Advice

Patients are non-infectious after five days of therapy with ERYTHROMYCIN.

Although the usefulness of chemoprophylaxis has not been well demonstrated, a 14-day course of ERYTHROMYCIN and CO-TRIMOXAZOLE for close contacts aged less than one year and for immunized close contacts under seven years may be beneficial.

Table 26.2 Incubation periods

	Incubation period	Prodromal period	Isolation period[1]
Short			
Gastro-enteritis	One to seven days	Nil	Until diarrhoea stops
Diphtheria	One to seven days	Nil	Until three throat swabs are negative (MC)
Influenza	One to seven days	Nil	Until apyrexial and feeling better
Meningo-coccal disease	One to seven days	Nil	Two days from start of treatment (MC)
Scarlet fever	One to seven days	Nil	Until rash fades and desquamation starts
Intermediate			
Measles	Seven to 14 days	Three to seven days	Five days from start of rash (seven days)
Pertussis	Seven to 14 days	Up to 21 days; usually five to seven days	Four to six weeks or for first two days of treatment with ERYTHROMYCIN (MC)
Polio	Seven to 14 days	Three to 36 days	Ten days (MC)
Tetanus	Seven to 14 days	Nil	Not required
Typhoid	Seven to 14 days	Nil. Diagnosis difficult in early stages of disease	Until three consecutive stool cultures are negative (MC)
Long			
Chicken pox	14-21 days	Nil to two days	Until lesions crusted, usually five to seven days (14 days)
Hepatitis A	15-40 days	Two to five days	Seven days from onset of jaundice (seven days)

Hepatitis B	60-180 days	Two to five days	Until no longer jaundiced
Mumps	14-21 days	Nil to one day	Until swelling subsides (nine days)
Rubella	14-21 days	Nil to two days	Nil, except from pregnant women for approximately seven days

[1] Information in parentheses refers to when the patient may return to a teaching institution in terms of regulation R2438 (30 October 1987) of the 1977 Health Act. MC refers to submission of a medical certificate and figures refer to the number of days after which a patient may return to a teaching institution.

Statutory notifiable diseases[1]

Acute flaccid paralysis
Acute rheumatic fever
*Anthrax
*Brucellosis
*Cholera
Congenital syphilis
*Diphtheria
*Food poisoning (out-breaks of more than four persons)
Haemophilus influenzae type B infections
*Haemorrhagic fevers of Africa (Congo fever, Dengue fever, Ebola fever, Lassa fever, Marburg fever, Rift Valley fever)
Lead poisoning
Legionellosis
Leprosy
Malaria
Measles
*Meningococcal infections
*Paratyphoid fever
*Plague
*Poisoning from any agricultural or stock remedy registered in terms of the Fertilizers, Farm Feeds Agricultural Remedies and Stock Remedies Act 1, 1947 (Act No. 36 of 1947)
*Poliomyelitis
*Rabies (specify whether human case or human contact)

[1] See page 319 for medico-legal aspects.

Tetanus

Tetanus neonatorum

Trachoma

Tuberculosis

(i) Pulmonary and other forms, except cases diagnosed solely on basis of clinical signs and symptoms.

(ii) In the case of any child younger than five years with a significant reaction following tuberculin testing.

*Typhoid fever

*Typhus fever (epidemic louse-borne typhus fever, endemic flea-borne typhus fever)

Viral hepatitis A, B, non-A, non-B and undifferentiated

Whooping cough

*Yellow fever

Source: *Government Gazette* No. R. 328 of 22 February, 1991

Notifiable diseases change from time to time. Remind yourself of new notifiable diseases by adding them to the above list.

Those diseases marked with an asterisk (*) must be notified immediately by telephone to the Medical Officer of Health for the area.

27 INJURIES

D H Bass, A J W Millar, J C Peter, H Rode
and S Cywes

Prevention

See Appendix 5, page 687.

Management of major injuries

Aims

Primary Survey

◆ Identify and correct life-threatening abnormalities.
◆ Resuscitate and stabilize vital functions.

Secondary Survey

◆ Determine full extent of all injuries.
◆ Definitive treatment in order of priority.

General principles

Successful management of the injured child requires:

◆ an organized approach combining diagnosis and treatment;
◆ a designated team leader who directs management and identifies priorities; and
◆ frequent review and documentation of the patient's response to treatment.

Primary survey and resuscitation

Resuscitation is described in Chapter 1. Where the injured child is concerned, bear the following in mind.

Airway and breathing

Impaired ventilation may be due to:

◆ aspiration, e.g. vomitus, foreign body;
◆ brain or spinal cord injury;

◆ chest injury, e.g. tension pneumothorax, flail segment; or
◆ dilatation of the stomach causing splinting of the diaphragm.

Avoid unnecessary movement of head until neck injury has been excluded.

Warning

When ventilation is assisted in a patient with chest injury, it is mandatory to insert a prophylactic intercostal drain on the side of the injury. See page 453.

Circulation

As soon as venous access is obtained, draw blood for:

◆ cross-matching, full blood count, urea and electrolytes, serum amylase (pancreatic injury);
◆ arterial blood gases.

Management

◆ Limit blood loss.
◆ Splint fractures.
◆ Elevate the bleeding limb.
◆ Apply direct pressure with a clean dressing (no tourniquets).

Circulatory shock following injury

Consider possible cause:

◆ concealed haemorrhage: usually abdominal;
◆ blunt chest injury: cardiac contusion, tension pneumothorax;
◆ spinal cord injury: present with a low blood pressure and warm peripheries; and
◆ brainstem injury: usually a terminal event.

Never attribute shock to minor or moderate head injury or bony injuries alone.

Failure to respond to fluid resuscitation

◆ Exclude non-haemorrhagic chest injury (tension pneumothorax, cardiac contusion).
◆ Exclude exsanguinating intra-abdominal haemorrhage requiring urgent laparotomy.

Acute gastric dilatation

Common in head, abdominal and multiple injuries. It is aggravated by assisted ventilation and causes respiratory embarrassment by splinting of the diaphragm. Aspiration of gastric contents is a hazard.

♦ Decompress the stomach.
♦ **Pass a nasogastric tube at an early stage.** See page 451.

Secondary survey

♦ Remove all clothing to avoid missing injuries.
♦ Avoid excessive heat loss by using ordinary blankets or warming blankets or overhead heaters.
♦ Monitor vital signs.
   Provide adequate analgesia (see Chapter 3).
♦ **AMPLE.** Obtain a brief history from a guardian or ambulance staff with reference to:
   A   Allergies.
   M   Medication. Past and present.
   P   Past medical history.
   L   Last meal, time of.
   E   Events surrounding the injury.

Head and neck

Cardinal features

♦ Soft-tissue injuries to face and scalp.
♦ CSF leak or bleeding from nose or ears.
♦ Level of consciousness: see Glasgow Coma Scale, page 665.
♦ Pupils: size and reaction to light.
♦ Limbs: movement, sensation and reflexes.

Urgent investigations

♦ Arterial blood gases if the level of consciousness (LOC) is decreased.
♦ X-ray cervical spine if unconscious or if there is a limited range of movement. A normal X-ray does not preclude spinal cord injury.
♦ Skull X-rays if fractures are suspected clinically.

Ominous features

Indications for a CT brain scan:

♦ Glasgow coma score of 12 or less.
♦ Generalized or focal seizures.
♦ Any focal neurological deficit.
♦ Abnormal flexor or extensor posturing.
♦ Progressive irritability or restlessness.
♦ Decreasing LOC or failure to improve over a 24 hour period.
♦ Cervical tenderness or limited neck movement.
♦ Evidence of spinal shock manifested by a low blood pressure, warm peripheries and absent anal sphincter tone.
♦ Depressed LOC and a skull fracture.

Management priorities

♦ Ensure adequate oxygenation, perfusion.
♦ CT brain scan if any ominous features noted.
♦ Abort seizures with rectal DIAZEPAM 0,2 mg/kg.
♦ Intubate and hyperventilate if coma scale <8.
♦ Limit IV fluids to two-thirds of daily maintenance for age. See pages 208-9.
♦ Early craniotomy or craniectomy is indicated only for intra-cranial haematoma, or compound depressed skull fractures.
♦ Spinal cord injury: decompress stomach and bladder. Institute assisted ventilation if the chest is involved. Log-roll.

Thorax

Cardinal features

♦ Visible rib-cage injuries, contusions, abrasions.
♦ Difficulty with respiration with cyanosis, dyspnoea, tachypnoea.
♦ Abnormalities of chest wall movement.
♦ Unilateral dullness or decreased air entry.
♦ Position of mediastinum determined by palpation of the trachea and the apex beat.
♦ Presence and quality of the heart sounds. Dull or muffled sounds indicate myocardial contusion or pericardial tamponade.

Urgent investigations

♦ Arterial blood gases.
♦ AP chest X-ray to exclude collections, contusions and the position and contour of the diaphragm.
♦ ECG and cardiac iso-enzymes.

Ominous features

◆ Progressive dyspnoea and mediastinal shift from a tension pneumothorax or ruptured diaphragm.
◆ Subcutaneous emphysema caused by rupture of a bronchus, the trachea, or the oesophagus.
◆ Circulatory shock that is resistant to resuscitation due to cardiac injury or tamponade.

Management priorities

◆ Ensure adequate oxygenation.
◆ Urgent drainage of large intrapleural collections.
◆ Adequate analgesia for multiple rib fractures.
◆ Ventilation for flail segment and respiratory failure.
◆ Urgent surgical repair of a ruptured diaphragm.
◆ Frequent chest physiotherapy for atelectasis.

Abdomen

Cardinal features

◆ Haemodynamic status, e.g. shock, anaemia.
◆ Abdominal wall bruising, abrasions, distension.
◆ Focal or generalized guarding, tenderness.
◆ Presence or absence of bowel sounds.
◆ Microscopic or macroscopic haematuria.
◆ Pelvic tenderness, induration or rectal bleeding.

Urgent investigations

◆ Full blood count, serum amylase (pancreatic injury).
◆ Chest X-ray, abdominal X-ray. Erect or shoot-through.
◆ Suspected urinary tract injury: intravenous pyelography (IVP) and urethrogram.

Ominous features

◆ Hypotension and abdominal distension: haemorrhage from liver, spleen.
◆ Increasing tenderness and/or peritonism: perforated viscus.
◆ Persistent macroscopic haematuria: renal injury.
◆ Failure to pass urine despite adequate resuscitation: injury to bladder, urethra.

Management priorities

◆ Frequent, regular clinical review.

◆ *Urgent laparotomy indicated for*
  ◇ Peritonitis or pneumoperitoneum (ruptured hollow viscus).
  ◇ Massive or ongoing haemorrhage requiring >40 ml/kg blood transfusion within 24 hours.
  ◇ Suspected renal pedicle injury.

Limbs and bony injuries

Cardinal features

◆ Pain, deformity, swelling.
◆ Limitation of movement.
◆ Features suggesting congenital bone disease, e.g. osteogenesis imperfecta.
◆ Distal neurovascular status, i.e. perfusion, muscular movements and sensation.
◆ Related soft-tissue wounds indicating compound fractures.

Urgent investigations

◆ X-ray of the affected limb in two planes. Always include joints above and below the fracture.
◆ Full blood count and ESR for suspected non-traumatic conditions such as osteitis and septic arthritis.

Ominous features

◆ Any sign of ischaemia distal to the fracture.
◆ Pain, swelling, pain on passive extension distal to the fracture: consider a compartment syndrome.
◆ Unstable pelvic fracture: exclude bladder, urethral or rectal injury by cysto-urethrogram and sigmoidoscopy.

Management priorities

◆ **Early reduction and immobilization** of fractures.
◆ **Early debridement** of soft tissue wound with IV antibiotic cover in compound fractures.
◆ **On-table angiography** for suspected vascular injury, reduction and immobilization of bony fracture followed by vascular repair.
◆ **Urgent fasciotomy** of all muscular compartments affected in suspected compartment syndrome.

The child and family

◆ Communicate openly and frequently.

◆ Avoid ill-founded optimism or prognoses.
◆ Provide the best emotional support possible.

Management of minor injuries

Simple lacerations

◆ Clean and debride meticulously.
◆ Provide adequate local anaesthesia (1-2% LIGNOCAINE).
◆ Close in layers without tension.
◆ Interrupted monofilament sutures to skin.
◆ Routine anti-tetanus prophylaxis with tetanus toxoid 0,5 ml IM.

Fingertip injuries

◆ Preserve maximal possible length.
◆ Principles as for simple lacerations.
  ◇ Avulsed fingertip: clean, dress with paraffin gauze and allow to granulate.
  ◇ Exposed bone: cut back to allow soft-tissue coverage.

Tongue lacerations

Repair under general anaesthetic if there is profuse bleeding; if the full thickness of tongue is involved; or if the child is unable to suck or feed.
  Use absorbable sutures.

Bites

◆ Most animal bites should be cleaned and sutured primarily.
◆ Neglected bites or those below the knee should be debrided and allowed to granulate.
◆ Consider the possibility of rabies and vaccinate if appropriate. See page 253.
◆ Indications for antibiotics: clinical evidence of sepsis or human bites (PENICILLIN).

Foreign bodies

◆ Soft-tissues: remove wherever possible.
◆ Inhaled: remove with bronchoscopy.
◆ Ingested: remove if lodged in the oesophagus, otherwise allow to pass *per rectum*. Intervention only for symptoms and signs of obstruction or perforation.

◆ Alkaline disc batteries: remove if in oesophagus. If in stomach or beyond, monitor progress by daily X-ray. Evacuation from stomach may be encouraged by oral MAGNESIUM SULPHATE and METOCLOPRAMIDE.

28 MALARIA AND PARASITIC DISEASES

M A Kibel

Malaria

Antimalarial medications available in southern Africa, and their dosages, are shown in Table 28.1. In South Africa CHLOROQUINE remains the preferred drug for both prophylaxis and treatment, but it must be born in mind that high grade CHLOROQUINE resistance is now very common across Africa. (See Table 28.2.)

Table 28.1 Available antimalarial medications

CHLOROQUINE SULPHATE (Nivaquine), CHLOROQUINE PHOSPHATE	Tablets each contain 150 mg of CHLOROQUINE base Syrup 5 ml = 0,33 tablet CHLOROQUINE PHOSPHATE injection contains 40 mg/ml.
QUININE	QUININE SULPHATE tablets 300 mg QUININE DIHYDROCHLORIDE injection 300 mg/ml.
PYRIMETHAMINE (Daraprim)	PYRIMETHAMINE tablets 25 mg Elixir 6,25 mg/5 ml This preparation is now never used on its own because of resistance.
PYRIMETHAMINE AND DAPSONE (Maloprim)	No longer recommended.
PYRIMETHAMINE AND SULFADOXINE (Fansidar)	PYRIMETHAMINE (25 mg) and SULFADOXINE (500 mg base) tablets
PRIMAQUINE PHOSPHATE (Primaquine)	Tablets 26 mg (approximately equal to 15 mg base). Available on special request from ICI Pharmaceuticals
PROGUANIL (Paludrine)	Tablets 100 mg
MEFLOQUINE (Lariam)	Tablets 250 mg

Prophylaxis

Protection against mosquito bites

Chemoprophylaxis is never completely protective and resistance to **all** available agents is increasing. Measures to prevent mosquito bites are therefore of prime importance. High risk groups (especially pregnant women, infants and young children) should if possible not enter highly endemic areas. **Protective measures can reduce risk.** Anopheles mosquitoes have nocturnal breeding habits, so be particularly careful between dusk and dawn. Exposure outside can be reduced by wearing clothing that adequately covers arms and legs. Repellant lotions and sprays can be used. The use of mosquito nets, and screening of windows and doors are especially important.

Chemoprophylaxis   2/1/6

This should preferably be commenced two weeks before entering a malarial area, continued once a week while in the area and for six weeks after leaving. If possible a test dose should be given one week before to assess tolerance of the drug or drugs. The choice and use of medications to prevent malaria remains a controversial issue as patterns of CHLOROQUINE resistance are changing rapidly. The current state of resistance should always be ascertained before entering a country or region. Table 28.2 shows suggested choices, and Table 28.3 dosages.

Prophylaxis during pregnancy

Pregnant travellers to malarious areas may take CHLORO-QUINE or CHLOROQUINE plus PROGUANIL with safety. PYRIMETHAMINE- and DAPSONE-containing preparations and MEFLOQUINE are not recommended.

Note

CHLOROQUINE may affect the taste of breast milk.

Prophylaxis in infancy

Infants under six weeks should not be given prophylaxis. Care should be taken not to overdose infants; they are especially susceptible to CHLOROQUINE toxicity.

Table 28.2 Choice of prophylactic medication

Areas with low CHLOROQUINE resistance (<1%)	CHLOROQUINE alone. This remains the first choice.
Areas of moderate CHLOROQUINE resistance (5-30%)	CHLOROQUINE plus PROGUANIL; or MEFLOQUINE. Give supply of Fansidar for self-treatment only if medical facilities are not immediately available. To be given as follows:

0-2 months: not recommended

5-10 kg:	½ tablet
11-20 kg:	1 tablet
21-30 kg:	1½ tablets
31-45 kg:	2 tablets
>45 kg:	3 tablets

High CHLOROQUINE resistance (>30%)	CHLOROQUINE plus PROGUANIL; or MEFLOQUINE or DOXYCYLINE for adults and children over eight years. Give supply of Fansidar, to be started should fever develop (dosages as above).

Table 28.3 Recommended dosages for prophylaxis

Age	CHLOROQUINE (Nivaquine) once weekly	PROGUANIL (Paludrine) daily	MEFLOQUINE (Larium) once weekly
0-6 months	2,5 ml	0,25 tab	not recommended
7-12 months	5,0 ml	0,25 tab	not recommended
1-3 years	7,5 ml	0,50 tab	not recommended
4-6 years	0,75 tab	0,75 tab	(15-19 kg) 0,25 tablet
7-10 years	1 tab	1 tab	(20-30 kg) 0,5 tablet
11-15 years	1,5 tabs	1,5 tabs	(31-45 kg) 0,75 tablet
16 years and over	2 tabs	2 tabs	(>45 kg) 1 tablet

Treatment

Mild to moderate attack (malaria contracted in CHLOROQUINE-sensitive area)

Management

CHLOROQUINE by mouth — dosage as per Table 28.4. May also be given by nasogastric tube to avoid the risk of vomiting.

Table 28.4 Chloroquine dosage

Age	First dose	Second dose (after six hours)	Second day	Third day
0-6 months	5 ml	2,5 ml	2,5 ml	2,5 ml
7-12 months	10 ml	5 ml	5 ml	5 ml
1-3 years	15 ml	7,5 ml	7,5 ml	7,5 ml
4-6 years	1,5 tabs	0,75 tab	0,75 tab	0,75 tab
7-10 years	2 tabs	1 tab	1 tab	1 tab
11-15 years	3 tabs	1,5 tabs	1,5 tabs	1,5 tabs
16 years and over	4 tabs	2 tabs	2 tabs	2 tabs

Note: 5 ml CHLOROQUINE syrup = 50 mg of CHLOROQUINE base
1 tablet = 150 mg of CHLOROQUINE base

Severe attack and cerebral malaria

Clinical presentation

Any of the following:

♦ any disturbance of consciousness except immediately after a seizure;
♦ hypoglycaemia (glucose <2,2 mmol/l);
♦ acidosis (pH <7,3);
♦ hyperparasitaemia – >20% in endemic areas
　◇ – >5% in non-immunes;
♦ renal failure;
♦ respiratory distress from
　◇ acidosis
　◇ pulmonary oedema
　◇ malaria lung (consider diagnosis);

◆ severe anaemia (Hb <5,0 g/dl); or
◆ persistent vomiting or diarrhoea.

Management

Give parenteral treatment, the options being CHLOROQUINE or QUININE.

◆ CHLOROQUINE IM 5 mg/kg. Repeat in six hours if necessary and follow by oral medication. CHLOROQUINE IV 5 mg/kg diluted to 0,5 mg/ml in saline at a rate not faster than 1 ml/minute, preferably with ECG and blood pressure monitoring. Repeat the dose in six to eight hours if necessary and follow with oral medication.
  OR
◆ QUININE DIHYDROCHLORIDE 10 mg/kg IV diluted to 0,5 mg/ml in saline at a rate not faster than 1 ml/minute with ECG and blood pressure monitoring. Repeat eight-hourly until the patient can take the drug orally.

Note

QUININE should be given as a first choice

◆ if the child has developed malaria while on prophylactic medication;
◆ if malaria has been contracted in a country of 'high' CHLOROQUINE resistance;
◆ if there has been no response to CHLOROQUINE within 36 hours of starting treatment.

In CHLOROQUINE-resistant cases, a second drug is recommended in addition to QUININE once parasitaemia is no longer detectable: CO-TRIMOXAZOLE, PYRIMETHAMINE/SULFADOXINE, or in children older than eight years, TETRACYCLINE.

Warning

CHLOROQUINE and QUININE should never be administered undiluted by the intravenous route

Ancillary management

◆ Watch for hypoglycaemia.
◆ Rehydration is important, but restrict fluids if unconscious.
◆ Anticonvulsants may be needed to terminate seizures.
◆ Low molecular weight DEXTRAN may be of value.

Plasmodium vivax, P. ovale and *P. malariae* **infections**

In the case of *Plasmodium vivax*, or *P. ovale* infections, PRIMAQUINE PHOSPHATE (0,3 mg/kg once daily for 14 days) must be added to eradicate the exo-erythrocytic stage after treating the acute attack with CHLOROQUINE. **G6PD deficiency is a contra-indication**. Discontinue if there is evidence of haemolysis, and do not use concurrently with SULFONAMIDES.

After the acute attack, continued prophylaxis is mandatory for those living in malarial areas.

Table 28.5 Important parasitic diseases
See Appendix 2 for dosages   Abbreviations: L = light infection H = heavy infection

Parasite or disease	Clinical features	Diagnosis	Treatment	Prevention
Amoebiasis *Entamoeba histolytica*	L: asymptomatic cyst passer. H: diarrhoea with mucus, blood and pus. Abdominal pain. Amoebic liver abscess.	Trophozoites in fresh stool or rectal smear. Cysts in stool. Complement fixation test.	METRONIDAZOLE or TINIDAZOLE	Good faecal disposal. Wash vegetables.
Bilharzia	Early: swimmer's itch; fever, urticaria, joint pains, tender liver. Later: nil or vague debility.	Eosinophilia; skin test; indirect fluorescent antibody test (IFAT); complement fixation test (CFT).	PRAZIQUANTEL or OXAMNIQUINE or NIRIDAZOLE	Short-term: avoid washing or swimming in infested streams, dams. Destroy snails with copper sulphate, Baylocide.
S. mansoni	Blood in stool; liver fibrosis or portal vein obstruction; ectopic sites – lungs, brain, spinal cord.	Viable ova in stool or rectal snip.		Long-term: provide rural communities with piped water toilets; cover or cement irrigation canals.

Parasite or disease	Clinical features	Diagnosis	Treatment	Prevention
S. haematobium	Terminal haematuria, obstructive uropathy; ectopic sites.	Viable ova in urine.	PRAZIQUANTEL or METRIPHONATE or NIRIDAZOLE	Educate community on disposal of excreta and cause of disease. Involve community in action.
S. mattheii (animal bilharzia)	Any of above; hybridizes with H. haematobium.	Ova in stool or urine.	PRAZIQUANTEL or METRIPHONATE or NIRIDAZOLE	
Giardiasis Giardia lamblia	L: asymptomatic cyst passers. H: foul-smelling loose stools. Malabsorption; abdominal pain.	Cysts, trophozoites in fresh stools. Duodenal aspiration. Enterotest capsule.	METRONIDAZOLE TINIDAZOLE	As for amoebiasis. Hygenic water supply.
Hookworm Ancylostoma duodenale	L: nil or mild abdominal discomfort. H: ground itch; severe anaemia; hypo-albuminaemia.	Eggs in faeces. Eosinophilia: mild to moderate.	MEBENDAZOLE or ALBENDAZOLE Treat anaemia.	Improve diet. Good faecal disposal. Wear shoes.

Parasite or disease	Clinical features	Diagnosis	Treatment	Prevention
Hydatid *Echinococcus granulosis*	Cysts in liver, lung, bone, brain. Symptoms depend on pressure effects.	Eosinophilia+++ Serological tests: CFT, IFAT, haemagglutination test (HT), enzyme-linked immunosorbent assay (ELISA), ARC5. Excision or biopsy of cyst.	Surgical	Prevent access of dogs to offal. Regular deworming of dogs twice-yearly with MEBENDAZOLE or PRAZIQUANTEL.
Pneumocystosis *Pneumocystis carinii*	Fever, cough, dyspnoea, lung infiltrates in immunocompromised host.	Sputum, bronchial brushings, lung biopsy.	CO-TRIMOXAZOLE or PENTAMIDINE	
Roundworm *Ascaris lumbricoides*	L: usually nil. Worms passed. H: cough, wheezing, pneumonitis; colic, obstruction. Worms in ectopic sites.	Worms in stool 10-15 cm long. Eggs in faeces. Eosinophilia high during migration.	PIPERAZINE or PYRANTEL or MEBENDAZOLE or ALBENDAZOLE	Good faecal disposal. Wash hands before eating food. Wash vegetables. Treat all children in household.

Parasite or disease	Clinical features	Diagnosis	Treatment	Prevention
Sandworm *Ancylostoma braziliensis/ caninum*	Intense itch, serpiginous lesions.	Physical features.	THIABENDAZOLE ointment (topical) or ALBENDAZOLE (oral)	Disposal of dog faeces. Avoid flesh contact with sand/soil.
Strongyloides stercoralis	L: Nil. H: Pruritic rash; may be recurrent. Bloody diarrhoea, anaemia (especially in immunodeficient individuals).	Eosinophilia +++ Larvae in fresh stool or duodenal fluid (Enterotest capsule).	MEBENDAZOLE or ALBENDAZOLE	As for hookworm. Special care with hygiene in immunocompromised children.
Tapeworm Beef tapeworm *Taenia saginata*	Usually none; may be mild abdominal symptoms.	Proglottid segments in faeces.	NICLOSAMIDE or MEBENDAZOLE or ALBENDAZOLE or PRAZIQUANTEL	Proper meat inspection for 'measles'. Adequate cooking. Freezing meat at –10°C for ten days kills the cysts.
Dwarf tapeworm *Hymenolepsis nana/diminuta*	L: Usually none. H: Auto infection – debility, weight loss.	Eggs in faeces.	NICLOSAMIDE or MEBENDAZOLE or ALBENDAZOLE or PRAZIQUANTEL	Proper meat inspection for 'measles'. Adequate cooking. Freezing meat at –10°C for ten days kills cysts.

Parasite or disease	Clinical features	Diagnosis	Treatment	Prevention
Pork tapeworm *Taenia solium*	Usually none; autoinfection Cysticercosis, brain, lungs, etc.	Proglottid segments in faeces. See page 326.	NICLOSAMIDE or MEBENDAZOLE or ALBENDAZOLE or PRAZIQUANTEL	As above. As above.
Thread or pinworm *Enterobius vermicularis*	L: nil. H: perianal itching. Insomnia. Vulvovaginitis.	Worm (10 mm) may be seen on perineum at night. Scotch tape preparation for ova.	MEBENDAZOLE or ALBENDAZOLE	Frequent washing. Keep finger-nails short. Treat all children in household.
Toxoplasmosis *Toxoplasma gondii*	**Congenital:** jaundice anaemia, hepato-splenomegaly, large or small head; retinopathy. **Acquired:** enlarged glands, spleen, myocarditis.	CFT, Dye test, IFAT.	PYRIMETHAMINE and SULFADIAZINE or SPIRAMYCIN (MCC permission).	Avoid contact with cat litter (especially during pregnancy).

Parasite or disease	Clinical features	Diagnosis	Treatment	Prevention
Visceral larva migrans *Toxocara canis* Dog roundworm	H: fever; cough; pneumonitis; hepato-splenomegaly. L: blindness if eye affected.	Eosinophilia +++ Serological tests; biopsy.	DIETHYLCARBAMAZINE or THIABENDAZOLE	Deworm pets. Avoid licking of face. Disposal of dog faeces.
Whipworm *Trichuris trichiura*	L: nil. H: bloody diarrhoea, anaemia. hypo-albuminaemia, rectal prolapse.	Typical ova in stool.	MEBENDAZOLE or ALBENDAZOLE	Wash hands. Wash vegetables. Good faecal disposal.

29 MALIGNANT DISEASES

C D Karabus and P S Hartley

Childhood cancer is relatively rare in South Africa (affecting possibly 1 300 children per year) and is only very occasionally seen by the average family physician.

♦ **Most childhood cancers are now curable.**
♦ The spectrum of cancer in childhood is totally different from that in adults.
  ◇ Leukaemia is much more common and the solid cancers seen are embryonal tumours and sarcomas, rather than the carcinomas seen in adults.
  ◇ More childhood cancers present in the first five years of life than in the period from five to 15 years of age, suggesting that prenatal influences are more important in the genesis of paediatric cancer than environmental carcinogens.
♦ The prognosis in children with cancer depends on the experience of a multidisciplinary treating team and demands accurate diagnosis and close co-operation between histopathologist, paediatric oncologist, surgeon and radiotherapist.
♦ Primary referral should be made to the paediatric oncologist who plays the central and co-ordinating role in the multidisciplinary team.

Types of childhood cancer

The relative incidence of cancer in childhood differs markedly from that in adults. Carcinoma of the breast, lung, bowel and genito-urinary organs are extreme rarities in the paediatric age group. Of the 1 856 children of all races registered at the Red Cross War Memorial Children's Hospital Oncology Centre between 1967 and 1993, leukaemia, brain tumours, lymphoma, neuroblastoma and Wilms' tumour accounted for nearly 80% of the total.

Clinical diagnosis

Early diagnosis improves the prognosis, particularly of solid tumours. However, because of the low prevalence of cancer in childhood, screening tests are not indicated. The 'early warning signs' of adult cancer, such as bleeding from orifices, changes in bowel habit or hoarseness are features of epithelial tumours (carcinomas) and are also not relevant in childhood.

Malignancy should be considered in children who present with the following cardinal features of cancer:

♦ pallor and purpura;
♦ unexplained prolonged fever;
♦ pain. This is often poorly localized and may present as a refusal to walk in a toddler. Persistent backache is a sinister symptom and may denote a spinal tumour;
♦ lymphadenopathy. It is often difficult to decide whether this is due to a common inflammation or a neoplasm. The child should be observed for no longer than four weeks and if there is no regression, biopsy is indicated. Supraclavicular adenopathy is frequently associated with intrathoracic or intra-abdominal tumours and should be investigated immediately;
♦ unexplained mass. An abdominal mass in a child under five is likely to be malignant. Other masses which are not typically benign should also be investigated;
♦ cranial nerve palsies, headache, vomiting or ataxia.

A child with suspected malignant disease should be referred immediately to a paediatric oncology centre. Invasive diagnostic procedures are best done at the cancer centre.

Acute leukaemia

The most common neoplastic disease in childhood is acute lymphoblastic leukaemia (ALL). With the development of new cytotoxic agents, effective prophylaxis against meningeal leukaemia and the more rational and intensive use of combination chemotherapy, the outlook for long-term survival and cure in ALL has improved dramatically. A five-year disease-free survival is to be expected and cure rates of 70% are being achieved. Such results are obtained only when treatment is initiated by, and continued in close association with a Paediatric Cancer Centre. The outlook for the child with leukaemia depends greatly on the experience of the medical personnel involved in the treatment.

Side-effects of cytotoxic therapy

General

◆ Bone marrow depression: this is common to most cytotoxic agents and is manifested by thrombocytopenia, anaemia and leukopenia. The blood count should be checked frequently and administration of cytotoxics delayed if platelets are less than $100 \times 10^9/l$, white cells less than $2 \times 10^9/l$ or granulocytes less than $1 \times 10^9/l$ (1 000/mm^3).

◆ Nausea and vomiting: this occurs with many of the medications and can be alleviated by ONDANSETRON (Zofran) IV or orally, GRANISETRON (Kytril) IV, DEXAMETHASONE IV, METOCLOPRAMIDE orally or CHLORPROMAZINE IV. CYCLIZINE suppositories may be useful. See Appendix 2 for dosages.

◆ Temporary alopecia: this is a common side-effect of therapy.

◆ Tissue necrosis and ulceration: this may result from extravasation of VINCRISTINE, MUSTINE, ACTINOMYCIN D and ADRIAMYCIN which must be given carefully and strictly intravenously.

Specific

◆ CYCLOPHOSPHAMIDE: haemorrhagic cystitis. Prevent by an IV fluid or oral intake of 3 l/m^2/24 hours and frequent emptying of the bladder.

◆ METHOTREXATE: photosensitivity, mouth ulcers.

◆ VINCRISTINE: constipation, abdominal and jaw pain, peripheral neuropathy.

◆ DAUNORUBICIN and ADRIAMYCIN: cardiomyopathy, uncommon if the cumulative dose does not exceed 500 mg/m^2. If mediastinal radiotherapy is also given, these cytotoxics should be limited to a maximum of 300 mg/m^2.

◆ ACTINOMYCIN D: stomatitis.

◆ ASPARAGINASE: anaphylaxis. Administer IM rather than IV and have parenteral corticosteroids and ADRENALINE available.

Warning

Stop therapy and telephone the Cancer Centre for advice if haemorrhagic cystitis, peripheral neuropathy, cardiomyopathy or fever occur.

Infection

Infection is a serious problem in the child with cancer and a major cause of morbidity and death. If fever develops, white cell and differential counts should be done immediately to determine whether neutropenia ($<1 \times 10^9$/l or $<1\,000$/mm^3) is present.

Bacterial infections

Septicaemia

Staphylococcus aureus or Gram-negative organisms such as *Pseudomonas aeruginosa*, *Escherichia coli* and *Klebsiella*. In children with indwelling venous catheters, *Staphyloccus epidermidis* is a common pathogen.

Pyrexia in neutropenic cancer patients

A cause for fever is frequently not found but urgent action must be taken in view of the serious potential of an infection.

Management

Culture blood, urine, and any infected lesions, and obtain a chest X-ray. Start IV antibiotics immediately, without waiting for culture results. Given the potential pathogens and current antibiotic sensitivity patterns, a combination of CEFTRIAXONE and AMIKACIN is used at the Children's Hospital. If *S. aureus* or *S. epidermidis* are suspected, CLOXACILLIN or VANCOMYCIN is added. The antibiotics must not be given together. Allow at least 15 minutes between infusions. Plasma AMIKACIN levels should be monitored. If a positive culture becomes available, the antibiotics may need to be changed, depending on the laboratory sensitivity tests.

Opportunistic infections

Pneumocystis carinii pneumonia and occasionally systemic fungal infections.

Viral infections

Viral infections include varicella, measles and interstitial pneumonia.

Prevention

In non-immune patients, exposure to measles should be treated with hyperimmune measles globulin 0,25 ml/kg IM. Varicella contacts are given zoster immune globulin 0,15 ml/kg IM. Prophylaxis is effective only if given within 72 hours of exposure.

Overt varicella and herpes simplex infections are effectively treated with ACYCLOVIR 10 mg/kg and 5 mg/kg respectively IV eight-hourly.

Interstitial pneumonia

This may result from measles, varicella or other viral infections and can also be caused by the protozoan *Pneumocystis carinii*. The earliest sign is an increased respiratory rate, followed rapidly by fever, non-productive cough and cyanosis. Little may be heard on auscultation.

Management

Immunosuppressed children with tachypnoea should be admitted and a chest X-ray taken. The arterial PaO_2 must be measured urgently and oxygen therapy started if indicated. Concomitant bacterial pulmonary infection may also be present and antibiotic therapy should be given to the neutropenic patient as described above. Specific therapy with CO-TRIMOXAZOLE in large doses (suspension 2,5 ml/kg/day or 1 paediatric tablet/kg/day in three divided doses) is administered for 14 days to eradicate a possible *P. carinii* infection. If varicella or herpes simplex is suspected as the cause of the pneumonia, ACYCLOVIR is used.

Terminal care

Once a cancer is no longer responsive to chemotherapy, it is seldom in the interest of the child to continue treatment. The situation and therapeutic options should be openly and fully discussed with the family (and the child, if old enough) and a joint decision made to discontinue specific curative therapy and treat only the symptoms. The family should be assured of the support and availability of the treatment team and seen frequently at the outpatient clinic. Children are happiest in their home environment and should remain there as long as possible, but for various reasons temporary or terminal admission to hospital may be necessary. Important aspects of care may include provision of a wheelchair for the child, sheepskins to lie on and meticulous attention to the mouth and pressure parts.

The staff at the cancer centre should be easily contactable at all hours. A centre which is unable to provide round-the-clock comprehensive terminal care should refer the child and family to a local hospice if one is available.

A major and most feared symptom of incurable cancer is pain. Pain is not difficult to manage and generally the amount and severity of pain suffered by a patient with cancer is inversely proportional to the quality of medical care.

Principles of pain management

♦ Drug therapy should be appropriate to the severity of the pain.
♦ Therapy should be given regularly, not as necessary.
♦ The correct dose of MORPHINE is one which abolishes pain.
♦ Adjuvants should be added as necessary, e.g. local radiotherapy for pain due to local bone infiltration, PREDNISONE for marrow infiltration, DEXAMETHASONE for raised intracranial pressure. Nonsteroidal anti-inflammatory agents (NSAID's) may be usefully added to MORPHINE for bone pain.

Analgesic step ladder

1. PARACETAMOL 30 mg/kg (or ASPIRIN 30-60 mg/kg, if the platelet count is normal) every four to six hours.
2. PARACETAMOL or ASPIRIN plus CODEINE PHOSPHATE every four to six hours.
3. MORPHINE SULPHATE 0,4 mg/kg orally or 0,2 mg/kg IV every four hours, increase by 50% or more with each subsequent dose until pain is controlled.

Once pain control has been achieved, the total daily amount of soluble MORPHINE is divided into 12-hourly (occasionally eight-hourly) doses and given as long-acting MORPHINE SULPHATE in a controlled-release form (MST Continus 10 mg or 30 mg tablets). Neither addiction nor respiratory depression are significant problems when used to produce analgesia. The main side-effect is constipation which should be treated appropriately. Urinary retention should be looked for if the child becomes restless, and it is managed by gentle bladder compression. Drowsiness and troublesome itching may occur initially.

30 MEDICO-LEGAL ASPECTS

*L S Smith**

> *'The simplest of medical tasks carries a risk . . .*
> *fortunately presenting relatively rarely . . .*
> *often predictable . . . and nearly always treatable . . .'*

Risks in paediatric practice have no less a litigation potential than in medical practice in general, making essential the knowledge of Common Law and Statutory medico-legal requirements relating to the treatment of children. This chapter provides a brief outline of those requirements about which health professionals are often uncertain, or unawareness of which results in preventable and time-consuming medico-legal issues. Subject matter is given in alphabetical order. See page 317 for definitions as applicable to different Acts. References appear at the end of the chapter.

Note: in the Statutes read 'his' as meaning both 'his' or 'hers', as stipulated by the Interpretation Act.

Affidavits

Must be factual, accurate, detailed and directed to the needs of the Court. Before preparing an affidavit which may involve the medical practitioner in litigation, the latter should consult his or her 'insurer', e.g. Medical Defence Union or Medical Protection Society. The State Attorney should be informed through the medical superintendent if the medical practitioner is a state employee in hospital practice, or through his or her superior if employed in other state departments.

AIDS

The duty rests with a medical practitioner of a patient with AIDS (acquired immune deficiency syndrome) to inform health

---

* Written in collaboration with Dr W Turek

workers at grave and clearly defined risk and sexual partners (if possible) accordingly. This should be done even where the patient after due counselling refuses to consent to such disclosure.

Refer to the Medical Practice Bulletin on Legal and Ethical Issues of the Medical Association of South Africa. (Supplement to the *S Afr Med J* December 1993;83).

Artificial insemination

The introduction artificially of a male gamete into the female internal reproductive organs, as well as the placing of the product of the union of a male and a female gamete outside the body into the uterus.

The child is the legitimate child of the husband and wife so inseminated, provided both consented to artificial insemination, and this will be presumed unless proven otherwise. (Ref. 6)

No right, duty or obligation arises between the child and the male gamete donor other than the husband. (Ref. 6)

Blood transfusion

A medical practitioner who plans to infuse blood must:

◆ **positively** identify the patient;
◆ **ensure** that blood is kept at 2-10 °C until immediately before transfusion;
◆ **retain** the blood container at 2-10 °C for 48 hours; and
◆ **report** an untoward reaction to the issuing Blood Bank expeditiously. (Ref. 11)

Certificates
General comment

The South African Medical and Dental Council may take disciplinary steps (over and above Court actions) in respect of the granting of certificates in a professional capacity, unless the med-

Warning

Exercise extreme care with regard to wording especially in sick leave, insurance, disability or any other certificates to be used for whatever purpose. (Ref. 13)

ical practitioner is satisfied from personal observation that the **facts** are correctly stated therein, or are qualified by 'as I am informed by the patient' or his or her other source of information.

Death

Natural causes

The medical practitioner who attended the patient before his or her death shall, if satisfied that death is due to natural causes, issue the prescribed certificate stating the cause of death.

If he or she did not attend any person before death but examined the corpse and is satisfied that death was due to natural causes, he or she may issue the prescribed certificate to that effect.

If a medical practitioner is of the opinion that death was due to other than natural causes, he or she shall not issue the prescribed certificate and shall inform a police officer as to his or her opinion in this regard. (Ref. 4)

Cot death

A non-natural death by definition for the purposes of the Births and Deaths Registration Act.

Stillbirth

If satisfied that the child was stillborn the medical practitioner who was present at the stillbirth or examined the corpse shall issue the prescribed certificate as to his or her opinion in this regard. If no medical practitioner was present or examined the child's corpse, the midwife or any person shall make a prescribed declaration to an authorized person. (Ref. 4)

Non-natural death

Not defined by law except for 'anaesthetic death'. For the purposes of a death certification, the following serves as a guideline of what **does not constitute a natural death:**

◆ due to trauma, i.e. any extrinsic, chemical or physical force directly or as a consequence thereof;
◆ when thought to be due to an act or omission on the part of any person;
◆ when uncertainty exists as to whether the cause of death was natural or unnatural. Not, however, where the cause is

thought to be due to natural causes, on definite grounds, but there is uncertainty as to the exact cause;

◆ when death occurs while under the influence of a local or general anaesthetic, or of which the administration of an anaesthetic has been a contributory cause, this is not deemed to be a death from natural causes as contemplated for the purposes of the Inquests Act and Births and Deaths Registration Act. (Ref. 13)

Notification of non-natural death: **any person** who has reason to believe that a person has died from causes other than natural causes shall notify the South African Police immediately unless the person has reason to believe this has already been done. (Ref. 12)

Birth notification

◆ A parent must register the birth of a live child with the authorized person within seven days of birth.
  ◇ In the absence of the parents, a person requested to do so by a parent shall register the live birth.
◆ If a child is born alive outside South Africa and one parent is a South African citizen, notice of birth **may** be given to a South African Mission or Regional Representative. (Ref. 4)
◆ Notice of birth of an abandoned child, which has not yet been given, shall be given after an enquiry in terms of the Child Care Act by the social worker or authorized officer concerned. (Ref. 4)

Child abuse

A dentist, medical practitioner, nurse or social worker who examines, attends or deals with any child whose condition gives rise to the suspicion of ill-treatment, or suffers from any injury, single or multiple, the cause of which might have been deliberate, or who suffers from a nutritional disease, shall immediately notify the Director-General of National Health and Population Development or his or her designate, i.e. the Regional Director of the Department of National Health and Population Development.

Should any of the aforementioned not do so, he or she shall be guilty of an offence. No legal proceedings shall lie against the person in respect of any notification given in good faith. (Ref. 5a)

Any person who examines, treats, attends to, advises, instructs or cares for any child in circumstances which ought to give rise to the reasonable suspicion that such a child has been ill-treated, or suffers from any injury, the probable cause of which was deliberate, shall immediately report such circumstances to a Police Official, a Commisioner of Child Welfare or a Social Worker. A Judge or Magistrate may prohibit any person from asssaulting or threatening the child or entering the premises where the child is. (Ref. 5b)

Consent

Consent must be obtained by the medical practitioner who undertakes a procedure, or it may be obtained under the latter's delegation if that person is competent to obtain the consent required by law.

Lawfulness of consent

♦ Consent shall be
  ◊ voluntary and without constraint;
  ◊ given by a person capable of forming intention, i.e. if intellectually of sufficient maturity to understand the implications of his acts and not mentally ill and not under the influence of drugs or alcohol;
  ◊ not be in conflict with good morals (*contra bonos mores*).
♦ Informed consent shall be based on an awareness of procedure, benefits, inherent risks, alternative methods, risks of not receiving treatment.
  ◊ 'Rule of thumb'. The more drastic the proposed procedure and potential risks, the more information the consentor should be given. Err always on the safe side. (Strauss SA – personal communication 1994)
♦ In case of conflict between husband and wife the husband's opinion is decisive in terms of common law.
♦ A woman shall be the guardian of her minor children born out of marriage
  ◊ equal to that of the father's common law rights;
  ◊ subject to a court order awarding sole guardianship to another person. (Ref. 6b)
♦ Consent shall be obtained by the medical practitioner who undertakes a procedure, or it may be obtained under the latter's delegation if that person is competent to obtain the consent as required by law.

Abortion

An abortion is defined as the abortion of a live foetus of a woman with intent to kill such a foetus. The latter is not defined but is regarded as the product of the union of gametes after implantation.

An abortion is lawful if:

♦ **pregnancy endangers life, or is a serious threat to physical or mental health**
Certification: two medical practitioners to certify accordingly.

♦ **pregnancy is the result of illegitimate carnal intercourse (mentally defective or mentally handicapped female)**
Certification: two medical practitioners (one a State Psychiatrist) certify that the woman, due to permanent mental handicap or defect, is unable to understand the consequences of coitus and to bear parental responsibilities.

♦ **pregnancy will result in a serious risk of a child being irreparably handicapped**
Certification: two medical practitioners certify on scientific grounds accordingly.

♦ **pregnancy is the result of rape or incest**
The pregnancy is the result of unlawful carnal intercourse, i.e. rape or incest.
Certification: two medical practitioners (one the District Surgeon who examined the victim) to certify that the pregnancy is due to rape or incest.
A magistrate must certify that he or she is satisfied that a complaint has been lodged with the police or that there was good reason why not so lodged; that unlawful carnal intercourse took place; and in case of alleged incest, that this constituted incest; and that pregnancy is the result of the unlawful carnal intercourse. This must be made available to the person authorizing the abortion, i.e. the Medical Superintendent.

Note

The two medical practitioners who issue certificates in the foregoing instances shall not be partners or have a common employer (except if State employees) and one of them shall have been registered as a medical practitioner for four years.

Medical examination of a minor: victim of violence or indecency

Who may consent

◆ Parent or guardian.
◆ Magistrate: if a parent or a guardian cannot be traced timeously; is a suspect in the case; unreasonably refuses consent; is mentally disordered; or is deceased.
◆ Commissioned Police Officer or Police Station Commander: if the magistrate is not available and the district surgeon or a registered medical practitioner declares under oath that to avoid defeating the purpose of the examination, the examination is necessary forthwith. (Ref. 7)

Medical treatment and procedures

Who may consent

Ad hoc transfer of parent's consent

The person to whom the parent's or guardian's power of consent has been transferred in writing, may give consent. (Ref. 5)

Arrested individual

No consent is necessary to draw blood for analysis if a district surgeon, a medical officer in hospital practice or a registered nurse is requested to do so by a police officer or a traffic officer. (Ref. 7)

Medical Superintendent

Case of urgency: when intervention is necessary to preserve the life or save the child from physical injury or disability and where it cannot be deferred for the purpose of consulting the person who is legally competent to consent.

Minister of Health

The Minister or his delegate, the Regional Directors of National Health and Population Development may consent if he or she considers the operation or treatment necessary and when the parent or guardian is not available, deceased, incompetent by reason of mental disorder or has acted unreasonably in refusing treatment. (Ref. 5)

Patient 18 years and older

Competent to consent to medical and surgical treatment without the assistance of a parent or guardian.

Patient 14 years and older

Competent to consent to medical treatment for himself or herself or his or her child, but the parent or guardian must give consent for procedures and surgical interventions.

Patient appears intoxicated

If admitted to hospital a medical practitioner may draw blood if he or she is of the opinion that the findings may be relevant to any later criminal proceedings. (Ref. 8)

Patient is a potential organ donor

Death must be certified by two Medical Practitioners, one of whom shall have been registered for five years. A parent or guardian may consent should the patient die. In the case of eye tissue, a death certificate only is required to establish the fact of death. If the organs are not replaceable by natural processes, donation is not permitted from a living child. (Ref. 11). See also Tissue donation on page 320.

If a patient is institutionalized in a mental hospital, consent may be given by a curator, parent, major brother or major sister in this order.

Post-mortem examination
Natural death

In hospital: parent, guardian or the medical superintendent may consent to a post-mortem if it is deemed necessary for scientific purposes.

In district: magistrate may consent. (Ref. 11)

In case of infectious communicable disease: Regional Director, National Health and Population Development. (Ref 10)

Non-natural death

See definition on page 307. Refer to South African Police. (Ref. 12)

Sterilization

The child is incapable or incompetent to give consent. In order for this to be done, certification, consent and certain other requirements have to be fulfilled.

Certification: 'a psychiatrist and another medical practitioner certify a child suffering from a hereditary condition of such a nature that if he or she were to procreate a child such child would suffer from a physical or mental defect of such a nature that it would be seriously handicapped or due to permanent mental handicap or defect is unable to comprehend the consequential implications of, or bear the parental responsibility for the fruit of coitus.' (Ref. 11)

Consent: parent or guardian consents, or if they are not traceable, the magistrate.

Authorization: the Minister or a medical officer in the Department of National Health and Population Development authorizes the sterilization in writing.

Warning

For the indications listed, sterilization may only be performed in a State institution or a specially authorized institution.

Disability grant

Any person 16 years and older who is unfit, owing to physical or mental disability, to obtain from any service, employment or profession the means to enable him or her to provide adequately for his or her maintenance is regarded as a disabled person for purposes of the Social Pensions Act. (Ref. 18)

Employment

No employer shall employ a person under 15 years of age or permit an employee to work from four weeks prior to and eight weeks after her confinement. If there is dispute in legal proceedings regarding the age of any person, then the district surgeon can be required to estimate the age and submit a certificate. (Ref. 3)

Genetic manipulation

Genetic manipulation outside the human body of gametes or zygotes is not permitted. (Ref. 11)

Guardianship and custody

The guardianship of the child of an unmarried minor mother rests in the guardian of the mother. The custody of the child rests in the mother of the child, although a Court may direct otherwise. (Ref. 6).

A mother of under 21 years of age (a minor) acquires the status of a major by marriage or by becoming an independent breadwinner, and then becomes both custodian and guardian. (Ref. 6)

Illegitimate child

The child shall be registered under the mother's surname or, with joint consent of the father and the mother, under the father's surname. (Ref. 4)

Liability

All employees of the State are covered by the latter in terms of the vicarious liability of the 'master', for any damages arising from the wrongful act of the employee. **However**, the employee may **forfeit** this cover if he or she:

◆ did not act in the **execution** of his or her official duties;
◆ exercised in **bad faith** or **exceeded** his or her power;
◆ made **excessive use of liquor or drugs** which resulted or contributed to liability;
◆ made an **admission of guilt** without prior consultation with the State Attorney;

◆ acted **recklessly** or wilfully; or
◆ failed to **comply** with or ignored standing instructions of which he or she was aware or could reasonably have been expected to be aware. (Ref. 9)

Nobody can afford to practise any form of medicine without adequate medical liability cover by his or her private or group insurer.

Judgement of negligence

This arises when a defendant and/or an accused failed to foresee and guard against the possibility of harm that the reasonable medical practitioner in a similar position would have foreseen and guarded against. Delictual claims of a minor lapse one year after majority attained.

> *Warning*
> Records should be kept till a lapse of this proviso.

Reasonable practitioner

If the defendant or accused is a general practitioner the test of the latter's action(s) is based on the anticipated actions of a reasonable general practitioner, i.e. that expected of an average general practitioner under similar circumstances and conditions. In the case of a practitioner who professes to have specialist skills in a branch of medicine, the test is that expected of the average specialist in that branch of medical practice.

Precautions in respect of prescribing

Before treatment is prescribed or a procedure carried out the following questions need to be answered in the affirmative.

◆ Is the drug or procedure the one of choice under the circumstances?
◆ Is its use indicated?
◆ Are the dangers and contra-indications known?
◆ Has an attempt been made to anticipate whether the patient may exhibit idiosyncrasy to the drug or procedure?

◆ Are the appropriate counter-reactants immediately available should an untoward reaction occur?
◆ Has cognisance been taken of the package insert in the case of medication?
◆ Is the other health professional to whom the administration of a drug or the carrying out of a procedure been delegated, competent and permitted to undertake the task?

Untoward reaction or mishap

◆ **Report** timeously and appropriately to insurer and/or superior any mishap affecting a patient or circumstances which could give rise to a complaint or claim.
◆ **Make and keep** accurate contemporaneous notes which must be legible, objective and worthy of independent scrutiny.
◆ **Carelessness in documentation** reflects on the credibility of the health professional and on the credibility of the recorder. The defendant's legal representatives are disadvantaged when these notes become the subject of court scrutiny.
◆ **Avoid** criticism of a colleague(s).
◆ **Do not admit legal liability** without prior reference to your 'insurer'.
◆ **Show** professional courtesy in all dealings.
◆ **Do not hesitate** to contact your insurer, e.g. Medical Defence Union or Medical Protection Society.

Motor vehicle accident claim

Form MMF1 (Multilateral Motor Vehicle Accident Fund Act) 'Medical Report' must be completed by the medical practitioner treating the injured child or the medical superintendent or his or her nominee with the consent of parent or guardian. Section 1 to 6 of the first part of the form must be completed by the applicant or legal representative before the medical practitioner completes all sections of the medical certificate.

Claims for minors do not prescribe until one year after the child gains majority (Multilateral Motor Vehicle Accident Fund).

Paternity

In legal proceedings, if either party refuses to submit himself or herself or the child to the taking of blood for paternity testing, it will be presumed that unless the contrary is proved, that refusal is aimed at concealing the truth concerning the paternity of the child. (Ref. 6)

Punishment

If a district surgeon or his or her assistant certifies that a juvenile is not fit to receive judicial whipping, the person charged by this Court to undertake the whipping must forthwith deliver this certificate to the Court. (Ref. 8)

Rape

Rape is defined as sexual intercourse with a female without her consent. Sexual intercourse with a female under 13 years of age constitutes rape. Intercourse with an unmarried female over 13 years and under 16 years with her consent is a sexual offence. (Ref. 17)

Terminology employed for medico-legal purposes

For purposes of the:

Age of Majority Act No. 87 of 1972

Major (person of age)

Any person of the age of 21 years, or declared a major in terms of the Age of Majority Act (No. 87 of 1972) or who has contracted a legal marriage.

Birth And Deaths Registration Act No. 5 of 1992

Birth

Birth means the birth of a child born alive.

Stillborn, stillbirth

Stillborn, in relation to a child, means that it has had at least 26 weeks of intra-uterine existence but showed no sign of life after a complete birth.

Child Care Act No. 74 of 1983 as amended

Child

Child means any person under the age of 18 years.

Medical officer

Medical oficer means a medical practitioner in the service of the State, including a provincial administration, or of a local authority.

Criminal Procedure Act No. 51 of 1977 as amended

Evidence of relationship on charge of incest

At criminal proceedings at which an accused is charged with incest:

1. It shall be sufficient to prove that the woman on whom or by whom the offence is alleged to have been committed, is reputed to be the lineal ascendant or descendant or the sister, stepmother or stepdaughter of the other party of the incest.
2. The accused shall be presumed, unless the contrary is proved, to have had knowledge, at the time of the alleged offence, of the relationship existing between him and the other party of the incest.

Evidence on charge of infanticide or concealment of birth

1. At criminal proceedings at which an accused is charged with the killing of a newly-born child, such child shall be deemed to have been born alive if the child is proved to have breathed, whether or not the child had an independent circulation, and it shall not be necessary to prove that the child was, at the time of its death, entirely separated from the body of its mother.
2. At criminal proceedings at which an accused is charged with the concealment of the birth of a child, it shall not be necessary to prove whether the child died before or at or after birth.

Criminal Law Amendment Act No. 4 of 1992

Minor

A person under 21 years of age and not married (see definition of a Major, page 317).

Health Act No. 63 of 1977

Notification of births

A local authority may request the Minister of Health to make regulations relating to the compulsory notification of live and stillbirths. This notification is in addition to registration of births and is not uniform throughout the country. The person responsible for the notification of a birth is usually the medical practitioner or midwife who was present at the birth.

Notifiable medical conditions

A list of conditions which must be notified to the Department of National Health and Population Development is published from time to time in the Government Gazette — see page 276. (See also Communicable diseases on pages 275-6.)

Notification to local authority of death from a notifiable medical condition

◆ When a notifiable medical condition is prevalent within the district of a local authority, any person who has reason to believe that any other person has died within such district, shall as soon as possible report accordingly to the local authority concerned, unless he or she has reason to believe that such a report has been or will be made by any other person or that the deceased was attended to by a medical practitioner during the illness immediately preceding his death.

◆ In every case of death from a notifiable medical condition, the medical practitioner who attended to the deceased immediately prior to his or her death, shall immediately notify the local authority concerned of the death and the cause thereof, and shall make the best arrangements practicable, pending the removal of the body, to prevent the spread of that condition.

◆ Any person who keeps any dead body in any room in which anybody lives, sleeps or works, or in which food is kept, prepared or eaten, or who keeps, except with the written authorization of the local authority concerned, the body of any person who is known to the first-mentioned person to have died of a communicable disease, for more than 24 hours in any place other than a mortuary or other place set apart for the keeping of dead bodies, shall be guilty of an offence.

Post-mortem examination of body of person suspected of having died of communicable disease or other medical condition

Whenever any person is suspected of having died of a communicable disease or other medical condition, and further information pertaining to the facts of such disease or condition is required in order to determine what steps, if any, may be necessary with a view to preventing the spread of such disease or the recurrence of such condition, and such information cannot be obtained except by means of a post-mortem examination of the body of the deceased person, the Director-General of National Health and Population Development or a magistrate for the district in which such a body is, may order that a post-mortem examination of such body be made by a medical practitioner and that such body, if buried, shall be disinterred for the purposes of such examination.

Mental Health Act No. 18 of 1973
Child

'Child' means any person under the age of 18 years: provided that any person detained in an institution who is over the age of 16 years may, with the approval of the Minister, be treated therein as a child up to an age recommended by the hospital board concerned.

Psychopathic disorder

'Psychopathic disorder' means a persistent disorder or disability of the mind (whether or not subnormality of intelligence is present) which has existed in the patient from an age prior to that of 18 years and which results in abnormally aggressive or seriously irresponsible conduct on the part of the patient, and 'psychopath' has a corresponding meaning.

Human Tissue Act No. 65 of 1983
Tissue donation

Any tissue from a living **minor** which is not replaceable by a natural process, or gamete shall not be used for the transplantation or the manufacture into any diagnostic or therapeutic product or for artificial insemination.

References of Acts and regulations:

Their purposes relevant to paediatrics
1. Abortion and Sterilization, 1975 as amended: conditions in

which abortion may be procured; permitting sterilization for persons incapable of consent.

2. Drug and Drug Trafficking, 1992: dealing in drugs in schools, primary and pre-primary schools. Prevention and treatment of drug dependency, 1992. Transfer of children to treatment or registered treatment centres.

3. Basic Conditions of Employment, 1983 as amended: conditions of employment of certain employees.

4. Births and Deaths Registration, 1992: registration of births and deaths; illegitimate, legitimate, live or stillbirths.

5a. Child Care, 1983 as amended: treatment, protection and welfare; adoption; maintenance of children; incidental matters.

5b. Prevention of Family Violence 1993: reporting of ill-treatment of children.

6a. Children's Status, 1982: paternity; guardianship; status of certain children; surrogate pregnancy; artificial insemination.

6b. Guardianship, 1993: guardship of minor children.

7. Criminal Law Amendment, 1992: medical examination of a minor: victim of violence or indecency; definition of minor.

8. Criminal Procedure, 1977 as amended: procedures leading up to, and in Court; blood sampling; safe-keeping of foreign bodies removed from persons suspected to be concerned with an offence; expert evidence; affidavits.

9. Exchequer, 1975: includes provision relating to claims against the State and persons in its service.

10. Health, 1977 as amended: includes provisions for Notifiable Medical Conditions; communicable diseases; exclusion from school for medical conditions; post-mortem examinations in case of communicable disease.

11. Human Tissue, 1983 as amended: donation of tissue, blood, gametes; post-mortem examinations; artificial insemination; inspectors of anatomy.

12. Inquests, 1959 as amended: inquiry into death from allegedly other than natural causes; reporting and investigating such deaths; procedures at inquest; medical assessors.

13. Medical, Dental and Supplementary Health Service Professions, 1974 as amended: control of medical, dental and supplementary health professions; registration; conduct; disciplinary matters.

14. Medicines and Related Substances Control, 1965 as amended: registration of medicines; prescriptions; scheduling.

15. Mental Health, 1975 as amended: reception; detention; treatment; certification of the mentally ill.
16. Nursing, 1978 as amended: control of registered; enrolled nurses; nursing assistants; midwives.
17. Sexual Offences, 1957: relating to sexual matters other than common law factors which amounts to an offence.
18. Social Pensions, 1973 as amended: pensions for blind, deaf, disabled and aged.
19. South African Medical Research Council, 1991: promotion of research.

Recommended reading

Medical Practice Bulletin: Legal and clinical issues. Supplement to *S Afr Med J* December 1993;83.

Quality health care in South Africa. Clinical therapeutic guidelines workshop. Supplement to *S Afr Med J* March 1994;84.

Strauss SA. *Doctor, patient and the law.* 3rd Ed. Pretoria: JL van Schaik, 1991.

Van Oostens FFW. The legal liability of doctors and hospitals for medical malpractice. *S Afr Med J* 1991; 80: 23-27.

D H Hanslo

General

Familiarity with laboratory routine ensures optimal results. It is best to consult beforehand about the availability of tests – particularly for new procedures, and specialized or after-hours investigations.

Request forms

Correct personal details and folder number of the patient are essential for computer registration of specimens, as well as for later retrieval of results. Wherever possible, use official patient stickers. Appropriate clinical information, including **length of illness** and any **antimicrobial therapy** given is very important when deciding on specific media or tests that may be required.

Provide separate forms for each different type of investigation that will need registration or referral to other laboratories, e.g. acid fast bacilli (AFB), and viral or fungal investigation in addition to routine culture.

Specimen collection and transport

Blood cultures, cerebrospinal fluids (CSFs) and normally sterile body fluids must be submitted in sterile containers. For other specimens, unsterile clean containers are suitable. Screw-caps are preferred as there is less chance of leakage.

Several varieties of swabs are commercially available. Fine wire ENT swabs are ideal for obtaining samples through small orifices, e.g. from middle ear, posterior nasopharynx, urethra, and vagina.

Transport media for swabs are preferable as they prevent dessication of the material on the swab and preserve less hardy organisms. Media containing charcoal (black) are especially useful for very fastidious organisms such as neisseriae or haemophili.

Special viral transport media which contain antibiotics, if available, should be used for viral culture specimens. All specimens for viral culture should be kept cold (0-4 °C) but not frozen. The preferred means of transport is on a melting ice and water mixture.

Ensure that all specimens are labelled with patient details and, where appropriate, with site. On no account should **any** microbiological specimen be wrapped in its request form as this practice poses an infection hazard during transport and sorting.

Regard **all** blood samples or heavily blood-stained body fluids as potentially contaminated with viruses such as Hepatitis B or HIV. When collecting blood, use gloves as a precaution against spillage. Clean off any blood that has spilled onto the specimen container with hypochlorite solution. Blood specimens must be transported individually in sealed plastic bags.

When transporting specimens by post, wrap the primary leak-proof container in sufficient absorbent packing (e.g. paper towelling) to absorb all liquid in case of spillage, and then place it in an outer rigid leak-proof container. The outer wrapper must be clearly labelled with both recipient's and sender's names and addresses. Indicate the nature of the contents and attach biohazard stickers as appropriate.

Blood culture

This is the single most important investigation in microbiology.

Collection should be an **aseptic** procedure to avoid specimen contamination.

Wash hands with soap and water, then dry. The wearing of gloves is recommended to protect in case of spillage. Identify the puncture site and clean with 10% POVIDONE IODINE solution in a circular motion, applying firm pressure to remove skin debris. Remove POVIDONE with 70% alcohol and **allow to dry.** Thereafter, do not palpate the puncture site unless sterile gloves are worn. Perform venepuncture. Ideally 3 ml of blood should be drawn per bottle; however, this is often impossible in young infants. If multiple bottles are to be inoculated, e.g. Aerobic and Anaerobic, divide the collected blood equally between them. Disinfect the top of each bottle with a swab soaked in 70% alcohol before inoculating. If blood is being collected for several investigations, always inoculate blood culture bottles first.

Shake the bottles gently to mix. Ensure that both are labelled, then send immediately to the laboratory, or hold in an incubator.

Cerebrospinal fluid (CSF)

Before proceeding, the patient should be correctly positioned and a sterile lumbar puncture pack should be available. Wash hands with soap and water, dry thoroughly with sterile paper or towel, and don sterile gloves.

Clean the puncture site with 10% POVIDONE IODINE, then remove with 70% alcohol and allow to dry. Aseptically tap CSF into two separate sterile tubes (ideally at least 1 ml into each), plus 0,1 ml into a fluoride tube for quantitative glucose estimation. Screw caps on firmly. Label tubes, and send immediately to the laboratory, or hold in an incubator.

◆ For possible viral meningitis: keep an aliquot of the CSF at 4 °C at all times.
◆ For possible TBM: a further 1-2 ml CSF is necessary for AFB culture. A second CSF sample is often needed to confirm the diagnosis – indicate that the fluid is specifically for AFB culture and/or other tests such as ADA, TB-antigen or gene detection.

Pus and aspirates

For abscesses or effusions, actual exudate or fluid aspirated into a syringe or collected in a sterile tube is preferable to a swab, especially where anaerobes are likely. Blood culture bottles are not recommended except in special circumstances, as this precludes direct microscopy, chemistry or subsequent AFB culture. Similarly, it is preferable not to send pus or fluid in swab containers.

Swabs

◆ For mucosal swabs collect material from any local lesion present, e.g. discharge, pustule, follicle, membrane.
◆ For skin lesions, first clean off any surface crust or exudate with unpreserved sterile saline. Collect material from the oozing base or edge of an ulcer.
◆ Swabs for viral culture are best sent in transport medium, on ice.
◆ To make a smear for microscopy, e.g. for meningococci, chlamydiae, or viral-infected cells, **roll the swab** on the centre of a clean glass slide. Label the slide and indicate which side has been used for the smear.

Serology

◆ Clotted blood is necessary for serological tests, i.e. **no anti-coagulant.** Submit in screw-capped tubes, in sealed plastic bags.

◆ Serological diagnosis of acute infections can be by demonstration of a specific IgM response (e.g. syphilis, rubella, cytomegalovirus (CMV)). In most cases, however, a follow-up 'convalescent' specimen ten to 14 days later is important to show evidence of seroconversion or a rising titre.

◆ If congenital infection is suspected, take blood from both the infant and the mother.

◆ As serological testing is a rapidly developing field and new techniques are freqently introduced, it is advisable to seek prior advice on the availability of tests or interpretation of results, especially when the infection to be investigated is uncommon.

Sputum

Sputa from children are often of poor quality. Postural drainage in the early morning can produce a suitable specimen. Alternately, enlist the aid of a physiotherapist to obtain an adequate sample.

◆ For AFB: submit two consecutive early morning sputa or gastric washings.

◆ For chlamydia: submit sputum or nasopharyngeal aspirate as is for direct immunofluorescent staining.

◆ For pneumocystis: broncho-alveolar lavage is the best sample, submitted as is for microscopy after special staining.

◆ For viral culture: nasopharyngeal or bronchial aspirates are best and should be kept cold (4 °C).

Stools

The equivalent of a teaspoonful of faeces is necessary for reliable culture. Submit in screw-capped container. Rectal swabs are not suitable as they do not provide sufficient material. Warm stools are only necessary if amoebiasis is suspected; for other stool pathogens and parasites the specimen may be allowed to cool. Keep viral specimens cold (4 °C).

Urine

At least 5 ml is required for reliable microscopy. Clean catch samples are suitable for very young infants, alternately supra-pubic aspiration should be attempted (see page 457). If urine is collected in a bag or bedpan, carefully decant into a conical-bottomed tube (used for centrifugation).

◆ For AFB: submit two consecutive total early morning urines.
◆ For schistosoma: submit a terminal sample of urine collected between 12h00 and 14h00.
◆ For viruses: keep specimen cold (4 °C). If available, use a viral transport medium.

Virology

Virus isolation is best achieved early in the clinical illness. Viruses are labile and special transport media are usually required, sent in an ice-water mixture to maintain the specimen at 0-4 °C.

Suitable specimens

◆ Respiratory: nasopharyngeal or tracheal or bronchial secretions, throat swab, blood for serology.
◆ CNS: CSF, stool or rectal swab, throat swab, blood for serology.
◆ Eye: eye swab, conjunctival smear (scraping).
◆ Skin lesions: vesicle fluid or swab, throat swab, stool or rectal swab, blood for serology.
◆ Myocarditis or myositis: throat swab, stool or rectal swab, blood for serology.
◆ PUO[1], possibly viral: throat swab, stool or rectal swab, urine, blood for serology.

Suitable viral transport media, as well as information regarding specimens, can be obtained from: Diagnostic Virology Laboratory, UCT Medical School (See Appendix 5, page 696).

---

[1] Pyrexia of unknown origin.

32 NEUROLOGICAL DISORDERS

P M Leary and J C Peter

Clinical diagnosis

History and examination

In most cases the history and the physical examination indicate the correct diagnosis. Examine the following in every child with a neurological problem: the state of consciousness, cranial nerve function, muscle tone and power, limb and trunk movements and tendon reflexes.

In infants palpate the anterior fontanelle and observe motor development. Note the state of primitive reflexes: Moro, grasp, tonic neck and protective. Record the presence of neck stiffness. Measure head circumference and relate to age. See pages 669-70. Note the shape of the skull and any skin lesions.

Investigations

- CSF: often assists diagnosis.
- X-ray skull: may show intracranial calcification, sutural diastasis or abnormal pituitary fossa.
- Ultrasound: feasible only when anterior fontanelle patent. Will demonstrate ventricular dilation, haemorrhage and structural abnormalities of the brain.
- CT scan: first choice investigation if clinical suggestion of hydrocephalus, subdural collection, abscess, haemorrhage, tumour or cerebral oedema.
- MRI scan: expensive. Will demonstrate intra-cerebral demyelination. First choice investigation if clinical picture suggests spinal cord lesion.
- EEG: demonstrates brain function and not anatomy. Wide application in diagnosis and management of seizure disorders.
- Nerve conduction studies, electromyography and muscle biopsy aid diagnosis in disorders of peripheral nerves and muscles.

◆ Electroretinography (ERG), visual evoked responses (VER) and brainstem auditory evoked responses (BAER) reflect the integrity of specialized sensory pathways.

Spinal dysraphism

Commonly lumbosacral.

◆ Skin-covered midline swellings, e.g. meningocoeles, lipomeningocoeles, lumbosacral lipomas, dermoids. Refer to a neurosurgical centre at six weeks of age.
◆ Partially-epithelialized or open midline lesions, e.g. myelo-meningocoele, myeloschisis. Nurse in a prone position. Cover neural plaque with sterile, saline-moistened dressing.

Refer to neurosurgical centre immediately so that the closure can be done within 36 hours of birth.

Dermal sinuses

Cutaneous communication with the CNS.

Diagnosis

Look carefully for a small pit in the midline or just off it, any-where from the external occipital protuberance to the coccyx. Very occasionally it may be found in the frontonasal area. Sus-pect with recurrent meningitis.

Management

All should be referred to a neurosurgical centre except those occurring in the natal cleft in the coccygeal area. Sacrococ-cygeal dermal sinuses seldom, if ever, communicate with the CNS and do not require investigation. **Do not probe.**

Craniosynostosis

Clinical presentation

Suspect with an abnormally shaped head. Confirm by skull X-ray.

Unisutural

Sagittal (scaphocephaly), coronal (anterior plagiocephaly), lambdoidal (posterior plagiocephaly).

Multisutural

Bicoronal, basal (brachycephaly).

Craniofacial abnormalities

Crouzon's disease and Apert's syndrome.

Refer before six months of age. Best repaired by combined plastic/neurosurgical procedure.

Note

Synostotic deformities can be corrected at any age. The unisutural disorders are most easily corrected before six months of age.

Microcephaly in the vast majority of cases is caused by primary brain growth failure and is rarely due to synostosis.

Hydrocephalus

This is present when the volume of CSF within the skull is increased.

Clinical presentation

Suspect if a child has a large head and any of the following: rapidly increasing head circumference, full fontanelle with wide sutures, squint or failure of upward gaze, drowsiness, vomiting and spasticity of the legs.

Management

Refer to a neurosurgical centre.

Blocked V-P shunt

Clinical presentation

◆ Before closure of sutures: as for hydrocephalus.
◆ After sutures closed (over 18 months): headache, drowsiness, vomiting, development of a squint and seizures.

Infected V-P shunt

Usually occurs within two or three months of shunt insertion or revision.

Clinical presentation

As for blocked shunt and pyrexia – stiff neck, redness of shunt tract and peritonism.

Management

Urgent referral to a neurosurgical centre.

Impaired consciousness

Disorders of consciousness range from reduced awareness of surroundings to total unresponsiveness to any stimuli (coma). The level of consciousness should be recorded in terms of response to simple stimuli. The Glasgow Coma Scale may be used for patients aged five years or older. See page 665.

Aetiology

Intracranial causes

Trauma. Meningitis. Encephalitis or encephalopathy. Brain abscess. Acute hydrocephalus. Cerebral oedema. Post-ictal state. Brain tumour. Blocked shunt.

Extracranial causes

Drugs and toxins. Hypo- or hyperglycaemia. Acid base derangement. Hypo- or hypernatraemia. Hypo- or hyperthermia. Liver failure. Uraemia. Hypoxia. Hypotension.

Management

- ♦ Ensure adequate airway.
- ♦ Assist ventilation if indicated.
- ♦ Set up IV line and infuse fluid as indicated by circulatory state.
- ♦ Establish the cause of the coma: clinical examination, skull X-ray, CT scan, blood glucose, urea, electrolytes, pH, PaO_2, $PaCO_2$, blood culture, specimens for viral culture, blood ammonia, blood and urine screen for toxins (see page 423), EEG.

Raised intracranial pressure

Intracranial pressure is influenced by the size of the calvarium, its contents, systemic arterial pressure and the efficiency of venous drainage. Raised intracranial pressure may develop slowly over weeks or within hours depending on the mechanism.

Aetiology

Hydrocephalus. Infection, e.g. meningitis, encephalitis, abscess. Subdural and extradural collections, e.g. effusion, haematoma, empyema. Cerebral oedema. Tumour. Benign intracranial hypertension.

Clinical presentation

Psychological withdrawal, headache, vomiting, seizures, unsteadiness and squint.

Bulging anterior fontanelle, papilloedema (rare in young children), stiff neck, deteriorating level of consciousness, third and sixth cranial nerve palsies, enlargement of head (in infancy), 'Crack-pot' sign (after infancy), radiological separation of sutures and demineralization of pituitary fossa.

Management

Warning

LUMBAR PUNCTURE SHOULD NOT BE PERFORMED WHEN THERE IS A DEPRESSED LEVEL OF CONSCIOUSNESS OR EVIDENCE OF RAISED INTRACRANIAL PRESSURE.

Urgent referral for investigation.

Cerebral oedema

Cerebral oedema exists when the water content of white and grey matter of the brain is excessive. This occurs when there is a loss of vascular autoregulation or capillary permeability and brain cell functions are impaired by hypoxia. There is an increase in intracranial pressure (ICP) with corresponding decrease in cerebral blood flow.

Aetiology

Meningitis, encephalitis, septicaemia, trauma, intracranial haemorrhage, anoxia (following cardiac arrest or near-drowning), status epilepticus, tumour, abscess, lead, carbon monoxide, hepatic coma, Reye's syndrome, hypertensive encephalopathy, steroid withdrawal.

Clinical presentation

Suspect in a child with clinical signs of meningitis or encephalitis whose state of consciousness is impaired. When ICP exceeds mean arterial pressure, cerebral perfusion ceases and brain death occurs.

Investigations

As for impaired consciousness.

Management

◆ Treat circulatory shock. (See page 7 as to how to improve cerebral perfusion.)
◆ Prevent cerebral vascular engorgement. Maximize venous drainage by elevating the head of the bed 30 degrees and placing the patient's head in neutral forward position.
◆ Intubate and commence artificial ventilation if the $PaCO_2$ exceeds 5,3 kPa (40 mmHg) and maintain $PaCO_2$ between 4-4,7 kPa (30-35 mmHg). See pages 2-3.
◆ Prevent and treat convulsions. Prevention: PHENYTOIN or PHENOBARBITONE in full therapeutic dose. Treatment: see page 338. Use THIOPENTONE SODIUM infusion if convulsions persist (see page 339).
◆ Treat fever. Monitor rectal temperature and maintain below 38 °C with PARACETAMOL, fanning and tepid sponging.
◆ Remove intracranial fluid. Give MANNITOL 0,25-0,5 g/kg IV. Repeat MANNITOL when there is a deterioration in the level of consciousness or the fontanelle tension increases. MANNITOL should not be given more than three times if there is no clinical response.
◆ Avoid fluid overload and hyponatraemia. Limit intravenous fluids to two-thirds maintenance requirements. Monitor serum electrolytes, urine output and concentration. Be on the look-out for the syndrome of inappropriate anti-diuretic hormone secretion (SIADH).
◆ DEXAMETHASONE is effective in reducing cerebral oedema in certain cases, such as tumours. It should be given six-hourly intravenously in a dose of 0,25 mg/kg/day. After

48 hours the dosage should be reduced and gradually tailed off over the next five days.

Imminent coning

Clinical presentation

◆ Trans-tentorial: deteriorating level of consciousness, ipsilateral third nerve palsy (dilating pupil) and contralateral weakness, progressing to bilateral dilated pupils, respiratory irregularity, hypertension and bradycardia.

◆ Foramen magnum: fluctuating level of consciousness, irregular breathing, apnoeic spells and episodes of decerebrate posturing.

Management

Aimed at a rapid reduction of intracranial pressure (ICP). Hyperventilation causes an immediate fall in ICP; MANNITOL takes about ten to 20 minutes and FUROSEMIDE (Lasix) about 30-60 minutes to have the same effect.

Proceed as follows:

Step 1. Hyperventilate with bag and mask if breathing is slow or irregular. Do not hyperventilate <4,0 kPa $PaCO_2$ (30 mmHg) for more than one hour. During IPPV keep $PaCO_2$ between 4,0-4,7 kPa (30-35 mmHg).

Step 2. Give MANNITOL 1 g/kg IV and FUROSEMIDE (Lasix) 0,5 mg/kg IV. Gradually reduce hyperventilation, starting about 15 minutes after the MANNITOL and assess effect.

Step 3. Give PHENOBARBITONE 15 mg/kg IV, if not previously given.

Step 4. Exclude causes which can be treated surgically, e.g. extradural haematoma.

Brain abscess

Table 32.1 Brain abscesses

Pathogenesis	Common site
Trauma	Site of trauma.
Middle ear disease	Temporal lobe and cerebellum.
Sinusitis	Frontal lobe.
Lung disease, cyanotic heart disease, bacterial endocarditis	Distribution of middle cerebral artery.

Clinical presentation

Presence of primary cause:

◆ general signs of infection;
◆ raised intracranial pressure;
◆ localizing neurological signs; and
◆ seizures.

Diagnosis

Suspect and refer for definitive diagnostic procedure, i.e. CT scan with contrast. Do not lumbar puncture.

Management

Surgical drainage and appropriate antibiotics.

Subdural empyema

Clinical presentation

Toxic febrile state, seizures, neurological signs and depressed level of consciousness.

Suspect in: pansinusitis, chronic ear disease, trauma.

Diagnosis

CT scan with contrast.

Management

◆ Antibiotics: PENICILLIN, CHLORAMPHENICOL, METRONIDAZOLE.
◆ Surgical drainage of sinus or middle ear. See Chapter 19 pages 188-98.
◆ Burrhole or craniotomy drainage of empyema.

Cerebral tumour

Peak incidence in childhood is between five and ten years. Site is 60% infratentorial.

Common tumour types

Infratentorial

◆ **Medulloblastoma**: arises from roof of fourth ventricle. Hydrocephalus occurs early. Malignant, 'seeds' to meninges.

◆ **Astrocytoma**: arises from cerebellar neuroglial cells. Often benign, cystic and completely resectable.
◆ **Brainstem glioma**: locally infiltrative, progressive cranial nerve and pyramidal tract involvement. Poor prognosis.
◆ **Ependymoma**: arises from wall of fourth ventricle, early obstruction.

Supratentorial

◆ **Glioma**: prognosis depends on histological grading.
◆ **Craniopharyngioma**: arises from embryonal remnants. Locally invasive; visual defects and hormonal changes.
◆ **Optic nerve glioma**: unilateral visual deterioration, exophthalmos.
◆ **Pineal region tumours**: Parinaud's syndrome (loss of conjugate upward gaze).

Clinical presentation

◆ Raised intracranial pressure (see page 331).
◆ Onset usually gradual.
◆ Local effects: ataxia, cranial nerve involvement, visual field defects.
◆ Hormonal and metabolic effects.

Management

Refer to a neurosurgical centre.

Seizure disorders

A seizure may be an isolated event in a child's life or may recur at varying intervals. The most likely cause in an individual child relates to that child's age. A clear distinction must be made between seizures and breath-holding attacks, night terrors, hysterical attacks and vasovagal syncope. A careful history and the absence of EEG abnormality usually serve to distinguish these entities from true seizure disorders.

Aetiology

Causes are listed according to age and order of frequency in Table 32.2.

Febrile seizures

Between 2 and 5% of children have one or more febrile seizures

Table 32.2 Aetiology of seizure disorders

Neonate (birth to one month)	Infancy and early childhood (one month to five years)	Childhood (after five years)
Perinatal anoxia	Acute infection Febrile convulsions Meningitis Encephalitis Abscess	Epilepsy Focal Simple partial Complex partial Secondarily generalized Generalized Absence Tonic/clonic Myoclonic
Cerebral trauma Haemorrhage Meningitis	Brain damage and defects Cerebral vein thrombosis Infantile myoclonic (West and Lennox-Gastaut)	Brain damage and defects Infection Meningitis Abscess Encephalitis
Metabolic Hypoglycaemia Tetany Hypomagnesaemia Uraemia Pyridoxine dependency Maternal drug withdrawal	Metabolic Hypernatraemia Hyponatraemia Hypocalcaemia Uraemia Amino or organic aciduria Toxins Brain Tumour Degenerative diseases	Metabolic Hypernatraemia Hyponatraemia Hypocalcaemia Amino or organic aciduria Toxins BrainTumour Degenerative diseases

between the ages of six months and four years. In most instances the attack occurs at the start of an intercurrent infection, is generalized in nature and lasts less than five minutes. Such seizures are described as 'simple' and carry a good prognosis.

Seizures are designated complex when there is a focal element, when the attack lasts for longer than 20 minutes, or when it recurs in the course of a single febrile episode. Such seizures carry a more guarded prognosis and call for on-going surveillance. The most appropriate prophylactic therapy for febrile seizures is rectal DIAZEPAM 5 mg administered when fever is first recognized and repeated at 12-hourly intervals.

Status epilepticus

Status epilepticus is present when one seizure follows another without any intervening period of consciousness. There is often an underlying aetiological factor of an infective, traumatic or metabolic nature which should, if possible, be eliminated. The risk of brain damage is markedly increased if status epilepticus continues for more than 30 minutes.

Treatment of seizures

◆ Ensure patent airway.
◆ Reduce body temperature if febrile: remove clothing, fan, tepid sponge.

If the seizure does not cease spontaneously within five minutes, initiate the following steps:

Step 1. Administer DIAZEPAM (Valium) rectally. 5 mg (1 ml) to infants under 10 kg weight and 10 mg (2 ml) to larger children. This will terminate most seizures within a few minutes. In certain circumstances (e.g. febrile seizures) rectal DIAZEPAM may be administered by suitably instructed lay persons while awaiting the arrival of the doctor. There is no danger of respiratory depression.

If the seizure does not cease after a further five minutes proceed to steps 2,3 and 4.

Step 2. DIAZEPAM (Valium) 0,3 mg/kg (maximum 10 mg) IV over two minutes is usually immediately effective. Transitory respiratory arrest may occur if the rate of IV administration is too rapid. Be prepared to assist ventilation. DIAZEPAM **must never be given IM.**

Step 3. Loading dose of PHENOBARBITONE 10-20 mg/kg IV or PHENYTOIN 15-20 mg/kg IV, if the patient has not already been receiving oral PHENOBARBITONE.

Note

◆ PHENYTOIN is an irritant to veins. Administer diluted in normal saline at 0,5-1 mg/kg/minute.

◆ Serum blood level one hour after initial dose is desirable to assess the need for further loading doses.
◆ Only one of these long-acting anticonvulsants should be used. If necessary the blood level may be pushed above the stated therapeutic level.

Step 4. Administer 2-4 ml/kg of 25% dextrose water intravenously. Fits due to hypoglycaemia will stop. Commence 5% dextrose water IV.

Oxygen: 100% by facemask.

Do appropriate biochemical investigations: e.g. blood for glucose, electrolytes, calcium, magnesium, toxicology and anticonvulsant levels and for toxicology studies if indicated.

If seizures do not cease after five minutes, proceed to:

Step 5. Repeat DIAZEPAM (Valium) 0,2-0,4 mg/kg intravenously or give: CLONAZEPAM (Rivotril).

◆ Infants 0,5 mg (1 ml), IV slowly.
◆ Children 1 mg (2 ml).

If seizures do not cease after a further 15 minutes proceed to steps 6 and 7.

Step 6. Admit to intensive care. Institute cardiac and BP monitoring. Select one of the following infusions:

◆ PHENYTOIN 15-20 mg/kg (if not previously used) as an infusion, diluted in normal saline at 0,5-1 mg/kg/minute.
◆ CLONAZEPAM (Rivotril) 0,05 mg/kg in 200 ml 5% dextrose water. Run initially at 10 drops (1 ml) per minute and then titrate according to response. In resistant cases the dose of CLONAZEPAM may be increased to 0,3 mg/kg.

Step 7. MANNITOL can be used to treat assumed cerebral oedema. Give 1 g/kg IV immediately as a single dose only.

If the seizure has not ceased within 60 minutes consider

Step 8. Intubation, ventilation and THIOPENTONE (Pentothal) infusion.

THIOPENTONE 1 g in 200 ml 5% dextrose water. Start infusion at three drops per minute and increase every five minutes, in increments of three drops, (6,9,12, etc.) until a response can be seen. Increase to 2 g in 200 ml infusion if problems with fluid volume are encountered.

Intubation and ventilation may be necessary.

Further management

Once seizures have been abolished, institute appropriate special investigations. Lumbar puncture may be indicated if physical signs suggest meningitis. Commence an anticonvulsant maintenance regime guided by age, nature of convulsions and special investigations.

Long-term therapy

Anticonvulsant medication may adversely affect intellectual function and development. Careful consideration is necessary before embarking on long-term therapy. A child who has had more than two non-febrile seizures within a period of weeks should be considered for long-term therapy. Choice of anticonvulsant is determined by the nature of seizures and cost of the drugs.

The goal of treatment should be full seizure control with a single anticonvulsant at a dose which causes minimal side-effects. It is usual practice to continue therapy for two years after the last seizure and then gradually wean over a period of months.

Table 32.3 Choice of anticonvulsant

Seizure	Anticonvulsant
Focal Simple partial Complex partial Secondarily generalized	CARBAMAZEPINE LAMOTRIGINE VIGABATRIN
Tonic/clonic	PHENOBARBITONE, CARBAMAZEPINE, SODIUM VALPROATE, PRIMIDONE, CLONAZEPAM, PHENYTOIN
Absence attacks (petit mal)	SODIUM VALPROATE, ETHOSUXIMIDE
Myoclonic and atonic	SODIUM VALPROATE, CLONAZEPAM, CLOBAZAM
Infantile spasms (West syndrome)	ACTH 40 units daily for 14 days.

See Appendix 2, 'Pharmacopoeia' for dosages and therapeutic serum ranges.

It is advisable to refer the child if good seizure control cannot be maintained and/or if significant adverse reactions develop to the drugs used.

Note

There is poor correlation between serum levels of SODIUM VALPROATE, CLONAZEPAM and ETHOSUXIMIDE and seizure control. The effectiveness of treatment with anticonvulsants should be gauged according to clinical criteria.

The floppy child

Tone is the resistance which a relaxed muscle shows to passive movement. The normal suppleness and ligament laxity of childhood should not be mistaken for hypotonia. Hypotonia may occur with or without paralysis.

Conditions affecting the lower motor neurone

◆ Spinal muscular atrophy, e.g. Werdnig-Hoffman, Kugelberg-Welander.
◆ Congenital myopathies, e.g. central core disease, nemaline myopathy, myotubular myopathy and mitochondrial disorders.
◆ Glycogen storage disease, e.g. Pompe's disease.
◆ Muscular dystrophies.
◆ Neuropathies, e.g. poliomyelitis, Guillain-Barré syndrome and peripheral neuritis.
◆ Dystrophia myotonica, myasthenia gravis, hypokalaemia and spinal cord transection.
◆ Infantile botulinism.

Conditions in which the lower motor neurone is intact

◆ Acute illness.
◆ Disorders of the CNS, e.g. mental retardation, Down's syndrome, hypotonic cerebral palsy, degenerative brain disorders, sequela to kernicterus and Prader Willi syndrome.
◆ Disorders of connective tissue, e.g. congenital laxity of ligaments, Ehlers-Danlos syndrome and Marfan syndrome.
◆ Metabolic, e.g. undernutrition, rickets and hypothyroidism.

Involuntary movements

Facial tics

Stereotyped repetitive facial movements, i.e. blinking, twitching. These increase with emotional tension, and reflect an anxiety state.

Spasmus nutans

Rhythmical head titubation (head nodding), torticollis and nystagmus. The cause is unknown, and the course is benign.

Sydenham's chorea

Rapid irregular non-repetitive quasi-purposive movements predominantly of limbs. Associated hypotonia and other signs of rheumatic fever.

Athetosis

Slow, coarse, writhing peripheral movements absent at rest but evoked by attempted voluntary movements. Indicate basal ganglion damage due to kernicterus, anoxia, toxin or drug.

Intention tremor

Coarse tremor, absent at rest and increasing in amplitude as limb approaches its goal. May be associated with gait and truncal ataxia. Indicative of cerebellar dysfunction.

Dystonia

'Frozen athetosis'. Wide amplitude writhing movements which involve mainly proximal joints and force the patient into bizarre postures. Most commonly seen as a toxic manifestation of treatment with phenothiazines and HALOPERIDOL. Opisthotonus, torticollis and deviation of eyes may also be seen. Rapid response to IV administration of BIPERIDEN (Akineton).

Myoclonus

Sudden shock-like mass contraction of muscles. In infants this is termed 'salaam spasms'. Older children may be thrown to the ground. Associated abnormal EEG. Suggests infantile myoclonic epilepsy, SSPE or other degenerative disease of CNS.

33 NEWBORN

V C Harrison

Assessment at birth

The Apgar assessment reflects the ability of a baby to breathe adequately after birth. It is done at one and five minutes of age and is scored from 0 to 10.

Table 33.1 Apgar Score

Sign	0	1	2
Heart rate	Absent	Under 100/min	Over 100/min
Respiratory effort	Absent	Weak, irregular	Strong, regular
Muscle tone	Limp	Some flexion	Active movement
Response to stimuli	None	Weak response	Cry
Colour	Blue or pale body	Pink body, blue extremities	Completely pink

Advantages

One minute: a high score (8 or more) implies good adaptation; whereas a low score (3 or less) indicates the need for resuscitation.

Five minutes: a low score reflects an inadequate response to resuscitation.

Prolonged depression increases the risk of death or cerebral damage.

Limitations

The score cannot identify the presence or absence of prenatal hypoxaemia. Consequently it cannot predict the outcome after birth.

Birth asphyxia and resuscitation

An infant who fails to breathe adequately after birth is considered to be asphyxiated.

◆ Anticipate the need for resuscitation in the following circumstances: preterm delivery, fetal distress, maternal sedation, e.g. general anaesthesia, PETHIDINE, MORPHINE.
◆ Ensure that the baby is kept warm at and after birth.
   ◇ Arrangements to create a warm birth environment at the home, hospital or clinic are important.
   ◇ A resuscitation table with overhead infrared heating or a wall-mounted panel heater is a minimal requirement for a health facility's delivery room.
   ◇ Dry the baby rapidly and use a clean dry warm towel to rewrap.
   ◇ Suction secretions from the nostrils and mouth.

Apgar Score of ≤3

Ominous signs include a slow heart rate (<100/min), apnoea and floppiness.

◆ Place a facemask ventilator (Samson, Laerdal, Ambu) firmly over the baby's nose and mouth.
◆ **Use only a neonatal ventilator to avoid excessive pressure.**
◆ Compress the bag as rapidly as possible and ensure that oxygen (if available) is flowing into the circuit (4 l/min).
◆ **Positive response:** the heart rate accelerates and the mucosae become pink.
◆ **Negative response within 30 seconds:** intubate the larynx with a 2,5 mm endotracheal tube. Attach this to the facemask ventilator and continue to expand the lungs.
◆ Establish that the tube is in the trachea by observing equal movements of the chest and by auscultating equal breath sounds of the lungs.
◆ Use external cardiac massage if a bradycardia (<100/min) persists. Place a hand around the chest and compress the mid-sternum against the vertebral column with the thumb (approximately 100 times/min). Continue to ventilate. Spontaneous breathing may be delayed despite an improvement in colour and heart rate. Although unusual this is probably due to a metabolic acidosis, oversedation or hypoglycaemia.

◆ Continue to ventilate the lungs and have an assistant inject the following mixture into the umbilical vein or a peripheral vein.

Neonatal NALOXONE	1,0 ml
Sodium bicarbonate 4,2%	2,0 ml
Dextrose water 5%	2,0 ml

By now the majority (99%) of infants with a low Apgar Score will be breathing satisfactorily.

◆ Anticipate a poor outcome if bradycardia (<60/min), pallor, gasping, apnoea, or floppiness persist despite adequate resuscitation.
◆ Continue ventilation until you can exclude treatable conditions such as pneumothorax or hypovolaemia.

Pneumothorax: X-ray of the chest.
  Management: chest drain.
Hypovolaemia: the venous packed cell volume (PCV) is <30.
  Management: correct with a rapid transfusion of blood or stabilized human serum (15 ml/kg).

◆ Discontinue resuscitation if these measures do not result in adequate breathing.

Apgar Score of 4-7

The infant usually makes some effort to breathe.

◆ Hold the facemask ventilator over the baby's nose and mouth so that oxygen can be inhaled.
◆ Flick the feet with a finger.

Adequate breathing: provide warmth and routine management.
Failure of adequate breathing within 15 seconds: expand the lungs using facemask ventilation. This is usually successful. If not then proceed as for a low Apgar Score.

Gestational age and intra-uterine growth

Term babies are between 37 and 42 weeks of gestation and can cope with extra-uterine life. Babies less than 37 weeks are preterm and those over 42 weeks are post-term.

NOTE: Read this figure in conjunction with Table 33.5 on physical maturity on page 375.

Figure 33.1 Ballard Scoring System for clinical assessment of maturation in newborn infants

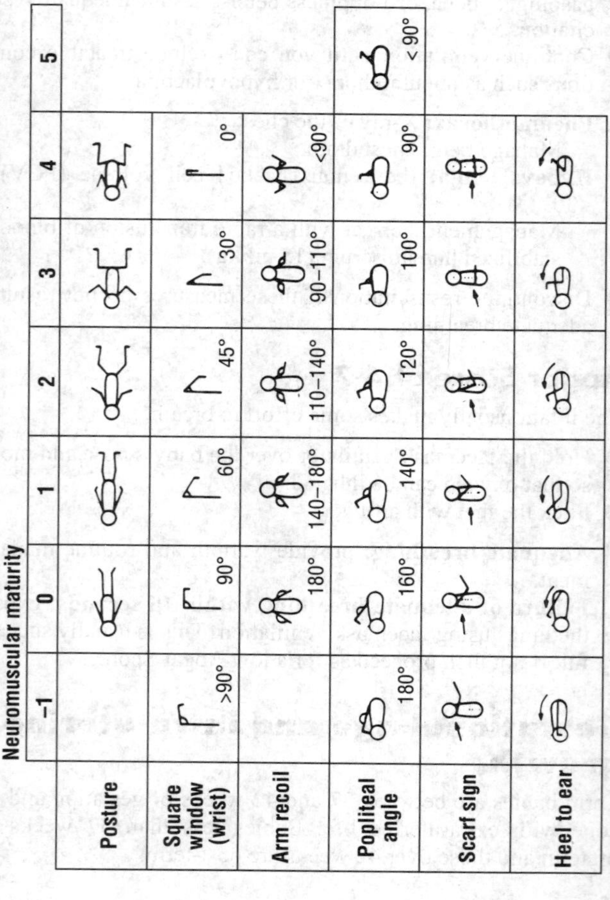

Neuromuscular maturity

	−1	0	1	2	3	4	5
Posture							
Square window (wrist)	>90°	90°	60°	45°	30°	0°	
Arm recoil		180°	140–180°	110–140°	90–110°	<90°	
Popliteal angle	180°	160°	140°	120°	100°	90°	<90°
Scarf sign							
Heel to ear							

Reprinted with permission from *J Paed* 1991; 119:417–423.

Gestation

Methods of assessment of gestational age

Menstrual history: when exact dates are known the duration of amenorrhoea is an accurate indication of gestation.

Examination of infant: various physical and neurological characteristics can be used to estimate gestation. They have been incorporated into methods such as the Ballard Score (see Figure 33.1) which is reasonably accurate (±2 weeks).

Intra-uterine growth

Weight (Appendix 4, Figure 9, page 674), head circumference (Appendix 4, Figure 10, page 675) and length (Appendix 4 Figure 11, page 676) at birth reflect the adequacy of intra-uterine growth. Most babies have a birthweight within the 90th and 10th percentiles on a growth chart. Their weight is appropriate for gestational age (AGA). Those under the 10th percentile are underweight for gestational age (UGA).

An equivalent depression of head circumference and length indicates prolonged fetal undernutrition. When only weight is diminished, the duration of undernutrition has been short. In some cases the weight is disproportionately less than head circumference and length but is not below the 10th percentile. This indicates a short period of intra-uterine 'wasting' and has the same implications as UGA.

Babies above the 90th percentile are overweight for gestational age (OGA). Most have diabetic mothers.

Risks: UGA and OGA babies

UGA

Sudden intra-uterine death, birth asphyxia, increased risk of congenital abnormalities, hypoglycaemia, retarded growth in childhood.

OGA

Sudden intra-uterine death, birth trauma, increased risk of congenital abnormalities, hypoglycaemia, hypocalcaemia, hypomagnesaemia.

Hypoglycaemia

Definition

A blood glucose level below 2,5 mmol/l indicates hypo-glycaemia.

Aetiology

Common causes

◆ **Decreased glycogen stores:** preterm baby, underweight for gestation baby, wasted baby.
◆ **Increased demands for glucose:** respiratory distress, hypothermia, infection.
◆ **Increased blood insulin level:** infant of a diabetic mother.

Rarer causes

Hepatitis, hypoxia and pancreatic cell hyperplasia.

Clinical presentation

◆ **Asymptomatic:** hypoglycaemia is detected on a low Dex-trostix or an alternative method when screening babies at risk.
◆ **Symptomatic:** lethargy, apnoea and seizures are important signs.

Management

Prevention

◆ Maintain the level of blood glucose above 2,5 mmol/l in babies at risk (see 'Common causes').
◆ Feed those who can tolerate milk by breast, bottle or naso-gastric tube within an hour of birth.
◆ Give 10% dextrose water by continuous intravenous infusion (60 ml/kg/day) to those who are unable to feed.

Treatment

Asymptomatic or symptomatic hypoglycaemia

◆ Give 10% dextrose water infusion intravenously to raise the level of blood sugar above 2,5 mmol/l as rapidly as possible.
◆ Ensure that oral feeding is established before discontinuing the intravenous fluid.

♦ HYDROCORTISONE 5 mg/kg may be given intravenously if dextrose alone fails to maintain a normal level of blood sugar.
♦ Use Dextrostix or an alternative method to monitor the level hourly until it is stabilized.
♦ Monitor blood glucose concentrations three-hourly for the next 24 hours.

Natural history

Hypoglycaemia is most likely to occur within six hours of birth. Thereafter the possibility declines and it is uncommon after 24 hours.

Complications

Symptomatic hypoglycaemia is associated with brain damage in more than 30% of cases.

Pitfalls

Ensure that oral feeding is established before an intravenous dextrose infusion is discontinued. Sudden withdrawal can result in hypoglycaemia.

Hypothermia

The peripheral temperature reflects a baby's metabolic state better than the rectal temperature. The latter falls only when various sources of heat production have been exhausted, e.g. brown fat, glycogen, food.

Peripheral temperature is measured with a low-reading thermometer in the axilla (normal 36,5-37 °C) or on the exposed skin of the abdomen (normal 36,2-36,8 °C). Levels below 36 °C indicate hypothermia.

Predisposing factors include: exposure to a cold environment, e.g. home delivery in winter and low birthweight.

Prevention

At birth

Ensure that birth takes place in a warm environment. Dry the baby with a warm towel and wrap in a second clean, dry, warm towel. Place the baby in a warm cot.

After birth

A term baby can usually maintain body temperature when

clothed, covered with two blankets and kept in a cot. The room should be free from draughts and the environmental temperature should not fall below 23 °C.

A baby of less than 1 800 g cannot maintain body temperature without additional warmth. Incubation provides the most effective control of body temperature and is used for an infant below this weight.

Alternative steps must be taken if incubators are unavailable.

◆ Warm the room (>28 °C).
◆ Keep windows and doors closed.
◆ Dress the baby warmly and cover the head with a thick woollen cap or wrap the baby in aluminium foil.

Diagnosis

Clinical observations and confirmation with a low thermometer reading.

Natural history

The newborn infant remains susceptible to cold at all times.

Complications

Hypoglycaemia, hyperbilirubinaemia, cold injury. The latter is characterized by lethargy, bradycardia, sclerema, and pulmonary haemorrhage.

Management

Heat the baby rapidly in a closed or open overhead infrared incubator. When rectal temperature (core) has reached 37 °C ensure a constant environmental temperature to prevent over-heating. Administer 10% dextrose water IV by constant infusion (80 ml/kg/day) to prevent hypoglycaemia during reheating.

Pitfalls

A severely cold baby can look deceptively healthy. The skin is pink because of trapped red blood cells which contain oxygenated haemoglobin.

Infection

Preterm babies are vulnerable and can suffer serious complications as they are unable to combat infection adequately.

Sources

Infection may be acquired before, during, or after birth.

Antenatal

Maternal infection can be transmitted to the fetus across the placenta. Important blood-borne diseases include syphilis, rubella, cytomegalovirus and toxoplasmosis.

Natal

Organisms may spread to the amniotic cavity through the cervix or can be acquired in the birth canal. Important agents include Group B Streptococcus, Gonococcus, *Herpes simplex* and Chlamydia.

The risk is increased by prolonged rupture of membranes (>24 hours), preterm labour, obstetric manipulations (e.g. Shirodkar suture).

Postnatal

Cross-infection may result from inadequate hand washing in a nursery or from contaminated feeds. Important organisms are *Staphylococcus aureus*, *Escherichia coli*, Streptococcus and Coxsackie virus.

Clinical presentation

Antenatal

Suspect infection when an unexplained stillbirth occurs, a congenital abnormality is detected, e.g. heart defect in rubella, or when characteristic clinical signs are seen at birth, e.g. hepatosplenomegaly, rash, pallor (syphilis).

Natal

The signs of infection occur soon after birth (<72 hours). Conjunctivitis (Gonococcus, Chlamydia) is common. Pneumonia and septicaemia (Group B Streptococcus) are less common.

Postnatal

Nursery-acquired infection presents after 72 hours of age. Conjunctivitis and oral thrush are common. Cord and skin infections (*S. aureus, E. coli*) are less common. Pneumonia, septicaemia, meningitis and urinary tract infection are uncommon.

Diagnosis

Clinical signs

Local infections such as conjunctivitis, omphalitis, skin pustules and thrush are obvious.

Systemic ones such as septicaemia are characterized by non-specific features. These include lethargy, poor sucking, unstable temperature, failure to gain weight, jaundice, hepatosplenomegaly, abdominal distension and vomiting.

X-ray

Patchy shadows occur in the lungs in pneumonia. Characteristic changes are seen in long bones in syphilis and rubella.

Laboratory

No single test gives a rapid and unequivocal diagnosis.

◆ **White cell count:** the total count may be raised ($>30 \times 10^9$/l) or lowered (5×10^9/l) in severe infection. Immature neutrophils (bands) are plentiful and the band to total neutrophil ratio exceeds 0,2.
◆ **IgM:** this antibody increases and a level over 30 IU/dl in the first 48 hours is significant.
◆ **Urine:** the antigen of Group B Streptococcus can be detected in urine in systemic infection.
◆ **Culture of bacteria:** the growth of an organism from blood, cerebrospinal fluid or urine provides evidence for infection. The inevitable delay makes this a retrospective diagnosis and treatment cannot be withheld if other features favour infection.
◆ **Identification of organisms:** the spirochaete can be demonstrated by dark ground illumination under the microscope. Chlamydia is identified by a rapid immunofluorescent stain and Candida can be seen on Gram's staining.
◆ **Virus identification:** the agent may be grown in tissue culture from blood, urine, throat swab, stool or cerebrospinal fluid. Viral particles, e.g. *Herpes simplex* can be detected in the spun deposit from vesicle fluid.

Important infections

The contaminated baby

Vaginal organisms may enter the amniotic cavity during pregnancy to cause inflammation in the placenta and membranes (chorio-amnionitis). Products of this reaction are swallowed by the fetus who is then at risk for infection. Chorio-amnionitis is most likely to occur in preterm labour and prolonged rupture of membranes (>24 hours).

Obtain a sample of baby's gastric fluid soon after birth in these circumstances. A count of more than five polymorphs per high power field indicates contamination. Bacteria may also be seen on a Gram's stain. A contaminated baby should receive antibiotics only when the risk of subsequent infection is high. Indications for antibiotic therapy include:

◆ contaminated babies under 1 500 g;
◆ those with Gram-positive cocci, as this may be Group B Streptococcus.

Conjunctivitis

Gonococcal conjunctivitis

The eyes are swollen and red and exude copious pus. Gram-negative diplococci may be seen in the discharge. Blindness may follow corneal ulceration.

◆ **Commence treatment immediately as the infection can result in blindness.**
◆ Instil PENICILLIN drops (20 000 units/ml) into the eyes at five-minute intervals for 30 minutes, then hourly for three days.
  ◇ If penicillin drops are unavailable, irrigation of the eyes with normal saline should be performed every five minutes for 30 minutes and then at hourly intervals for as long as necessary to eliminate the purulent discharge
◆ Give IM PROCAINE PENICILLIN (page 648) for seven days.
  ◇ Give intravenous penicillin for seven days in septicaemic patients.
  ◇ Penicillinase-producing strains should be treated with CEFTRIAXONE (page 581).
◆ Ensure that the mother and her sexual partner(s) are investigated and treated.

Non-gonococcal conjunctivitis

Many organisms can cause conjunctivitis. Most do not produce copious pus.

◆ Swab the conjunctivae for culture and for an immunofluorescent chlamydia stain.

◆ Instil CHLORAMPHENICOL ointment into the eyes three times a day for five days.

◆ Suspect chlamydia infection if there is no response to CHLORAMPHENICOL or if the immunofluorescent stain is positive. Treat chlamydia with ERYTHROMYCIN eye drops and with oral ERYTHROMYCIN suspension for a week.

Ocular prophylaxis

Ophthalmic ointments containing ERYTHROMYCIN, TETRACYLINE, CHLORAMPHENICOL or 1% SILVER NITRATE are all useful.

Meningitis

In bacteraemia, organisms may cross the blood-brain barrier to cause meningitis. Alternative sources include local abnormalities such as a meningomyelocele.

In the early stage, the non-specific features of sepsis prevail. Neurological signs are ominous and include a tense fontanelle, squinting, seizures, increased tone and coma.

◆ Obtain cerebrospinal fluid by a lumbar puncture. The fluid may be hazy and may contain organisms which can be detected on a Gram's stain. The diagnosis is confirmed by culture.

Treatment

CEFTRIAXONE is the drug of choice. It crosses the blood-brain barrier readily and is effective against most organisms which are implicated.

The Group B Streptococcus is common and AMPICILLIN is added to the regimen when this organism is identified. Treatment is needed for 14 to 21 days.

Omphalitis

Initially the skin at the base of the cord is red. It later becomes oedematous and pus may ooze from the cord. The risk of peritonitis or septicaemia is high. Omphalitis is caused by a variety of organisms.

◆ Obtain a swab for culture before starting treatment. CEFTRIAXONE given for seven days is the antibiotic of choice.

Septicaemia

Bacteria can enter the blood from a colonized area or from a local infection. The preterm baby is particularly susceptible and shows non-specific features of sepsis. Late signs are ominous and include hypothermia, bleeding, sclerema and prolonged blanching of the skin on compression. Meningitis and osteomyelitis are likely complications.

◆ A positive blood culture confirms the diagnosis. Treatment must not be delayed if reasonable clinical and laboratory evidence is present. CEFTRIAXONE is given for 14 days. The type of organism and its sensitivity will determine the necessity for additional or alternative antibiotics.

Group B Streptococcus is a common organism, and other likely bacteria include *E. coli* and Klebsiella.

The following complications may need to be treated:

◆ hypothermia: heated crib or incubator;
◆ hypoxaemia: oxygen, ventilation;
◆ anaemia: packed red blood cell transfusion;
◆ shock: stabilized human serum;
◆ thrombocytopaenia: platelet transfusion; or
◆ metabolic acidosis: sodium bicarbonate 4,2%.

Skin pustules

Purulent or clear vesicles may occur at any site, have a narrow red base and contain Gram-positive cocci. *S. aureus* is usually cultured.

CLOXACILLIN suspension, the antibiotic of choice, is given for seven days.

◆ Skin sepsis is contagious and precautions must be taken to prevent the spread of infection. Hand washing is essential.

Syphilis (congenital)

See page 262.

Thrush

Candida involves the mouth or buttock area. White plaques adhere to the inner cheeks, lips and the tongue and the underlying mucosa is red. Most napkin rashes are associated with Candida although the fungus may not have initiated the problem. The area may be red or excoriated or it may be peppered with punctate ulcers.

◆ Treat oral thrush with NYSTATIN drops: 1 ml into the mouth after each feed for a week.
◆ Treat a napkin rash with NYSTATIN ointment: apply this to the buttocks after each napkin change.
◆ Seek a source of infection such as the mother's nipples or vagina. The fungus may also contaminate bottles, teats, dummies, hands or gripe water.
◆ Boil dummies, teats and bottles, discard gripe water and treat maternal thrush if applicable.

Tuberculosis
See pages 562-7.

Urinary tract infection
See page 488.

Organisms frequently seed out in the urinary tract in bacteraemia. An underlying abnormality such as hydronephrosis may also result in infection. Non-specific signs such as failure to thrive or jaundice predominate.

Diagnosis depends on the growth of a single organism, usually *E. coli* from a 'clean catch' or suprapubic specimen of urine. The bacterial count must exceed 100 000 organisms per mm^3.

◆ CEFTRIAXONE provides adequate therapy in most cases and the subsequent choice of an antibiotic depends on sensitivity results. Treatment is needed for ten to 14 days.
◆ Check the urine for infection at intervals over the next three months.
◆ Request an ultrasound examination of the urinary tract to exclude underlying abnormalities.

Jaundice
Jaundice is the most common problem in the first week of life.

Physiological jaundice
The serum level of unconjugated bilirubin rises in all babies after birth. In many (45%) it may be sufficiently high to be clinically evident. This physiological event has never been adequately explained.

Diagnosis

- ♦ Jaundice seldom appears before the second or third day.
- ♦ It rarely lasts for more than ten days.
- ♦ The maximum level of bilirubin is usually below 250 μmol/l.
- ♦ Only the unconjugated fraction of bilirubin is increased.
- ♦ The baby thrives and shows no signs of illness.
- ♦ Treatment is unnecessary.

Pathological jaundice

Jaundice is considered to be pathological if it:

- ♦ appears within 24 hours of birth;
- ♦ exceeds 250 μmol/l;
- ♦ persists for more than ten days; or
- ♦ is mostly conjugated.

Table 33.2 Hyperbilirubinaemias

Unconjugated hyperbilirubinaemia	
Excessive haemolysis	**Defective conjugation**
ABO incompatibility	Prematurity
Rhesus disease	Infection
Familial spherocytosis	Hypoxaemia
G6PD deficiency	Hypoglycaemia
Enclosed haemorrhages	Hypothyroidism
Polycythaemia	

Conjugated hyperbilirubinaemia	
Hepato-cellular disease	**Bile obstruction**
Syphilis	Bile duct atresia
Other congenital infections	Cystic fibrosis
Galactosaemia	Choledochal cyst
α-antitrypsin deficiency	

Mixed unconjugated and conjugated hyperbilirubinaemia
Congenital infections
Postnatal infections
Severe Rhesus disease

The jaundice may result from an increase in unconjugated or conjugated bilirubin or in a combination. In most cases (99%) it is associated with unconjugated hyperbilirubinaemia. Conjugated hyperbilirubinaemia is always pathological but rare. Important causes are listed below.

Early onset jaundice: within 24 hours

This is likely to be caused by haemolytic disease of the newborn (ABO, Rh) and the following should be performed immediately:

◆ check the mother's blood group;
◆ check the level of bilirubin three-hourly;
◆ start phototherapy.

If mother's group is O, then ABO incompatibility is the most likely cause.

The following investigations are important:

◆ blood groups of mother and baby — for incompatibilities;
◆ direct Coombs test — for antibodies on infant's red blood cells;
◆ cord blood bilirubin level — for haemolysis before birth;
◆ haemoglobin and packed cell volume – for anaemia;
◆ reticulocyte count – for increased production of red cells;
◆ peripheral blood smear – for abnormally shaped cells; and
◆ maternal immune antibodies – for maternal sensitization.

Further tests are rarely required, but in unusual cases the following may be helpful:

◆ red cell enzymes;
◆ haemoglobin electrophoresis; or
◆ osmotic fragility of red blood cells.

Excessive jaundice: after 48 hours

A level of unconjugated bilirubin which exceeds 250 μmol/l needs investigation.

◆ Check the blood groups of mother and baby to exclude incompatibility.
◆ Examine baby to exclude an obvious infection or enclosed haemorrhages.
◆ Collect a specimen of urine for group B streptococcal antigen test to exclude infection.
◆ Check the packed cell volume to exclude polycythaemia (PCV >70).

Figure 33.2 Unconjugated bilirubin: term infants

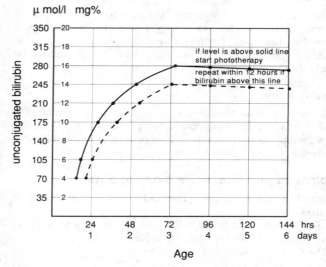

Figure 33.3 Unconjugated bilirubin: preterm infants

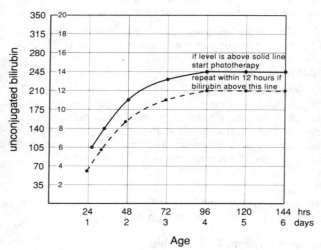

Term baby

In most cases a cause will not be found for the jaundice. It is considered to be an exaggeration of physiological hyperbilirubinaemia. Treatment will depend on the level of bilirubin (see Figure 33.2 on page 359) which should be checked daily.

Preterm baby

In the absence of an obvious cause, the jaundice is considered to be due to immaturity of the conjugating mechanism in the liver. Phototherapy is needed and is commenced at lower bilirubin levels than in term babies (see Figure 33.3 on page 359).

Prolonged jaundice: more than ten days

A term baby rarely remains jaundiced for more than a week to ten days.

Likely causes are: breast milk jaundice, urinary tract infection, hypothyroidism, bile duct atresia and hepatitis

The following steps should be taken:

◆ determine whether or not the baby is breast-fed;
◆ collect urine to exclude infection and also test for reducing substances to exclude galactosaemia; and
◆ measure the conjugated fraction of bilirubin.

If none of these are applicable then ensure that the infant's thyroid function is normal by obtaining a blood level of TSH and T4.

Breast milk Jaundice

Some breast-fed infants remain yellow for several weeks. This usually follows an exaggerated physiological jaundice in the first week. It is thought to be due to milk glucuronidase causing an excessive absorption of bilirubin in the gut, thereby raising serum unconjugated bilirubin. The level of bilirubin rarely exceeds 200 µmol/l and treatment is unnecessary.

Note

Before giving the baby the label of 'breast milk jaundice' ensure that a urinary tract infection has been excluded.

Conjugated hyperbilirubinaemia

This implies an obstruction to the outflow of bilirubin from the liver. It may result from swelling of liver cells caused by a hepatitis or from the absence of bile ducts. In severe haemolytic disease and infection, the unconjugated and conjugated fractions may be raised. The level of total serum bilirubin (TSB) gives no indication of the amount of conjugated bilirubin. Serum conjugated bilirubin concentrations must be measured in the following circumstances:

◆ Jaundice associated with illness such as hepatosplenomegaly, rashes, pallor, e.g. syphilis.
◆ Signs of bile obstruction such as pale stools and dark urine.
◆ Jaundice which persists for more than ten days.

Important investigations include:

◆ serum IgM – to detect infection;
◆ X-ray long bones – to detect congenital syphilis;
◆ stool –to detect bile pigments;
◆ urine – to detect bilirubin and to exclude infection;
◆ ultrasound scan of the liver – to assess the status of bile ducts.

Additional studies are needed in obscure cases. They include a liver biopsy and a radionucleide liver scan. See also page 548.

Complications

If unconjugated bilirubin crosses the brain barrier it can cause an encephalopathy. Signs vary from lethargy and poor sucking to opisthotonus, hypertonia, pyrexia and convulsions when kernicterus (yellow-stained ganglia) has occurred. Late manifestations include learning disabilities, mental retardation, deafness and cerebral palsy.

The possibility of damage is increased by:

◆ an excessive blood level of unconjugated bilirubin (>350 µmol/l);
◆ prematurity, particularly in babies under 1 000 g;
◆ drugs – especially sulphonamides; and
◆ severe hypoxaemia and acidosis.

These factors can be prevented or minimized by avoiding risk factors such as sulphonamides, preventing haemolytic disease caused by Rhesus sensitization and by treating unconjugated hyperbilirubinaemia promptly with phototherapy.

Management of jaundice

Prevention of Rhesus disease

Give anti-D globulin to each Rhesus-negative mother who delivers a Rhesus-positive infant. If given within 72 hours of birth, this will prevent her developing anti-D antibodies.

Repeat the treatment after every pregnancy if there are no maternal Rhesus antibodies and the infant is Rhesus-positive. If delays are experienced in obtaining the blood groups of babies, give the anti-D regardless of the infant's blood group.

Any factor which can cause a significant transfer of blood from the fetus to the mother warrants the use of anti-D globulin during pregnancy.

These include: abortion, ectopic pregnancy, antepartum haemorrhage, amniocentesis and external cephalic version.

Phototherapy

Fluorescent light at 400-500 nm wavelength alters the molecular structure of unconjugated bilirubin and renders it water-soluble and non-toxic. The indications for phototherapy in term and preterm babies are shown in Figures 33.2 and 33.3 (page 359). During treatment ensure that the baby's temperature is normal, that the intake of fluid is adequate and that the eyes are protected from intense light. In haemolytic disease the response is unpredictable and serum bilirubin should be checked several times a day. In conditions other than haemolytic disease the expected decrease in bilirubin is 60 µmol/l per day during continuous exposure to light.

Technique

A small baby is treated in an incubator, a large one in a cot. Undress the baby and cover the eyes with gauze pads. These are kept in place with micropore plaster or a commercial cloth harness. Position the phototherapy unit about 50 cm above the baby.

Complications

Rashes, loose stools, thirst, hypo- or hyperthermia.

Pitfalls

◆ Ensure that eye pads are positioned correctly. They may obstruct nasal breathing if too tight or if dislodged.

◆ Light tubes lose their effectiveness after approximately 1 500 hours. Change them if light intensity cannot be measured.
◆ Severe and undetected anaemia may develop in haemolytic disease.

Exchange transfusion

This procedure is now seldom required because of phototherapy and anti-D globulin.

Indications

At birth

Hydrops foetalis. Severe anaemia (Hb <10 g/dl) due to haemolysis.

Within 24 hours

A rise in serum bilirubin which exceeds 17 μmol/l/hour despite phototherapy.

After 24 hours

Fullterm infant: unconjugated bilirubin >350 μmol/l in Rh disease; >420 μmol/l in others. Preterm infant: unconjugated bilirubin >300 μmol/l.

Note

Lower levels (subtract 50 μmol/l from above) may have to be used when risk factors such as sulphonamides, extreme prematurity and severe asphyxia are present.

Technique

◆ Use whole blood (Group O Rh negative) which is less than 72 hours old. Warm the pack to 37 °C in a blood warmer or waterbath.
◆ Restrain the baby's limbs and monitor the temperature, heart rate, respiration and colour.
◆ Fill a size 8F catheter with heparinized saline and introduce it into the umbilical vein. Advance the catheter until a free flow of blood is obtained. Connect two two-way taps in series to the catheter and a 20 ml syringe. Attach tubes from the blood pack and disposal bag to the side arms of the taps.
◆ Perform a 160 ml/kg exchange in 10 to 20 ml aliquots over 60 minutes. Use smaller volumes for sick or very small

Recognizable syndromes

Table 33.3 Incidence, features and outcome[1]

Type	Incidence	Neonatal features	Outcome
De Lange	1 in 10 000	Short stature, microcephaly, weak cry, hypertonicity, hirsutism, long curly eyelashes, thick eyebrows, coarse hair, short nose, crescentric downcurving mouth.	Severe mental retardation
Down's	1 in 2 000 <25 yrs 1 in 50 >45 yrs	Hypotonic, small ears, small stature, small head, flat occiput, slanted eyes, epicanthic folds, single palmar crease, short fingers sandal gap, congenital heart lesion 50%.	Mental retardation, recurrent infections deafness, male azoospermia (female fertile), 50% die in childhood.
Fetal alcohol	Variable	Growth retardation, microcephaly, micro-phthalmia, small palpebral fissure, upturned nose, hypoplastic philthrum and maxilla, congenital heart disease.	Mental retardation, small stature.
Kline-felter	1 in 1 000 males	Small testes.	Gynaecomastia, mental retardation. 25% infertility.
Russel-Silver		Small stature, hemihypertrophy, small triangular face, thin lips, mouth down-turned corners, clinodactyly, cryptorchidism, hypoglycaemia.	Slow growth, normal intelli-gence.
Trisomy 18	1 in 4 000	Growth retardation, small mouth, micrognathia, fingers: Index overlaps third, fifth overlaps fourth. Hypotonia,	Severe mental retardation. Most die within 18 months.

Type	Incidence	Neonatal features	Outcome
		hypoplastic nails, rocker-bottom feet, ventricular septal defect, cryptorchidism.	
Trisomy 13	1 in 5 000	Microcephaly, microphthalmia. Colomboma of iris, cleft lip and palate, thin ribs, ventricular septal defect.	Severe mental retardation. Most die within 18 months
Turner's	1 in 3 000 females	Female, small stature, lymphoedema, web neck, puffy hands and feet, wide-spaced nipples, cubitus valgus. Cardiovascular defects 20%.	Short, sterile. Some are mentally retarded or deaf.

[1] Further information on genetic conditions or services is obtainable from University Departments of Human Genetics or the Subdirectorate: Genetic Services of the Department of National Health and Population Development.

Table 33.4 Distinguishing features of common diseases

	Hyaline membrane disease	Wet lung syndrome	Meconium aspiration	Congenital pneumonia
X-ray chest	Diffuse granular appearance with air bronchograms	Hilar streaking, over-inflation	Patchy shadowing, over-inflation	Patchy shadows
Gastric fluid shake test	Negative	Positive	Positive	Positive
Pus/bacteria	Absent	Absent	Absent	Present
Urine Latex test Group B Streptococcus	Negative	Negative	Negative	Positive if Group B Streptococcus

infants. These infants should receive a constant infusion of glucose and calcium by separate IV lines to prevent hypoglycaemia and hypocalcaemia, particularly after the exchange. When the catheter has been removed, cover the umbilicus with a dry sterile dressing. Antibiotic prophylaxis is not recommended unless the exchange has been repeated.

◆ Phototherapy should be used after the exchange.
◆ Commence nasogastric feeding with milk if bowel sounds are present and monitor blood glucose and bilirubin six-hourly.

Respiratory distress

Definition

Respiratory distress is characterized by two or more of the following signs: persistent tachypnoea (>60/min), rib and sternal recession, expiratory grunting, central cyanosis in room air.

Causes

Common diseases are: hyaline membrane disease, aspiration pneumonia (meconium or bacteria) and wet lung syndrome.

Less common ones are: pneumothorax and patent ductus arteriosus.

Rare causes include: diaphragmatic hernia and congenital heart disease.

Diagnosis

Diseases cannot be distinguished by clinical signs, and the following tests are most helpful:

◆ X-ray chest
◆ Gastric fluid – Shake test for surfactant.
　　　　　　　　 – Gram's stain for pus/bacteria.
◆ Urine　　　　 – Latex test (Wellcome) for Group B Streptococcus.

Management

Provide the distressed infant with adequate oxygen, warmth and energy, prevent acidosis and prevent and treat infection.

Oxygen

◆ Place a perspex hood over the baby's head and ensure that

the lips and tongue remain pink by regulating the concentration of oxygen in the hood. A gas blender can be used for this purpose.

♦ Measure the saturation of oxygen in the baby's blood with a pulse oximeter. A reading of between 89 and 92% will ensure a normal arterial oxygen tension (PaO$_2$ 7-12 kPa, 50-90 mmHg). Adjust the concentration of oxygen in the hood to achieve this level.

♦ If oxygen monitors are unavailable use the least amount of oxygen which will keep the baby's mucosae pink. **Attempt to reduce the concentration every few hours.**

Warning

Oxygen is potentially harmful to small babies, especially those less than 1 500 g. When saturation readings exceed 92% the arterial tension may be sufficiently high to cause eye damage (retrolental fibroplasia). If prolonged oxygen therapy is necessary, transfer the baby to a centre where monitoring is available.

Assisted ventilation

Ventilatory assistance is needed if a satisfactory oxygen saturation cannot be maintained.

Continuous Positive Airway Pressure (CPAP)

The infant inhales oxygen under pressure (0,7 kPa, 5 cm H$_2$O) through nasal prongs.

Indications

Use CPAP if oxygen saturation remains less than 89% in a hood concentration of 80%.

Intermittent Positive Pressure Ventilation (IPPV)

A respirator is used to ventilate the lungs through nasal prongs or an endotracheal tube.

Indications

Use IPPV if CPAP fails to raise oxygen saturation above 89%, or if the baby develops apnoea.

Warmth

Place the baby in an incubator or open crib with heater and maintain skin temperature between 36,2 and 36,8 °C. This avoids an increase in the metabolic demands of respiratory distress.

Energy

Ensure that the blood sugar is maintained within a normal range (>2,5 mmol/l). A 10% dextrose or Neonatalyte solution is given intravenously through a peripheral vein. The flow rate (60 ml/kg/day) is controlled by an infusion pump. Nasogastric feeding with full strength milk can usually be commenced after 24 or 48 hours if bowel sounds are audible and meconium has been passed.

Acidosis

A metabolic acidosis can be prevented by adequate oxygenation and by adding a small quantity of sodium bicarbonate to the 10% Dextrose solution (10 ml 4,2% $NaHCO_3$ to 200 ml 10% Dextrose water).

Metabolic acidosis may also be corrected according to the formula:

$$mmol\ bicarbonate = base\ deficit \times wt\ in\ kg \times 0,6$$

It is wise to give only half the calculated amount of 4,2% sodium bicarbonate initially and then to reassess the situation. Do not use 8% sodium bicarbonate. It has a very high osmolality.

A severe respiratory acidosis ($PaCO_2$ >10 kPa, 75 mmHg) implies inadequate ventilation and is an indication for CPAP or IPPV.

Antibiotics

Treat an obvious or suspected pneumonia with an antibiotic. CEFTRIAXONE is a suitable choice. It is given once a day by intramuscular or intravenous injection and will destroy most of the bacteria which are likely to be implicated.

Hyaline membrane disease

Immature lungs lack surfactant. They are therefore unstable during expiration. The alveoli collapse and need considerable pressure for reinflation. Surfactant production is inhibited by hypoxaemia, acidosis and hypothermia. The more asphyxiated or shocked an infant, the more severe is the respiratory distress.

Clinical presentation

Hyaline membrane disease is likely to occur in the appropriately-grown preterm baby. Respiratory distress is apparent at birth and persists. Chest movement is impaired and the baby grunts to keep the alveoli inflated during expiration. Other features of organ immaturity may be present: oedema, ileus and jaundice are common. Abnormal neurological signs such as seizures may result from intraventricular bleeding.

Management

◆ Atelectatic alveoli can be re-expanded by SURFACTANT.
◆ Indications: use SURFACTANT for the distressed infant who requires assisted ventilation (IPPV).
◆ Dose: 100 mg/kg. Instil this dose into the trachea in four equal amounts. It may be injected through a 5F feeding catheter which is inserted just beyond the tip of the endotracheal tube. Alter the baby's position after each portion and ventilate the lungs mechanically to disperse the drug.
◆ Response: oxygen and pressure requirements decrease. Repeat the treatment within six hours if the response is inadequate.

Outcome

Most babies recover within a week and the survival rate exceeds 95%.

Complications

Pneumothorax, patent ductus arteriosus, bronchopulmonary dysplasia.

Pitfalls

Group B Streptococcus pneumonia can mimic the clinical and radiological features of hyaline membrane disease. Be sure to exclude this diagnosis.

Wet lung

Lung fluid is cleared from the interstitial space into veins and lymphatics within 30 minutes of birth. A delay in resorption decreases lung compliance.

Clinical presentation

This condition affects some babies who are delivered before term by Caesarian Section. Respiratory distress is present at birth: is not as severe as hyaline membrane disease; and resolves within 24 to 48 hours.

Treatment

Oxygen if needed.

Meconium aspiration

Meconium is expelled *in utero* as a result of hypoxia. It may be inhaled before or after birth to obstruct bronchi and cause pneumonitis. This results in atelectasis and hyperinflation of alveoli.

Clinical presentation

Term babies and those who are wasted or underweight for gestation are susceptible. Respiratory distress is present from birth and the chest is overexpanded and hyper-resonant. The umbilical cord, skin and nails may be stained with meconium. Other complications of hypoxaemia may be present.

Management

◆ Many cases can be prevented if meconium is cleared from the nasopharynx before the onset of breathing. Use a 10F end-hole catheter to suction meconium from the mouth and pharynx when the head is delivered.
◆ After birth, wash out meconium from the stomach with 2% sodium bicarbonate.

Intubation

This is recommended if thick meconium extends to the vocal cords. Insert an endotracheal tube into the larynx, instil 1 ml normal saline and remove by suction. Repeat until secretions are clear.

Complications

Pneumothorax, pulmonary hypertension, secondary infection.

Pitfalls

Air leaks are common but difficult to diagnose from clinical signs. Suspect a pneumothorax if the infant deteriorates.

Congenital pneumonia

Bacteria may enter the lungs before or after birth. The Group B Streptococcus is the most common organism. It colonizes the vagina in 15% to 30% of pregnant women and can be transferred to the fetus. Many infants are contaminated but few develop infection.

Clinical presentation

Preterm babies are vulnerable. Respiratory distress is present at birth or may occur within 72 hours of delivery. The signs can mimic hyaline membrane disease and additional investigations are essential to establish the diagnosis, e.g. Latex urine test. Systemic signs of infection may predominate. They include lethargy, unstable temperature, prolonged blanching of the skin on compression and bleeding.

Treatment

If an organism has not been identified, CEFTRIAXONE is suitable and AMPICILLIN is added if Group B Streptococcus is suspected.

Pneumothorax

Alveoli can rupture in any type of respiratory distress, particularly if high pressures are generated by assisted ventilation. Stiff lungs cannot collapse and the entrapped pleural air may compress the heart and blood vessels.

Clinical presentation

Hyper-resonance and decreased air entry may be detected but are usually not obvious. Consider the diagnosis in a baby with deteriorating respiratory distress. Signs include a displaced apex beat and cyanosis, apnoea, pallor, hepatomegaly and poorly palpable pulses.

Diagnosis

Use a fibrescope to transilluminate the chest. A diffuse glow will be seen on the side of the pneumothorax. If the infant's condition permits further delay, obtain an X-ray of the chest to confirm the diagnosis.

Treatment

Use a narcotic, e.g. MORPHINE to sedate the infant before incising the skin in the anterior axillary line. Use fine forceps to dissect the underlying tissues until the pleural surface is seen. Rupture the sac and insert a 10F pleural catheter. This is immobilized and attached to an underwater drain.

Natural history

Resolution with drainage.

Complications

Pneumopericardium, pneumomediastinum, cardiac tamponade.

Pitfalls

Clinical signs may not be obvious. Confirm suspicion by transillumination and X-ray.

Patent ductus arteriosus

The ductus may remain patent after birth. This often occurs in preterm babies who have hyaline membrane disease. It results in shunting of blood. The direction of the shunt depends on the pressures in the heart and great vessels.

Clinical presentation

Suspect a patent ductus in the following circumstances: the peripheral pulses are bounding and easily palpable, a systolic murmur is audible, assisted ventilation is needed for more than 48 hours, or signs of heart failure are present, i.e. tachycardia, hepatomegaly, oedema.

Diagnosis

The clinical features are usually sufficient to make a diagnosis but confirmation can be obtained by ultrasonography.

Treatment

◆ Restrict the intake of fluid to 80 ml/kg/day.
◆ Use a diuretic: FUROSEMIDE 1 mg/kg.
◆ Correct anaemia if the PCV is less than 30.
◆ Intravenous INDOMETHACIN 0,2 mg/kg. This is given once a day over 30 minutes and repeated for five days. (The intravenous product is not available commercially in RSA. Consult a pharmacist.)
◆ Surgical ligation: this is rarely needed and is considered if heart failure cannot be controlled or the infant is ventilator-dependent because of the shunt.

Natural history

Closure usually occurs when the primary disease, e.g. hyaline membrane disease, has resolved.

Complications

Heart failure.

Pitfalls

A heart murmur is often absent. Concentrate on the character of the peripheral pulses.

Note

For other forms of congenital heart disease in newborns see Chapter 11 pages 101-3.

Seizures

Idiopathic epilepsy and febrile convulsions do not occur in the newborn and grand mal seizures are most uncommon.

Clinical presentation

The manifestations of seizures can be subtle, especially in the preterm baby and include: apnoea, lateral deviation of the eyes or flickering of the eyelids, exaggerated chewing or sucking, pedalling of arms and legs and clonus. Clonus may be confined to a limb (focal) or involve two or more (multifocal). Tonic and myoclonic seizures are uncommon and usually imply wide-spread derangement of the brain.

Common causes

Seizures which occur within 48 hours of birth are likely to be due to hypoxic ischaemic encephalopathy, hypoglycaemia, intracranial haemorrhage.

Those which occur later may be associated with meningitis, hypocalcaemia and hypomagnesaemia.

Diagnosis

Obtain heel blood to exclude hypoglycaemia (Dextrostix reading or an alternative method). Determine the level of serum calcium and magnesium. Do a lumbar puncture cautiously if bleeding or infection is suspected. Request an ultrasound examination of the brain if there is a likelihood of hypoxia or bleeding.

Management

Non-specific treatment

◆ Arrest the seizure immediately by giving PHENOBARBITONE, the drug of choice: dose 20 mg/kg. Route: IV. Prescribe an oral maintenance dose of 5 mg/kg/day.
◆ Ensure that the airway is clear, that oxygenation is adequate and that body temperature is normal. Useful anticonvulsants include PHENYTOIN and DIAZEPAM.

Intractable seizures

Add 0,5 mg CLONAZEPAM to 50 ml 5% dextrose water in a Buretrol. Route: IV. Rate: two drops per minute (60 drops/min dropper). PYRIDOXINE 50 mg (intravenous) should also be given. It will correct seizures due to PYRIDOXINE deficiency or dependency.

Specific treatment

◆ Hypoglycaemia: Dextrose 10% IV.
◆ Bacterial meningitis: CEFTRIAXONE.
◆ Hypocalcaemia: 10% calcium gluconate.
  2 mg/kg. Slow IV infusion.
◆ Hypomagnesaemia: 50% magnesium sulphate 0,2 ml/kg IM.

Prognosis

The outlook is good for hypocalcaemia, hypomagnesaemia and

primary subarachnoid bleeding. It is poor for hypoglycaemia, hypoxic ischaemic encephalopathy, intraventricular haemorrhage and meningitis.

Maturity rating	
score	weeks
-10	20
-5	22
0	24
5	26
10	28
15	30
20	32
25	34
30	36
35	38
40	40
45	42
50	44

Table 33.5 Physical Maturity

	-1	0	1	2	3	4	5
Skin	sticky, friable, transparent	gelatinous, red, translucent	smooth, pink, visible veins	superficial peeling &/or rash, few veins	cracking, pale arena, rare veins	parchment, deep cracking, no vessels	feathery, cracked, wrinkled
Lanugo	none	sparse	abundant	thinning	bald areas	mostly bald	
Plantar surface	heel-toe: 40-50 mm: -1 <40 mm: -2	>50 mm no crease	faint red marks	anterior transverse crease only	creases anterior 2/3	creases over entire sole	
Breast	imperceptible	barely perceptible	flat areola, no bud	stippled areola, 1-2 mm bud	raised areola, 3-4 mm bud	full areola 5-10 mm bud	
Eye / Ear	lids fused loosely: -1 tightly: -2	lids open, pinna flat, stays folded	sl. curved, pinna: soft, slow recoil	well-curved pinna; soft but ready recoil	formed and firm instant recoil	thick cartilage, ear stiff	
Genitals: male	scrotum flat, smooth	scrotum empty, faint rugae	testes in upper canal, rare rugae	testes descending, few rugae	testes down, good rugae	testes pendulous, deep rugae	
Genitals: female	clitoris prominent, labia flat	prominent clitoris, small labia minora	prominent clitoris, enlarging minora	majora & minora equally prominent	majora large, minora small	majora cover clitoris & minora	

34 NUTRITION AND NUTRITIONAL DISORDERS

H de V Heese and A Sive

Optimal nutrition supplies enough nutrients to promote normal growth, neurological development, health and well-being. Nutritional requirements change with age, especially during early infancy when growth is most rapid. One can estimate the normal nutritional needs at any age from the recommended dietary intake (RDI), but allow for deviation from the recommended norms in patients with specific nutritional problems.

Energy and nutrient intake

Recommendations

The recommended energy and protein intakes for age are shown in Table 34.1.

Table 34.1 Recommended dietary intake of energy and protein

Age	Energy/kg/day*		Protein g/kg/ day*
Preterm	546-630 kJ	(130 -150 kcal)	3,5
Term	420-500 kJ	(100-120 kcal)	2,5-4
0-6 months	460-500 kJ	(110-120 kcal)	2,2-3,5
6-12 months	440 kJ	(105 kcal)	2,0
1-3 years	420 kJ	(100 kcal)	1,8
4-6 years	360 kJ	(85 kcal)	1,5
7-12 years	270-340 kJ	(65-80 kcal)	1,0-1,2

* 1 kcal = 4,2 kJ

Energy is derived from macronutrients, such as protein, carbohydrate and fat in the diet. Calculate the total energy by adding the energy content of these dietary constituents (Table 34.2).

The diet must also supply sufficient vitamins, minerals and trace elements as shown in Tables 34.3, 34.4 and 34.5. For fluid requirements see pages 208-9.

Table 34.2 Approximate energy value of foods

Constituent	Energy
Protein	17 kJ/g (4 kcal/g)
Carbohydrate	17 kJ/g (4 kcal/g)
Fat	38 kJ/g (9 kcal/g)

Warning
Unless the total energy intake is adequate, the protein in the diet is used to provide energy, and will not be available for anabolism.

Exceptions and additions

Adequate quantities of balanced meals will generally supply all the nutrients necessary for growth but there are a number of exceptions.

Fluoride

Administer fluoride (Zymafluor or Listerfluor from the early neonatal period).

Fluoride content of water <0,3 ppm

◆ Birth to one year: 0,25 mg (1 tab./day of Zymafluor or Listerfluor crushed, mixed and given with milk or water or food in a spoon, or five drops Listerfluor or four drops Zymafluor).
◆ One to two years: 0,25 mg (1 tab./day, crushed, mixed and given with milk or water or food in a spoon, or five drops, i.e. 0,2 ml of fluoride solution (Listerfluor)).
◆ Two to three years: 0,5 mg (2 tabs./day, or ten drops of fluoride solution).
◆ Three to 13 years: 1 mg (4 tabs./day).

Table 34.3 Recommended dietary intake per day of vitamins

	A μg*	D μg**	E mg	C mg	Thiamine mg	Niacin mg***	B₆ mg	Folate μg	B₁₂ μg
	Fat soluble			Water soluble					
0-6 mths	350	10	3	30	0,3	5	0,3	50	0,3
6-12 mths	350	10	4	35	0,4	6	0,6	50	0,5
1-3 yrs	400	10	6	40	0,7	9	0,9	75	0,7
4-6 yrs	500	10	7	45	0,9	11	1,1	100	1,0
over 7 yrs	700-1 000	10	10	50	1,2	15	1,6	150	1,4

* 1 μg Vit A = 1 Retinol equivalent (RE) = 3,3 IU
** 10 μg cholecalciferol = 400 IU Vit D
*** 1 mg niacin = 60 mg dietary tryptophan

Table 34.4 Recommended dietary intake per day of selected minerals and trace elements

	Na# mg	K*† mg	Ca mg	Mg mg	Fe mg	I_2 µg	Zn mg	Cu* mg	Se* µg	Mn* mg	F* mg	Cr µg
0-6 mths	245	825	400	50	10	40	5	0,6	10	0,6	0,5	40
6-12 mths	335	700	600	70	15	50	5	0,7	15	1,0	1,0	60
1-3 yrs	500	800	800	85	15	70	10	1,0	20	1,5	1,5	80
4-6 yrs	700	1 100	800	120	15	90	10	1,5	20	2,0	2,5	120
over 7 yrs	1 200	2 000	800	200	15	120	10	2,0	30	3,0	2,5	200

* Estimated safe and adequate daily intakes

\# 1 g NaCl = 17 mmol of Na⁺

† 1 g KCl = 13 mmol of K⁺

Fluoride content of water 0,3-0,7 ppm

Omit fluoride until two years and thereafter administer half of the dose. See page 377 for information on water fluoride content.

Fluoride content of water >0,7 ppm

Omit fluoride.

Preterm infants

Recommended energy requirement per day is increased to 550-630 kJ/kg/day (130-150 kcal). Metabolic bone disease of prematurity is prevented by adding vitamin D 800 IU/day, calcium 2 mmol/day and phosphate 0,5 mmol/day, to each 100 ml of breast milk. Use CALCIUM GLUBIONATE syrup (Calcium Sandoz) 1 ml six-hourly. If special preterm milks are used, omit the calcium and phosphate supplements. Additional iron supplements vary with birth weight: 2 mg/kg/day for infants from 1,5-2,0 kg, 3 mg/kg/day between 1,0 and 1,5 kg and 4 mg/kg/day below 1,0 kg. In infants with a gestational age of less than 34 weeks on breast milk, add 3 mmol/kg/day of sodium.

Warning

The amount of vitamin D and iron in special preterm and other formulae may not be adequate to prevent the onset of nutritional rickets and iron deficiency anaemia. Always calculate the total **amount** ingested.

Parenteral nutrition

Prevent potential deficiencies of zinc, copper, manganese, selenium, chromium and molybdenum with a trace element mixture. See Table 34.4 for recommended dietary intakes.

Undernutrition

Document the nutritional status of all children routinely by plotting weight, height and head circumference on growth charts (G in GOBI FFF). Undernutrition will then be detected early. Specific nutritional deficiencies manifest as changes in the skin, hair, nails, mucous membranes, bones and lymphoid tissue.

Assess the cause of malnutrition not only in terms of the availability of food but also as a consequence of parental ignorance, neglect or cultural beliefs.

Protein energy malnutrition

Protein energy malnutrition (PEM) includes the entities of underweight for age (UWFA), marasmus, kwashiorkor and marasmic-kwashiorkor. They are separated by the presence or absence of oedema and by the child's weight as a percentage of the expected weight for age (taken as the 50th centile).

Table 34.5 Classification of protein energy malnutrition (Wellcome)

	60-80% expected weight	<60% expected weight
No oedema	Underweight (UWFA)	Marasmus
Oedema	Kwashiorkor	Marasmic-kwashiorkor

Note: Kwashiorkor may occur even if the child's weight is greater than 80% of expected weight.

UWFA and uncomplicated undernutrition

Children without nutritional oedema, signs of specific nutritional deficiencies and complicating illnesses usually improve when the dietary energy intake is increased. There is often a lag phase before they start gaining weight. Increase the intake of energy gradually over seven to ten days until 840 kJ (200 kcal)/kg/day is reached or until the child gains weight at a rate of 20-30 g/kg/day. Milk forms the basis of the diet, which can be complemented with cereal, vegetable oil or mixed foodstuffs. Diets consisting mainly of maize should be supplemented with dried beans, dried peas or milk powder. The energy content of the diet can be increased with sugar and/or vegetable oil (e.g. sunflower seed, peanut) using up to 5 g per 100 ml and 5 ml per 100 ml of milk respectively. Ensure that fat does not supply more than 50-55% of total calories. Limit protein intake to 3-3,5 g/kg/day.

Treat underlying infections and infestations and correct any specific nutritional deficiencies. Admit children who fail to thrive despite dietary supervision to hospital for trial feeding.

Severe malnutrition and kwashiorkor

The metabolic and biochemical consequences of kwashiorkor result from deprivation over a long period. There is usually some adaptation to this deprivation. Kwashiorkor is often complicated by diarrhoea, pneumonia, septicaemia, tuberculosis or other infections. Complications require specific investigations and therapy.

Clinical presentation

Kwashiorkor and marasmic-kwashiorkor are characterized by growth retardation, oedema and hypo-albuminaemia. The children do not look thin. The nails are pale and the skin shows areas of increased and decreased pigmentation which sloughs mainly in the nappy area. There is reddish discoloration of the hair, which is thin and brittle. The abdomen is protuberant but there is no ascites. The liver is enlarged, firm and has a well-defined edge. They are apathetic when left to themselves and irritable when handled. In contrast, children with marasmus look emaciated, do not have the skin, hair or mental changes associated with kwashiorkor and preserve serum protein concentrations.

All children with significant PEM have atrophic lymphoid tissue indicative of diminished cellular immunity. This is clinically manifest as small tonsils and impalpable or inappropriately small lymph nodes.

Osteopenia but not radiological rickets is a feature of PEM. Overt rickets may occur during refeeding.

Diagnosis

Clinical in the first instance. Only proceed to biochemical measurements if you suspect other causes of generalized oedema or failure to thrive. Where facilities exist, blood culture is mandatory to identify covert infections.

Management

If possible, admit the mother with the child and involve her from the start in the treatment and rehabilitation of her child and in the instruction in the basic principles of child health, nutrition and, where appropriate, vegetable gardening. Adhere to the principles listed below when treating children with kwashiorkor.

Fluids

Iatrogenic fluid overload is a hazard. Avoid intravenous fluids except in severe dehydration. When intravenous fluids are indicated, keep the maintenance component below 80 ml/kg/day (the younger the patient, the smaller the volume of intravenous fluid). Increase oral fluid volumes from 80-100 ml/kg/day on day 1 to 120-150 ml/kg/day by day 5 depending on the child's ability to tolerate the feeds.

Protein and energy

Limit the feeds to milk for the first five days. Lactose-free preparations (e.g. soya formulae) are preferred. Introduce solids such as cereal, mince and vegetables from day 6. Supplements of Caloreen (maximum 10 g per 100 ml milk) and Liprocil or sunflower oil (5 ml per 100 ml milk) are useful for increasing the energy content of the diet but are costly. In general, the more severe the disease, the more gradually should you proceed with the nutritional rehabilitation.

Antihelminthics

Deworm with PIPERAZINE, MEBENDAZOLE or ALBENDAZOLE and treat Giardia infestations with METRONIDAZOLE where parasites are endemic.

Minerals and electrolytes

Give oral potassium chloride at a dose of 6 mmol/kg/day (0,5 g/kg/day) until oedema has resolved. In renal failure, withhold potassium or give smaller doses. Oral magnesium chloride $6H_2O$ 0,24-0,3 mmol/kg/day (50-60 mg/kg/day) is also recommended from day 1 for seven days. Note that magnesium chloride may cause acidosis in malnourished children.

Vitamins

Start 10 ml/day of a multivitamin syrup for at least three months. Vitamin A deficiency varies from area to area but all children should receive oral 100 000 IU of vitamin A on admission. Parenteral vitamin K at a dose of 2-3 mg is given to patients with a bleeding tendency or a low prothrombin, expressed as a raised International Normalized Ratio (INR) exceeding 2.

Haematinics

Start oral FOLATE 5 mg/day with feeds from admission and continue for 21 days. Withhold iron until oedema has resolved. Thereafter give oral ferrous sulphate 6 mg elemental iron/kg/day for 12 weeks. Thereafter check for iron insufficiency during follow-up and treat appropriately (see page 240).

Blood transfusion is used only when severe anaemia (Hb <6 g/dl) is associated with life-threatening infections.

Trace elements

When oedema is resolved, use an oral trace element mixture providing 1,55 μmol/ml (100 μg) elemental zinc/kg/day and 0,025 μmol/ml (2 μg) elemental selenium/kg/day for one month. Continue supplementation with the mixture for generalized trace element deficiency (Table 34.6 page 391), but at double the dose for zinc and selenium for a further period of four to six weeks. If facilities are available, measure trace element concentrations at 30 days and 90 days.

Pitfalls

♦ Do not attempt to **rapidly** correct the biochemical abnormalities and nutritional deficits. This usually does more harm than good.

♦ Rickets may develop during rapid growth in the recovery periods. Treat with additional vitamin D 400 IU per day.

♦ Daily intake of large supplements of trace elements for prolonged periods could have deleterious effects.

♦ Trace element solutions are unpalatable. Mask the taste with sweeteners (e.g. methyl cellulose base with succhaine or saccharine, dicyclamate and raspberry).

♦ Trace element supplementation in incorrect proportions causes competition for absorption and paradoxical deficiency of one or more of the other trace elements.

Investigations

Where facilities are available, the following investigations may be helpful to identify infection.

♦ **Full blood count:** a haemoglobin concentration below 7,5 g/dl which falls further during treatment often indicates unrecognized infection. A low white cell count in the face of infection suggests inadequate immunity and overwhelming sepsis.

◆ **Bacteriology:** where facilities exist, blood culture is mandatory. Culture urine and stool if you suspect sepsis. Infection frequently occurs in the absence of clinical signs, e.g. fever.

◆ **Chest X-ray:** since the clinical signs may be minimal, the chest X-ray is useful for diagnosing pneumonia and excluding tuberculosis.

◆ **Mantoux:** malnutrition induces immunosuppression and the tuberculin test can be negative in the face of active TB. Start antituberculous therapy on clinical suspicion and a suggestive chest X-ray. If the child has TB, the Mantoux should become positive within four to six weeks of refeeding. Stop treatment if it remains negative. If available, a candida skin test may be used as a control for anergy.

Common complications

Infections

Children hospitalized for PEM frequently have septicaemia, pneumonia, tuberculosis, urinary tract infections, or infections at another site. Failure to respond to the diet indicates infection until disproved. The usual signs may be absent. Patients who appear systemically ill or have extensive weeping skin lesions on admission should be started on antibiotics. Where laboratory services are limited use 'prophylactic' antibiotics. Septicaemia is invariably Gram-negative, usually *E.coli*. For prophylaxis use CO-TRIMOXAZOLE. Change to CEFOTAXIME (alternate agents AMPICILLIN plus GENTAMICIN) if infection is suspected or proven in a severely ill patient. Treat documented and culture-proven infections appropriately.

Diarrhoea

Diarrhoea is the most common presenting complaint. Correct fluid balance carefully. See page 206. Lactose intolerance is common. Start lactose-free feeds (soya milks) from the beginning. Introduce cow milk feeds early and usually by day 10. Identifiable pathogens in the stool are relatively uncommon, but they should be treated when found. Treat persistent diarrhoea as described on page 217.

Hypothermia

Use a low-reading thermometer to measure rectal temperature. A rectal temperature less than 35 °C is not uncommon and if not recognized and corrected may lead to unexpected death. It is often associated with septicaemia. Prevent further heat loss by nursing the child in a warm environment (27 °C), using a 'space blanket' or aluminium foil and supplying adequate feeds.

Warning

Avoid hot water bottles, and use heating blankets with caution.

Hypoglycaemia

Hypoglycaemia (a blood sugar of less than 2,2 mmol/l) varies from area to area for unexplained reasons, but it carries a poor prognosis. Correct with 20% intravenous glucose and prevent recurrence with regular feeds.

Cardiac failure

Suspect cardiac decompensation if the heart size is normal on chest X-ray. The cardiac shadow is invariably small in malnutrition. Cardiac failure sometimes occurs five to seven days after starting treatment. It may be precipitated by excessive sodium and fluid intake. Treat with DIGOXIN and diuretics. The condition carries a poor prognosis.

Anaemia

A normochromic, normocytic anaemia caused by protein deficiency is common. Other specific anaemias (megaloblastic and hypochromic microcytic) will occur during recovery if supplements, such as FOLIC ACID and iron, are omitted.

Bleeding

Purpura is common. Patients with a more severe bleeding diathesis usually have disseminated intravascular coagulopathy and should be treated accordingly. See page 242.

Tremor

The 'kwashi-shakes' of unknown pathogenesis sometimes occur during recovery and may last for months. They resolve without treatment.

Unexpected death

Patients sometimes die unexpectedly four to seven days after admission, following apparent clinical improvement. The cause is usually unknown.

Long-term care

Although serum protein concentrations return to normal within one month of refeeding, physiological resolution is not attained till much later. A prolonged period (at least three months) of supervised feeding and parental education is required to prevent relapse. Refer all children on discharge to the community nutrition or social care services for ongoing care.

Vitamin A deficiency

Vitamin A is essential for the integrity of epithelial cells. Deficiency varies from area to area.

Clinical presentation

Examine the skin carefully for dryness and plugging of the hair follicle with keratin. Test visual acuity in poor light and examine the conjunctiva for xerosis and Bitot's spots. In advanced disease, corneal xerosis, keratomalacia and finally corneal ectasia and phthisis bulbi are present. The eye signs of vitamin A deficiency are exacerbated by measles, which has a high morbidity and mortality in vitamin A-deficient subjects.

Treatment

◆ Treat clinical deficiency with oral vitamin A 100 000 IU/day for three days.
◆ In areas of high prevalence, 200 000 IU of oral vitamin A at six-monthly intervals will eliminate xerophthalmia.
◆ Give all patients with measles 200 000 IU of oral vitamin A on admission and 200 000 IU a day later.

Vitamin C deficiency

Scurvy because of nutritional deficiencies is now rare, even in developing countries. It may occur where the vitamin C in milk, orange and other fruit juices or food is destroyed by a misinformed parent in attempts to sterilize the infant's food.

Clinical presentation

Consider the diagnosis in malnourished children with bleeding under the mucous membranes and perifollicular haemorrhages. A pseudoparesis as a result of subperiosteal bleeding suggests the diagnosis in an irritable infant lying in the 'frog position'.

Diagnosis

X-rays of the long bones show typical signs. See page 462.

Treatment

The therapeutic dose of vitamin C is 250 mg six-hourly for three days followed by a multivitamin syrup 10ml/day for three or more months and a diet sufficient in ascorbic acid.

Advice

Remember that vitamin C is important for promoting the absorption of iron from cereal diets.

Vitamin D deficiency

Vitamin D-deficient rickets results from a failure to mineralize the bone matrix at the growth plate. Vitamin D deficiency rickets occurs during periods of rapid growth, i.e. in children under two years and during puberty, where it may be limited to selected populations. Deficiency occurs because of lack of vitamin D intake or exposure of the infant to sunlight.

Clinical presentation

The wrists and costochondral junctions are widened. Chest deformity, bossing of the skull and craniotabes may be present. Hypotonia and sweating are usual. Children suffer repeated chest infections. Bowing of the limbs occurs in toddlers and other children.

Diagnosis

X-rays reveal osteopenia with cupping, fraying and flaring of the epiphyses. See page 474. Check for hypophosphataemia and elevated alkaline phosphatase levels. Hypocalcaemia is variable.

Treatment

Treat vitamin D deficiency rickets in the older child with 5 000

IU of oral vitamin D per day for four to six weeks. In the preterm infant rickets occurs not only as a result of vitamin D deficiency but also from calcium and phosphate insufficiency. In the older child, rickets may result from a deficient intake of calcium (lack of milk in the diet). The preventative treatment is described on page 380 and in established rickets is as for the older child.

Folic acid deficiency

Clinical presentation

Suspect the diagnosis when a megaloblastic anaemia with hyper-segmented polymorphs is found in a child with malnutrition or malabsorption. Children on an unsupplemented goat milk diet (usually for allergy) are at special risk from deficiency.

Diagnosis

There is a reticulocyte response within a day of starting therapy.

Treatment

Give 5 mg of FOLATE daily for three weeks to correct the deficit.

Niacin deficiency

Maize lacks the essential amino acid tryptophan, a precursor of niacin. An unsupplemented diet leads to pellagra.

Clinical presentation

Typical pigmented desquamating lesions on the sun-exposed areas of the skin. Apathy rather than dementia is seen in children, and diarrhoea may be accompanied by cheilosis, a sore tongue and dysphagia.

Treatment

NICOTINIC ACID 100 mg orally four-hourly for three days. Supplement the diet with animal protein, beans or peas.

Trace element disorders and deficiencies

Isolated trace element deficiencies are rare. Suspect deficiency in situations which predispose to deficiency; these include protein energy malnutrition, prolonged hyperalimentation, malabsorption, prematurity and living in specific geochemical environments. Non-specific signs such as growth failure, listlessness, apathy, anaemia and skin changes accompany nearly all trace element deficiencies.

Diagnosis of trace element deficiency

To diagnose zinc, copper, and selenium deficiency, measure the plasma concentrations. For manganese measure the whole blood concentration.

Note

Contamination of specimens is a major source of error. Contact the laboratory before you take the blood specimens. Clean the skin with 70% alcohol in double-distilled de-ionized water. Use disposable steel needles and plastic syringes to take the blood and store the samples in polystyrene tubes. Avoid glass which is heavily contaminated with zinc. Interpret copper concentrations in association with caeruloplasmin levels. Reference values for age (see page 686).

Zinc deficiency

The clinical picture of deficiency is best illustrated by acrodermatitis, an autosomal recessive condition manifesting shortly after weaning.

Clinical presentation

Dermatitis especially of the extremities; oral, anal and genital lesions; dystrophic nails and alopecia are usual. Other signs include chronic diarrhoea, malabsorption and steatorrhoea. Immuno-incompetence predisposes to frequent infections. Pure zinc deficiency associated with geophagia results in stunting of growth and testicular atrophy.

Diagnosis

Measure serum zinc and serum alkaline phosphatase concentrations (which are low in zinc deficiency and rise with treatment).

Treatment

◆ Correct suspected or proven zinc deficiency with 1-2 mg/kg/day of oral elemental zinc. In preterm infants, give 0,5

mg/kg/day. Doses of 25-50 mg/kg/day are required for acro-dermatitis enteropathica. (Note: 1 mg elemental zinc = 4,4 mg zinc sulphate, 2,1 mg zinc chloride or 3,4 mg zinc acetate.)
♦ Continue treatment until alkaline phosphatase concentrations return to normal.

Table 34.6 Trace element mixture formula

	Weight of constituents mg/4 ℓ	Elemental content	
		µmol/ml	µg/ml
Zinc acetate 2H₂O	1 360	1,549	100,26
Copper sulphate 5H₂O	320	0,320	20,36
Chromic chloride 6H₂O	3,6	0,003	0,18
Manganese sulphate 4H₂O	96	0,108	5,91
Sodium selenite	17,6	0,025	2,01

Other constituents
Citric acid 16 g, sodium citrate 28 g, saccharine sodium 2,64 g, sodium cyclamate 54 g, raspberry no.1 essence 16 ml and methylcellulose base* to 4 litres

*Methycellulose base:

    Methylcellulose   28 g
    Distilled water to 4 litres

Dose: 1 ml per kg per day to a maximum of 20 ml per day.

Copper deficiency

Clinical presentation

Consider copper deficiency in preterm infants with bone de-mineralization, periosteal reactions or fractures associated with a hypochromic anaemia, neutropenia and oedema. A severe form of copper deficiency occurs in Menke's disease, an X-linked recessive condition manifesting in infancy.

Diagnosis

Serum copper, caeruloplasmin and neutrophil levels are low. X-ray of the long bones shows osteopenia.

Treatment

0,2 ml/kg/day of a 0,5% copper sulphate solution given for 14-21 days or until anaemia, neutrophils and serum copper correct.

Generalized trace element deficiency

Treatment

When generalized trace element deficiency is suspected, use a mixture of trace elements. See Table 34.6 page 391.

This trace element mixture is administered at a dose of 1 ml/kg/day to a maximum of 20 ml/kg/day, and provides approximately 1,55 μmol/ml (100 μg/ml) of elemental zinc, 0,32 μmol/ml (20 μg/ml) of elemental copper, 0,003 μmol/ml (0,18 μg/ml) of elemental chrome, 0,108 μmol/ml (6,0 μg/ml) of elemental manganese and 0,025 μmol/ml (2,0 μg/ml) of elemental selenium.

E B Hoffman

Acute pyogenic osteomyelitis and acute septic arthritis

Osteomyelitis is an infective metaphyseal disease. In the neonate and infant the growth plate is not a barrier to infection and the epiphysis is destroyed, which has crippling consequences, especially in the hip. In the older child the pus decompresses subperiosteally which leads to sequestrum formation and chronic osteomyelitis.

Septic arthritis is due either to primary synovial involvement or is secondary to metaphyseal involvement in the infant or an intra-articular metaphysis as in the hip.

The average age incidence at which both conditions occur is seven years.

Aetiology

Osteomyelitis

◆ Neonates: 75% *Staphylococcus aureus* (possibly CLOXA-CILLIN resistant if previously hospitalized); 25% β-haemolytic streptococci.

◆ Infants and older children: *S. aureus*. All are sensitive to CLOXACILLIN, resistant to PENICILLIN.

Septic arthritis

◆ Six months to two years: most common organism *Haemophilus influenzae*. Others include *S. aureus*, streptococcus and pneumococcus.

◆ Over two years: *S. aureus* is the most common organism. Others include pneumococcus and streptococcus.

Clinical presentation

The child is ill and may be septicaemic. 75% of neonates appear to be relatively asymptomatic on presentation.

Local findings in the neonate and infant include pseudoparalysis and swelling. In the older child, refusal to bear weight and metaphyseal tenderness are common.

Peripheral joints have a palpable effusion in septic arthritis. In the hip joint, diagnosis can be difficult. A decreased range of movement (ROM) is classically present, but in the septicaemic, confused child and in the infant, the ROM can be normal.

Investigations

◆ The total and differential WBC count may be normal. The ESR is usually raised.
◆ Blood culture is positive in about 50% of patients.
◆ Radiographic investigations are of no help in the older child. In the neonate, metaphyseal rarefaction and hip subluxation are always initially present.
◆ Isotope bone scan: very helpful for localizing sites around the hip and in the pelvis, spine and in the foot.

Management

Admit the patient to hospital.

Treatment with antibiotics

Osteomyelitis

CLOXACILLIN 200 mg/kg/day IV for 48 hours (a higher dosage than generally recommended) followed by oral FLUCLOXACILLIN 100 mg/kg/day for six weeks. Add FUCIDIC ACID 30 mg/kg/day for possible resistant staphylococcus in a previously hospitalized neonate.

Septic arthritis

CLOXACILLIN as for osteomyelitis. In the age group six months to two years add AMPICILLIN 150 mg/kg/day IV, followed by AMOXYCILLIN 75 mg/kg/day orally for three weeks if *H. influenzae* is cultured. If streptococcus or pneumococcus is cultured, continue with AMOXYCILLIN or PENICILLIN.

Open surgical drainage

Imperative in all cases of septic arthritis and in 90% of osteomyelitis. Exceptions include the pelvis and vertebrae and early cases without swelling, which can be observed. Surgical intervention in these cases is indicated if there is no response in the temperature and local signs.

Angular kyphos

Spinal tuberculosis with destruction of contiguous vertebrae is the most common cause. The main differential diagnosis is congenital kyphosis due to a hemivertebra or an unsegmented bar. If this is not clear on routine radiography, then tomography should be employed.

Spinal tuberculosis

Conservative treatment with RIFAMPICIN, ISONIAZID and PYRAZINAMIDE for nine months. Surgery is indicated if three or more vertebrae are destroyed or if paralysis occurs. It is important to differentiate spinal tuberculosis from pyogenic spondylitis. In pyogenic disease, pain is a prominent symptom, whereas in tuberculosis the more commonly presenting feature is deformity. On radiographic examination, sclerosis is more a feature in the pyogenic form and destruction the dominant feature in tuberculosis. There is also a rapid response to oral FLU-CLOXACILLIN in the pyogenic disease.

Congenital kyphosis

Early surgery to prevent progression.

Club foot (congenital talipes equinovarus)

The foot has a fixed equinus, hindfoot varus and forefoot adduction and supination deformity. The majority of cases are idiopathic, but one should rule out underlying arthrogryposis and myelomeningocoele.

Refer for evaluation and management. Treatment is by serial weekly plaster moulding.

The majority of cases require a posterior release or a more extensive posteromedial release.

Congenital dislocation of the hip

Neonatal screening

Allows early diagnosis, easy treatment and has a good prognosis.

◆ **Ortolani test:** identifies a dislocated hip which locates with a 'clunk' on abduction.

◆ **The Barlow test:** identifies a dislocatable hip that dislocates on posterior and adductor force. Eighty percent of Barlow-positive dislocatable hips will stabilize at three weeks.

Diagnosis

Essentially clinical. Radiographic investigations are only helpful after the age of six weeks.

Management

Refer patients with dislocated hips and dislocatable hips which have not stabilized by three weeks immediately for evaluation and treatment by means of a Pavlik harness. Treatment after six months of age is more complicated and may entail open reduction.

Warning

There are also hips which dislocate late between four months to one year. Suspicious hips, i.e. patients with a positive family history, breech delivery, dislocatable hips which have become stabilized and patients with postural foot deformities such as calcaneovalgus and metatarsus adductus should be followed up three-monthly until the patient walks at one year and the acetabular index on radiographic investigation has shown improvement.

Flexible or postural flat foot

This is a condition with a benign natural history which usually resolves spontaneously by eight years. The patient has no longitudinal arch when standing, probably due to ligamentous laxity. A good arch develops when attempting to stand on tiptoe, due to the muscle power which comes into play. The majority of patients wear off the lateral aspect of the heel of the shoe, which is normal.

Differential diagnosis

Mobile flat foot but paralytic as seen in cerebral palsy, myelomeningocoele and poliomyelitis. Fixed deformity flat foot of congenital vertical talus or rocker-bottom foot in the neonate or tarsal coalition in the adolescent.

Management

The natural history of a flexible flat foot is not influenced by treatment. Intervention is only indicated to prolong shoe life if there is excessive medial shoe wear. The best treatment is probably a custom-built interchangeable arch support.

Note

Conditions mentioned in the differential diagnosis can be improved with surgery.

Genu varum and valgum

Bowlegs and knock-knees are physiological variations of the normal. The normal infant has bowlegs from birth to the age of two years and then develops knock-knees. The latter is maximal at three-plus years and corrects to normal at seven years. The main differential diagnosis is rickets.

Diagnosis

Radiographic investigations are indicated if rickets is suspected or if the intermalleolar distance exceeds 7 cm in genu valgum, is unilateral, or if genu varum persists after the age of two years where Blount's disease must be excluded.

Management

Refer for an opinion and corrective osteotomy in Blount's disease, a residual deformity in healed rickets, and in the rare case in which the physiological genu varum does not resolve by three or four years. Persistent physiological genu valgum after the age of eight years is treated with stapling of the distal femoral epiphysis at about 12 years.

Intoeing

Assess the torsional profile with the patient supine with the hips extended and knees flexed at 90°.

Metatarsus adductus is the most common cause in the first year. Ninety per cent resolve within the first year of life without treatment.

In the second year medial tibial torsion is the most common cause.

After the third year, increased femoral neck antetorsion (anteversion) is the most common cause.

Management

Medial tibial torsion and femoral neck antetorsion have a benign natural history and spontaneous resolution occurs by the age of eight years in 95% of cases. Parents need reassurance as only 1% of cases will require surgery for cosmetic and not functional reasons.

Perthes' disease

The patient presents with a painful limp between five and ten years of age. Abduction and internal rotation are limited.

Diagnosis

The diagnosis is radiological. Perthes' disease is an idiopathic avascular necrosis of the femoral head which progresses through three stages. During the avascular stage the femoral head appears sclerotic on radiographs with or without a sub-chondral fracture; during the revascularization stage the femoral head appears fragmented; and the final stage is that of re-ossification or healing.

Management

Refer suspected or confirmed cases for specialized management. The principle of treatment is to protect the head from collapsing during the avascular and fragmentation stage. Initially the patient is admitted for traction to overcome the irritability which is followed by abduction plasters to ensure containment of the head until healing occurs. The average duration of treatment is one year.

Prognosis

The prognosis of the disease depends on the age of presentation and the amount of femoral head involved.

Scoliosis

Postural scoliosis

This is due to leg length discrepancy and it disappears on sitting.

Structural scoliosis

Idiopathic

The adolescent form is the most common type and occurs largely in girls (90%) at about the age of ten years. Treatment is by means of bracing, or fusion if not adequately controlled by bracing.

Paralytic

As a complication of cerebral palsy, poliomyelitis and myelo-meningocoele. Treatment is by bracing or fusion.

Congenital

Hemivertebra or an unsegmented bar. Treatment is by early fusion to prevent progression.

Neurofibromatosis

Treatment is by fusion.

Slipped upper femoral epiphysis (SUFE)

Clinical presentation

SUFE presents with a painful limp and pain in the anterior thigh, which is often referred to the knee. Average age incidences are 12 years in girls and 14 years in boys. The cause is usually idiopathic. Presentation before the age of ten years or after 16 years may be due to a hormonal cause such as hypopituitarism.

Diagnosis

A pathognomic sign is that when the hips are flexed, they rotate externally. Antero-posterior and lateral radiographs are diagnostic.

Management

The preferred treatment is pinning *in situ*.

Note

Bilateral SUFE occurs in 20% of patients, and both hips should be X-rayed.

Transient synovitis of the hip (irritable hip)

Clinical presentation

The average age incidence is six years. The patient presents with a painful limp, is not systemically ill, and has a limitation of movement usually at the extremes of abduction and internal rotation. The main differential diagnosis is from a septic arthritis. Although the ESR and temperature can be raised, the patient is not as systemically ill as in septic arthritis.

Diagnosis

The diagnosis is one of exclusion and is based on the rapid resolution of the condition without specific treatment.

Management

Admit the patient to hospital for bed rest and traction.

36 PHARMACOLOGY

Principal Pharmacist and staff of the Pharmacy,
Red Cross War Memorial Children's Hospital

The child is not a small adult and the smaller and younger the child, the more cautious one must be in the use of medications. Hepatic and renal immaturity compound the unique problems that exist in the neonatal period and medicine clearance, for example DIGOXIN and AMINOGLYCOCIDES, may be very low, especially in preterm infants. Neonatal physiology and the capacity to handle medications alters markedly with advancing gestational and postnatal age. This necessitates individualized dosage with monitoring of serum levels so as to avoid over- or underdosage. CHLORAMPHENICOL overdosage results in the 'grey baby syndrome' characterized by the development of regurgitation of feeds, abdominal distension and a shock-like state and an ashen colour.

Certain preparations may not be suitable for particular age groups.

SULPHONAMIDES in the newborn displace bilirubin from albumin, and kernicterus may result. TETRACYCLINES produce permanent discoloration of teeth if given before 12 years of age. Phenothiazine anti-emetics such as PROCHLORPER-AZINE (Stemetil) are very likely to produce extrapyramidal side-effects, even at low dosage.

Topical preparations may be absorbed in significant amounts, particularly when applied to areas where the skin is excoriated or has been burned, resulting in systemic side-effects. Examples of these are steroids used for eczema and nappy rashes and HEXACHLOROPHENE in the neonate (neurotoxic).

Dosage

Dose should be calculated according to body weight, or, where critical, to surface area (e.g. cytotoxics). See page 664.

Reduce dose in:

♦ patients with renal disease if medicine is excreted by kidneys. See page 501;

◆ patients with liver disease, if medicine is metabolized by liver;

◆ if dehydrated;

◆ obese children: use dose for age rather than weight, as fat plays little part in medicine metabolism;

◆ where paediatric dose or child's weight is unknown, Catzel's percentage method may be useful. This should not be used for narcotics such as MORPHINE and CODEINE and bronchodilators such as AMINOPHYLLINE. In these instances the mg/kg of body mass dosage should be used. Under two weeks of age the correct mg/kg dosage should be obtained from the manufacturer's literature as neonates have impaired renal and hepatic excretion.

Table 36.1 Percentages of adult doses by age

Age	% of adult dose	Age	% of adult dose
Birth	10%	7 years	50%
2 months	15%	10 years	60%
4 months	20%	11 years	70%
12 months	25%	12 years	75%
18 months	30%	14 years	80%
3 years	33$\frac{1}{2}$%	16 years	90%
5 years	40	20 years	100

Prescribe the **minimum** number of preparations necessary for each patient. **Mixing medicines may be dangerous.** For example:

THEOPHYLLINE + ERYTHROMYCIN = Enhanced THEOPHYLLINE level

THEOPHYLLINE + CIMETIDINE = Enhanced THEOPHYLLINE level

When in doubt, consult a reference such as *Daily Drug Use:* author — Joe Talmud (Cape Town, Tincture Press, 1991). See also the *South African Medicines Formulary* produced by the Department of Pharmacology at the University of Cape Town, which is available from the Medical Association of South Africa, Publications Division, Private Bag X1, Pinelands 7430.

When using intravenous preparations one must be aware that some preparations are physically incompatible if given together. For example:

◆ BENZYLPENICILLIN and GENTAMICIN.
◆ AMPICILLIN and DOPAMINE.
◆ AMPHOTERICIN B and a number of substances, e.g. AMIKACIN, calcium chloride or gluconate, GENTAMICIN, PENICILLIN G.
◆ SODIUM NITROPRUSSIDE and all other drugs.

Do not put medications in blood transfusion bottles (except DESFERRIOXAMINE).

Allergic medicine reactions (serum sickness)

Allergic medicine reactions occur most frequently after a second exposure to the medicine. Reactions may vary from mild rash to fever, anaphylaxis and Steven Johnson syndrome.

The most common offenders causing allergic reactions are PENICILLINS and SEMI-SYNTHETIC PENICILLINS, with PROCAINE PENICILLIN having the highest incidence. Some cross-reaction (approximately 10%) is seen with CEPHALOSPORINS.

All vaccines and antitoxins based on animal serum have the potential to produce reaction in some individuals.

The most common cause of allergic pulmonary reaction is NITROFURANTOIN. PHENOTHIAZINES may cause cholestatic reactions, while SULPHONAMIDES, ISONIAZID, VALPROIC ACID and PYRAZINAMIDE may cause hepatocellular reactions. RIFAMPICIN has a high incidence of adverse effects (nausea, vomiting) if treatment is resumed after a break. SULPHONAMIDES and BARBITURATES may cause Steven Johnson syndrome.

It should be noted that these instances are far from exhaustive and that any medicine could be responsible for an allergic reaction in sensitive individuals. Bear in mind also that patients may be allergic to colouring, flavouring and preservatives.

In areas where PENICILLIN is administered by injection, a supply of ADRENALINE, PROMETHAZINE and HYDROCORTISONE should be available. See page 27 for anaphylaxis.

Antibiotic injections

Table 36.2 Table of diluents and stability of solutions

Important

1 Date, time of preparation and amount of diluent added must be written on the vial.
2 Most antibiotics requiring mixing before use do not contain a bacteriostatic. Contamination is a risk when vials are used repeatedly. Avoid puncturing the rubber cap more than necessary by using the lowest practical strength available, irrespective of stability.

Antibiotic	Diluent and concentration	Stability and remarks
AMIKACIN (Amikin)	Ready-prepared solutions Check strengths Conc.: 50 mg/ml, 125 mg/ml, 250 mg/ml	Check expiry date on vial.
AMPICILLIN	Water for injection For IV use. 250 mg vial: dilute to 5 ml 500 mg vial: dilute to 10 ml	Concentrated solutions unstable. Use immediately – discard remainder. IV infusions – use within four hours and change if solution becomes cloudy.
CEFAMANDOLE (Mandokef)	Water for injection 1 g vial: add 3,5 ml Conc.: 250 mg/ml	Room temp.: 24 hours. Refrigerator: 96 hours.
CEFOTAXIME (Claforan)	Water for injection 500 mg vial: add 3,6 ml Conc.: 125 mg/ml 1 g vial: add 7,2 ml Conc.: 125 mg/ml	Preferably freshly prepared. May be refrigerated for 24 hours if dosage is small.
CEFOXITIN (Mefoxin)	Water for injection 1 g vial: add 9,5 ml Conc.: 100 mg/ml	Freshly prepared solutions.
CEFTAZIDIME (Fortum)	Water for injection 500 mg vial: add 4,5 ml 1 g vial: add 9 ml 2 g vial: add 18 ml Conc.: 100 mg/ml	Preferably freshly prepared. Stable at 25°C for 18 hours or seven days in refrigerator.

Antibiotic	Diluent and concentration	Stability and remarks
CEFTRIAXONE	IV Water for injection 250 mg vial: add 5 ml 500 mg vial: add 5 ml 1 g vial: add 10 ml IM 1% LIGNOCAINE 250 mg vial: add 2 ml 500 mg vial: add 2 ml 1 g vial: add 3,5 ml	Preferably freshly prepared. Stable for 24 hours if refrigerated.
CEPHRADINE (Cefril)	Water for injection 250 mg vial: For IM inj.: add 1,2 ml Conc.: 250 mg/1,4 ml For IV inj.: add 5 ml 500 mg vial: For IM inj.: add 2 ml Conc.: 500 mg/2,4 ml For IV inj.: add 5 ml 1 g vial: For IM inj.: add 4 ml 1 g/4,8 ml For IV inj.: add 10 ml	Refrigerator: 24 hours. IV infusions remain stable for eight hours. Solution has a straw to yellow colour.
CHLOR- AMPHENICOL (Chloromycetin succinate)	Water for injection 1 g vial: add 10 ml Conc.: 100 mg/ml	Room temp.: 30 days.
CHLOR- AMPHENICOL (Kemicetine succinate)	Water for injection 1 g vial: add 3,2 ml Conc.: 250 mg/ml or: add 9,2 ml Conc.: 100 mg/ml	Room temp.: 30 days
CIPRO- FLOXACIN (Ciprobay)	Ready-prepared solution 100 ml vial Conc.: 2 mg/ml 50 ml vial Conc.: 2 mg/ml	Administer over 30-60 minutes by infusion.

Antibiotic	Diluent and concentration	Stability and remarks
CLINDAMYCIN (Dalacin C)	Ready-prepared solution Conc.: 150 mg/ml IV — must be diluted to a concentration of not more than 6 mg/ml in the Buretrol	Check expiry date on ampoule.
CLOXACILLIN (Orbenin, Prostaphlin A)	Water for injection 250 mg vial: add 1,8 ml Conc.: 125 mg/ml 500 mg vial: add 1,6 ml Conc.: 250 mg/ml	Refrigerator: four days.
CO-TRIMOXAZOLE (Septran, Bactrim)	Ready-prepared ampoules. TRIMETHOPRIM 80 mg and SULPHAMETHOXAZOLE 400 mg/5 ml *For infusion only*	Prepare infusion dilution immediately before use. Infuse within eight hours. *Refer to manufacturers' instructions.*
ERYTHRO-MYCIN (Erythrocin IV)	Water for injection. 1 g vial: add 20 ml Conc.: 50 mg/ml *Do not proceed without referring to manufacturers' instructions*	Concentrated solution. Refrigerator: 14 days. Diluted solution: administer within eight hours. *Beware when using dextrose solutions*
FUSIDIC ACID (Fucidin)	Dissolve 500 mg in 50 ml special buffer solution provided Dilute further to 250-500 ml with sod. chloride 0,9% or 5% dextrose water.	Fresh solutions to be used within 24 hours. If cloudy — discard. Infuse over two to four hours.
GENTAMICIN (Cidomycin, Garamycin)	Ready-prepared solutions — check strengths. 2 ml vial (Paed.): 10 mg/ml 2 ml vial (Adult): 40 mg/ml	Check expiry date on vial.

Antibiotic	Diluent and concentration	Stability and remarks
NETILMICIN (Netromycin)	Ready-prepared solution Conc.: 25 mg/ml, 100 mg/ml	Check expiry date on vial.
PENICILLINS		
PENICILLIN G or **CRYSTALLINE PENICILLIN** or **BENZYLPENICILLIN** or **SODIUM PENICILLIN** (Crystapen, Novopen)	Water for injection 1 million unit vial: 250 000 U/ml: add 3,6 ml 500 000 U/ml: add 1,6 ml 5 million unit vial: multidose 250 000 U/ml: add 17,8 ml 500 000 U/ml: add 7,8 ml 2 million U/5 ml: add 10,4 ml 5 million U/10 ml: add 7,8 ml See package for other dilutions	Refrigerator: seven days. 100 000 U/ml: add 9,6 ml Refrigerator: 14 days (buffered).
PROCAINE PENICILLIN (Novocillin)	Ready-prepared suspension 10 ml vial Conc.: 300 000 U/ml	Check expiry date on vial. Shake thoroughly before use. IM only.
BENZATHINE PENICILLIN (Bicillin LA, Penilente LA)	Water for injection 1,2 million unit vial 2,4 million unit vial Tap vial lightly before adding water. Single dose: add 3,5 ml Shake 4 ml injection	Refrigerator: seven days. IM only.
BENZATHINE PENICILLIN FORTIFIED (Penilente forte)	Water for injection Tap vial lightly before adding water. Single dose: add 1,4 ml Conc.: 600 000 U/ml Multidose: add 6,5 ml Conc.: 600 000 U/ml	Refrigerator: seven days. IM only.

Antibiotic	Diluent and concentration	Stability and remarks
PIPERACILLIN SODIUM (Pipril)	Water for injection. IV 2 g vial: add at least 10 ml 4 g vial: add at least 20 ml IM 2 g: add 4 ml. Water for injection or 0,5% LIGNOCAINE	Refrigerator: 48 hours.
RIFAMPICIN	Water for injection 600 mg vial: add 10 ml Dilute to 500 ml with 5% dextrose water.	Shake vigorously for 30 - 60 seconds. Discard unused portion. Infuse over three hours.
STREPTO-MYCIN	Ready-prepared solution 1 g in 3 ml	Check expiry date on vial.
TOBRAMYCIN (Nebcin)	Ready prepared solution. Check strengths. Conc.: 10 mg/ml 40 mg/ml	Check expiry date on vial.

Intravenous injections
Precautions and injection sites
General Comments

1. Check patient's name and identity, name of medication, dosage, volume and, finally, route to be administered, with a second person.
2. **Do not mix two or more antibiotics.**
3. If more than one antibiotic is due at the same time, they must be given with an interval of 15 minutes between each administration.
4. Before giving injection:
   ♦ Check that intravenous infusion is running satisfactorily.
   ♦ Clean injection bulb site with alcohol swab.
   ♦ Use the smallest needle available to avoid leakage from the bulb after injection (i.e. 0,45 x 16).
5. If medication is to be given in the Buretrol, the amount of fluid with the medication must be decided on by the doctor

and sister according to the concentration that is required per volume. Label Buretrol with medication, time and desired flow rate.

6. When a doctor orders a Schedule 6 or 7 medication, he must check and sign the Drug Register with the sister.

7. Only doctors may give the following intravenous medications into the bulb:

MORPHINE SULPHATE
PETHIDINE
DIGOXIN (Lanoxin)
AMINOPHYLLINE
DIAZEPAM (Valium)

8. Dilution of medication is facilitated by injecting medication slowly with intravenous running slowly.

Table 36.3 Intravenous injections – antibiotics

Antibiotic	Injection site		
Generic name (Trade name)	Into bulb	Into Buretrol	Into vacolitre
AMIKACIN (Amikin)	No	Yes	No
AMPICILLIN (Penbritin)	Yes	No	No
CEFAMANDOLE (Mandokef)	Yes	No	No
CEFOTAXIME (Claforan)	Yes	No	No
CEFOXITIN (Mefoxin)	Yes	Yes	No
CEFTAZIDIME (Fortum)	Yes	Yes	No
CEFTRIAXONE (Rocephin)	Yes	Yes	No
CEPHRADINE (Cefril)	Yes	No	No

Antibiotic	Injection site		
Generic name (Trade name)	Into bulb	Into Buretrol	Into vacolitre
CHLORAMPHENICOL (Chloromycetin)	Up to 2 ml	Over 2 ml	No
CIPROFLOXACIN (Ciprobay)	No	Yes	Yes
CLINDAMYCIN (Dalacin C)	No	Yes	No
CLOXACILLIN (Orbenin, Clocillin)	Yes	No	No
CO-TRIMOXAZOLE (Bactrim, Septran)	No	Yes	No
ERYTHROMYCIN (Erythrocin)	No	Yes	Yes
FUSIDIC ACID (Fucidin)	No	Yes	No
GENTAMICIN (Cidomycin, Garamycin)	Yes	Yes	No
PENICILLIN G or **CRYSTALLINE PENICILLIN** or **BENZYLPENICILLIN** or **SODIUM PENICILLIN** (Crystapen, Novopen)	Up to 2 ml	Over 2 ml	No
PIPERACILLIN (Pipril)	Yes	Yes	No
RIFAMPICIN (Rimactane)	No	Yes	No
TOBRAMYCIN (Nebcin)	Yes	Yes	No

Table 36.4 Intravenous injections — general

Generic Name (Trade Name)	Into bulb	Injection site Into Buretrol	Into vacolitre
ADRENALINE	Yes	No	No
AMINOPHYLLINE	Refer to page 596	Refer to page 596	No
ATROPINE	Yes	No	No
CALCIUM GLUCONATE	Yes	No	Yes
CHLORPROMAZINE (Largactil)	No	Yes	Yes
DEXAMETHASONE (Decadron Shock Pak)	Yes	No	No
DEXTROSE 50%	Yes	Yes	Yes
DIAZEPAM (Valium)	Yes Doctor or trained paediatric sister only	Yes Doctor or trained paediatric sister only	Yes Doctor or trained paediatric sister only
DIGOXIN (Lanoxin)	No	Doctor only	No
FUROSEMIDE (Lasix)	Yes	No	No
HEPARIN	Yes	Yes	Yes
HEXOPRENALINE (Ipradol)	Yes	Yes	No
HYDROCORTISONE (Solu-Cortef)	Yes	Yes	No
INSULIN	Never	Yes	Yes
ISOPRENALINE (Imuprel)	Never	Yes	Yes

Generic Name (Trade Name)	Injection site Into bulb	Into Buretrol	Into vacolitre
MAGNESIUM SULPHATE	No	No	Yes
PHENO-BARBITONE	Yes – but with sufficient fluid to produce 1:10 dilution.	No	No
PHENYTOIN SODIUM	See page 623		
POTASSIUM CHLORIDE	Never	Yes – but with sufficient fluid to produce 1:50 dilution.	Yes
SODIUM BICARBONATE	Yes	Yes	Yes

Table 36.5 Therapeutic ranges of commonly used medications*

Medication	Therapeutic levels
Anti-convulsants	
CARBAMAZEPINE	8-12 µg/ml (10-40 µmol/l)
CLONAZEPAM	20-80 µg/ml
ETHOSUXIMIDE	40-100 µg/ml (300-700 µmol/l)
PHENOBARBITONE	15-40 µg/ml (65-172 µmol/l)
PHENYTOIN	10-20 µg/ml (40-80 µmol/l)
PRIMIDONE	5-12 µg/ml (23-55 µmol/l)
VALPROATE	50-100 µg/ml (300-700 µmol/l)
Cardiovascular	
DIGOXIN	0,8-2 ng/ml
LIGNOCAINE	1,5-5 µg/ml
Immunosuppressant	
CYCLOSPORIN	250-1 000 ng/ml

Respiratory
THEOPHYLLINE

General	10-20 µg/ml
Neonatal apnoea	5-12µg/ml

Antibiotic	Trough level	Peak level
AMIKACIN	<5 µg/ml	>30 µg/ml (1 hr post)
GENTAMICIN	<2 µg/ml	>10 µg/ml (1 hr post)
TOBRAMYCIN	<2 µg/ml	>10 µg/ml (1 hr post)
VANCOMYCIN	5-10 µg/ml	20-40 µg/ml (2 hrs post)

---

* Note: levels provided may differ between laboratories. They are also influenced by sample time and other factors such as age, prematurity. The clinical response of the patient should be considered.

37 POISONING AND POISON INFORMATION CENTRES

Staff of the Poisons Information Centre

This chapter deals only with the emergency management of poisoning and includes some guidelines on symptoms and diagnosis of specific poisoning. Snake, scorpion and spider bites are discussed elsewhere. See Chapter 7, page 70. For detailed information on management of poisoning by specific substances, appropriate textbooks as well as pharmacists and/or a regional Poison Information Centre must be consulted. See Appendix 5, page 686.

Definitions

Poisoning: ingestion or inhalation of, or eye, skin or mucous membrane contact with, a potentially hazardous substance in a dose large enough to cause harm.

Acute poisoning: exposure to a single large dose or the cumulative effect of subtoxic doses taken within 24-36 hours.

Chronic poisoning: repeated exposures to subtoxic doses over a long period of time.

Aetiology
Some causes of poisoning in childhood

Medicines, household products, toiletries, insecticides, rodenticides, fungicides, herbicides, fuels, paints and painting supplies, hobby and do-it-yourself hardware products, plants and noxious gases.

Contributory factors

Socio-economic, housing and education, age and quality of child-minders.

Prevention of poisoning

Meticulous attention to the storage of potential toxins in sites not accessible or visible to an intrepid, ingenious, and inquisitive child.

Epidemiology

Accidental poisoning occurs in children under the age of five; the peak incidence is in the two to three year age group.

Intentional poisoning with one or more drugs is more common in older children, and the psychological and legal implications must be addressed.

Diagnosis

Consider poisoning whenever there is a history of exposure to a toxic substance. Include poisoning in the differential diagnosis of:

♦ sudden onset of unexplained illness in a previously healthy child;
♦ unexplained drowsiness, stupor, coma, ataxia, irritability or acidosis; or
♦ vomiting and diarrhoea after the ingestion of food.

Management of the poisoned patient

The following principles of management apply in all cases, and where possible, **must** be implemented **simultaneously**, as speed is a crucial factor in the treatment of poisoning.

Exclude life-threatening emergencies

Do immediate brief screening general examination to exclude:

♦ respiratory inadequacy: observe the respiratory rate and depth, presence of cyanosis. See page 683;
♦ circulatory failure: BP, pulse. See pages 99 and 683;
♦ depressed level of consciousness. See pages 331 and 665; and
♦ uncontrolled continuous seizures. See page 338.

Ask relevant questions to exclude these emergencies and advise as necessary if consulted by telephone.

Exclude and treat airway obstruction

Note any presence of dyspnoea, dysphonia, hoarseness, stridor, intercostal retraction, cyanosis, snoring, tachypnoea. See Chapter 1 for management of airway obstruction and page 516 for sizes of endotracheal tubes.

Exclude and treat hypoxaemia

Administer oxygen and assist ventilation after clearing the airway. If respiration is inadequate, if cyanosis is present or in cyanide poisonings, assist ventilation with a bag and mask by mouth-to-nose or mouth-to-mouth respiration or by mechanical ventilation. See Chapter 1.

Exclude and treat shock

For diagnosis and treatment of shock see page 7.

Exclude and treat hypoglycaemia

Draw blood for a blood glucose concentration (Dextrostix) and treat hypoglycaemia if present. Give GLUCOSE intravenously, 50% dextrose water 1 ml/kg, diluted to 25% solution. If life-threatening hypoglycaemia is present and an intravenous line cannot be established, 50% dextrose water 2 ml/kg, diluted 1:1 may be administered via a nasogastric tube with patient in left lateral position to avoid aspiration. See page 451. Maintain glucose administration to prevent reactive hypoglycaemia.

Control convulsions

Toxin-induced convulsions are usually brief, but if seizures persist see page 336. Ensure facilities are available to support and maintain respiration should respiratory arrest occur.

Control pain

Control severe pain with IV MORPHINE (**except** in scorpion- and snakebite). See page 37. Monitor for respiratory depression. If it occurs, stop or reduce dose of MORPHINE, administer NALOXONE HYDROCHLORIDE 0,01 mg/kg/per dose and provide ventilatory support.

Establish type of toxin and assess risk to patient

The decision to admit and treat the patient depends on the nature of the toxin and the risk of serious effects on the patient. The cause and the risk must be established as soon as possible from the history and physical examination.

On occasions certain special investigations and toxicology screening may help in establishing the diagnosis, but these procedures should **never** delay the induction of emesis, gastric lavage, administration of ACTIVATED CHARCOAL or local decontamination, where indicated.

History

Establish the type, amount, uses and nature of toxin, route and time of exposure, subsequent clinical course and treatment administered. Elicit information on medicines available in the home or at the site of probable exposure.

Ask for the container and remnant of suspected toxin and any vomitus subsequent to exposure. Keep for medico-legal or toxicological examination if indicated.

The risk of poisoning by any potentially toxic substance is a function of its inherent toxicity and the amount taken.

Significant poisoning due to low inherent toxicity is unlikely after ingestion of:

♦ insoluble chemically inert substances, e.g. rubber, plasticine;
♦ products for use in eye or cosmetics for use on skin (**except** those with ETHANOL);
♦ single episodes of ingestion of contraceptive or corticosteroid tablets;
♦ MERCURY from the bulb of **one** clinical thermometer; or
♦ toilet soaps, hair shampoos except anti-dandruff formulations.

Significant poisoning due to high inherent toxicity is likely after ingestion of:

♦ medicines, antiseptics and disinfectants;
♦ industrial, agricultural and hardware products;
♦ insecticides and rodenticides, both household and agricultural;
♦ cosmetics with ETHANOL, e.g. perfumes, after-shave lotions;
♦ anti-dandruff shampoos;

♦ household cleaners, swimming pool chemicals, bleaches, drain cleaners;

♦ fuels and petroleum distillates, e.g. KEROSENE, MINERAL TURPENTINE; or

♦ noxious fumes, e.g. CARBON MONOXIDE.

There is a high risk to the patient if he or she has taken a substance with a significant inherent toxicity. The stated amount taken may be inaccurate, but it is better to err on the side of caution. The risk to the patient is also influenced by the presence or absence of vomiting, treatment given and time after exposure.

Some toxins exhibit effects only after a latent period. These include alcohols, anticholinergics, ASPIRIN, enteric-coated slow-release tablets, glycols, iron-compounds, PARACETAMOL, PARAQUAT.

Button-battery ingestion causes severe local trauma if the battery is retained in any part of the gastrointestinal tract, most common site being the oesophagus.

Physical examination

Exclude conditions unrelated to poisoning, e.g. head injury etc. In most cases a tentative diagnosis can be reached on the history and physical findings. This allows one to decide whether or not to empty the stomach.

See table 37.1 on page 419 for a list of some findings which may be associated with specific toxins in acute or chronic toxicity. It is important to note that the list is **not** complete and neither the presence or absence of any of these findings is diagnostic, as many toxins cause similar symptoms.

Toxicology screening

This can be a useful adjunct in some cases, provided indications and limitations are clearly understood. Treatment should never be deferred until toxicology is available.

Consult centres responsible for toxicology testing in your area for details of tests available, type and method of collection of specimen, clinical data required and interpretation of results.

Specific blood levels of some toxins are important in directing therapy, e.g. alcohols, DIGOXIN, IRON, LEAD and other heavy metals, PARACETAMOL, PARAQUAT, PHENYTOIN, salicylates, THEOPHYLLINE.

Table 37.1 Signs associated with specific toxins

General signs

Hyperpyrexia	Antihistamines, ATROPINE, chlorophenoxy compounds, dinitrophenols, salicylates, tricyclic antidepressants
Hypothermia	Barbiturates, ETHANOL, MEPROBAMATE, opiates, phenothiazines
Loss of appetite	Chronic poisoning with TRINITROTOLUENE
Weight loss	Chronic poisoning with ARSENIC, chlorinated hydrocarbons, dinitrophenols, LEAD, MERCURY, thyroid

Odours

Acetone(sweet)	ISOPROPYL ALCOHOL, lacquer, METHANOL, salicylates
Bitter almonds	Apricot pips, CYANIDE
Garlic	ARSENIC, organophosphates, SELENIUM, THALLIUM
Moth balls	Camphor products
Wintergreen	METHYL SALICYLATE

Ocular signs

Blurred vision	ATROPINE, botulism, ETHANOL, organophosphates
Lacrimation	Irritants, organophosphates
Miosis	Muscarinic mushrooms, opiates, organophosphates, phenothiazines
Mydriasis	Antihistamines, ATROPINE, CARBON MONOXIDE, COCAINE, ETHANOL, tricyclic antidepressants
Nystagmus	Barbiturates, ETHANOL, PHENYTOIN
Papilloedema	Chronic poisoning with LEAD

Skin signs

Alopecia	Chronic poisoning with arsenic, LEAD, MERCURY, SELENIUM, THALLIUM
Burns .	Corrosives (acids, alkalis)
Cyanosis (without respiratory depression), e.g. methaemoglobinaemia, sulphaemoglobinaemia	ANILINE, antimalarials, chlorates, PHENACETIN, NAPHTHALENE in patients with G6PD deficiency, nitrites, NITROBENZENE
Desquamation/bullae	Barbiturates, borates. Chronic poisoning with ARSENIC, VITAMIN A
Red flushed colour	Anticholinergics, antihistamines, ATROPINE, atropine-containing plants, borates, tricyclic antidepressants, rarely CARBON MONOXIDE
Sweating	Organophosphates, nitrates, muscarinic mushrooms, salicylates

Oral/oesophageal signs

Burns/stomatitis	Corrosives (acids, alkalis, chlorophors, solvents), iodines, PARAQUAT, phenols, THALLIUM
Dysphagia	Local lesions (as above), botulism, button batteries, paralytic shellfish poisoning, phenothiazines with associated dystonic movements
Dry mouth (in absence of dehydration)	ATROPINE, antihistamines, anticholinergics
Excessive salivation	Local lesions, organophosphates, muscarinic mushrooms, STRYCHNINE
Gingivitis	Chronic poisoning with heavy metals
Gum lines	Chronic poisoning with heavy metals

Intestinal signs

Abdominal pain	Corrosives (acids, alkalis, solvents), heavy metals, iron compounds, phenols, plant irritants, salicylates

Constipation	Chronic poisoning with opiates, LEAD
Diarrhoea/vomiting	Almost all poisons, but excessive vomiting/diarrhoea may be food poisoning
Haematemesis/melaena	Anticoagulants (COUMARIN, PHENINDIONE, BRODIFACOUM), corrosives, iron compounds, salicylates, THEOPHYLLINE

Cardiovascular signs

Bradycardia	CLONIDINE, DIGOXIN, nitrites, opiates, organophosphates
Hypertension with a normal/slow pulse	Ergot derivatives, PHENYLPROPANOLAMINE
Hypertension with tachycardia	ADRENALINE, antihistamines, EPHEDRINE, NICOTINE, tricyclic antidepressants
Hypotension with bradycardia	Barbiturates, benzodiazepines, CLONIDINE, CYANIDE, METHYLDOPA, monoamine oxidase inhibitors, organophosphates, RESERPINE
Hypotension with tachycardia	Amatoxin-containing mushrooms, nitrates and nitrites, numerous plant toxins, phenothiazines, tricyclic antidepressants
Tachycardia	ATROPINE, CAFFEINE, beta adrenergics, iron compounds, THEOPHYLLINE, tricyclic antidepressants

Central nervous system signs

Ataxia	Antidepressants, antihistamines, barbiturates, ETHANOL, LEAD
Convulsions or seizures	AMPHETAMINE and other stimulants, CAMPHOR, carbamate insecticides, CARBON MONOXIDE, ETHYLENE GLYCOL, organophosphates, METALDEHYDE, STRYCHNINE, THEOPHYLLINE. May be a sign of serious toxicity or anoxia in many types of poisoning
Dystonic movements	METOCLOPRAMIDE, phenothiazines, PHENYTOIN, tricyclic antidepressants

Muscle fasciculation	LITHIUM, organophosphates
Muscle rigidity	STRYCHNINE
Muscle weakness	Carbamates, organophosphates, plant paralysers
Overactivity/ restlessness	ATROPINE, EPHEDRINE, phenothiazines, THEOPHYLLINE
Paraesthesiae	Chronic poisoning with CARBON TETRACHLORIDE, GASOLINE, heavy metals, HEXANE

Respiratory signs

Dyspnoea	Petroleum distillates, especially KEROSENE
Respiration: depressed	Many drugs or toxins cause central depression of respiration, e.g. ETHANOL, opiates, sedatives, tricyclic antidepressants. Drugs causing failure of ventilatory muscles, e.g. neuromuscular blocking agents, organophosphates
Respiration: increased	CARBON MONOXIDE, CYANIDE, hydrocarbons, salicylates

Simple laboratory or special investigations

BLOOD

Anion gap metabolic acidosis	Lactate accumulation due to anaerobic metabolism in hypoxia, shock, impaired hepatic lactate metabolism. Non-lactate anion gap acidosis with ETHYLENE GLYCOL, METHANOL, salicylates
Acid base imbalance with osmolar gap	ETHYLENE GLYCOL or METHANOL, especially when associated with large anion gap
Fluid and electrolyte imbalance	Any severe poisoning may cause derangements
Hyperkalaemia	Alpha adrenergics, beta blockers, DIGOXIN, FLUORIDE, oleanders
Hypokalaemia	CAFFEINE, SALBUTAMOL, salicylates, THEOPHYLLINE, thiazide diuretics
Hypocalcaemia	Glycols, oxalates

Hyperglycaemia	CAFFEINE, THEOPHYLLINE
Hypoglycaemia	Antidiabetic agents, hepatic failure
Methaemoglobinaemia	ANILINE, nitrates, nitrites, PHENACETIN

X-RAYS

| Abdomen or chest | Radio-opaque substances, e.g. button batteries, or CALCIUM, enteric coated, iron, POTASSIUM or SODIUM tablets. Signs of pneumonitis with aspiration of toxin especially petrochemical products |

ECG CHANGES

Bradycardia or AV block	DIGOXIN, oleanders, organophosphates
Sinus or supra-ventricular tachycardia	Adrenergics, e.g. EPHEDRINE, anticholinergics, e.g. ATROPINE and antihistamines, cellular hypoxia, e.g. CARBON MONOXIDE, xanthines, e.g. THEOPHYLLINE and CAFFEINE
Ventricular tachyarrythmias	CAFFEINE, DIGOXIN, FLUORIDE, phenothiazines, THEOPHYLLINE, tricyclic antidepressants
QRS and/or QT prolongation	ARSENIC, FLUORIDE, LITHIUM, MAGNESIUM, phenothiazines, QUININE, tricyclic antidepressants

Decontaminate the patient

Decontamination procedures prevent aggravation of injury due to prolonged contact with acids, alkalis or inhalational toxins, and they reduce absorption from the site of exposure.

Avoid splashing yourself and helpers with irrigating fluid. Wear gloves and protective clothing.

Do not re-use irrigation fluid, and do not use acid, alkaline or neutralizing agents.

Skin decontamination

Remove contaminated clothing, rinse and wash whole body with fresh running water and ordinary soap. Repeat washing three times, using fresh running water each time.

Eye decontamination

Continuously irrigate eye with fresh normal saline or running tap water for 15-20 minutes.

Bowel decontamination of ingested toxins

♦ Administer a diluent such as a cup of water or milk as a first aid measure unless oral fluids are contra-indicated due to a depressed level of consciousness, rapidly deteriorating consciousness, seizures or ingestion of petroleum distillates.

♦ If significant toxicity is expected, empty the stomach either by **emesis** or **gastric aspiration** or **lavage** unless contra-indicated.

♦ Give ACTIVATED CHARCOAL unless contra-indicated.

♦ Administer saline cathartics when indicated.

♦ Whole bowel irrigation.

Emesis

Contra-indications

♦ Poisoning by petroleum distillates (KEROSENE and like substances).

♦ Ingestion of corrosive acids or alkalis or co-ingestion of sharp objects.

♦ An unconscious patient, rapidly deepening depression of level of consciousness, e.g. CHLORAL HYDRATE, continuous seizures, poisoning with cyanide derivatives, tricyclic antidepressants.

♦ Children less than six months old as they have inadequate gag reflexes.

Dangerous

♦ In poisoning with agents causing central nervous system excitement and convulsions, e.g. CAMPHOR, STRYCHNINE. Gastric lavage after control of convulsions may be preferred.

♦ Repeated vomiting which may have already emptied the stomach.

Unnecessary

◆ When the time lapse after ingestion is greater than three or four hours, unless ingested drug (e.g. CARBAMAZEPINE) or subsequent treatment (e.g. ingestion of milk or cream) is known to delay gastric emptying.
◆ When a non-toxic substance is ingested.

Method of induction of emesis

◆ Agent of choice is **syrup** of IPECACUANHA (containing 1 mg emetine alkaloids per ml). Strong salt solutions must **never** be used to induce vomiting as they may lead to hypernatraemia.
  Note: Different preparations of IPECACUANHA vary in concentration of emetine alkaloids.
◆ Dose of IPECACUANHA: 1 mg/kg plus 15 ml/kg clear fluid.
◆ Vomiting should occur within 30 minutes. If no vomiting occurs the dose may be repeated **once** only. If there is still no vomiting (e.g. after significant ingestion of a strong anti-emetic substance such as CHLORPROMAZINE) do **not** give a third dose. Empty the stomach by gastric lavage.

Gastric aspiration or lavage

Contra-indications

◆ Ingestion of corrosive acids or alkalis.
◆ Co-ingestion of a sharp object.

Dangerous

◆ In poisoning by petroleum distillates. (If used as a fluid vehicle for a highly toxic substance such as PARATHION, gastric lavage may be used.
◆ Poisoning with ingested cyanide derivatives. **Urgent priority** is increased inspired oxygen concentration and administration of cyanide antidote kit.
◆ Poisoning by convulsants before seizures have been controlled.

Unnecessary

◆ When time lapse is greater than four to six hours after ingestion in circumstances not associated with prolonged gastric emptying time.

◆ Where patients are alert and have an active gag reflex, unless emesis has failed and the need to remove the toxin is urgent.

Method of gastric lavage

Size of tube

◆ Nasogastric tube: the nostril is the only limiting size. Usually size 8-12 F.
◆ Orogastric tube: 24-32 F.

Aspirating syringe to fit the tube

◆ **Place patient** in left lateral head-down position to prevent aspiration. **Extend** the head. In patients with no gag reflex, intubation is advocated.
◆ **Mark distance** on tube from mouth or nostril to epigastrium. **Pass** tube either through mouth over tongue or through nostril, along back wall of pharynx into oesophagus. **Do not** use force if obstruction is encountered before mark is reached. **Withdraw** tube somewhat and try again.
◆ **Place end of tube** in glass of water. **Beware:** bubbling on expiration indicates that the tube is in the lungs.
◆ **Aspirate gastric contents, examine** for pills or evidence of toxin and **save** first sample of aspirate for toxicology if indicated.
◆ **Instil lavage fluid:** aliquots of 5 ml/kg body weight, 0,45-0,9% saline warmed to body temperature. **Leave** lavage fluid in place for one minute, drain by gravity for five minutes. If drainage takes longer, assist with gentle suction on the tube.
◆ **Repeat** process until lavage fluid is clear.
◆ Pinch off the lavage tube prior to rapid withdrawal to minimize aspiration.

Administer ACTIVATED CHARCOAL

ACTIVATED CHARCOAL is advocated in many cases even where time lapse exceeds four to six hours. It may be used as a single dose or as repeated doses, e.g. in CARBAMAZEPINE, PHENOBARBITONE or THEOPHYLLINE ingestions.

Contra-indications

◆ Ingestion of corrosive (caustic) agents.
◆ Ineffective in ingestion of petroleum distillates (KEROSENE), which produce chemical pneumonitis.

◆ Ingestion of PARACETAMOL. (CHARCOAL interferes with action of specific antidote ACETYLCYSTEINE.)
◆ Ineffective in poisoning by BORIC ACID, CYANIDE, DDT, ETHANOL, FERROUS SULPHATE, METHANOL, many heavy metal toxins and water-insoluble substances.

Method of administration

◆ Empty stomach unless contra-indicated.
◆ Single dose: 1 g/kg in 50-100 ml of water.
◆ Serial doses: 0,5-1 g/kg every two to four hours.
◆ If the patient will not drink the dose within 15 minutes, administer by nasogastric tube.

Administer laxatives or saline cathartics

Routine use is debatable. If time lapse after ingestion of an ORGANOPHOSPHATE precludes emesis, saline cathartics in conjunction with ACTIVATED CHARCOAL may be useful.

Doses:

◆ SODIUM SULPHATE or MAGNESIUM SULPHATE 250 mg/kg, as a 10% solution.

Contra-indications

◆ Ingestion of, or rectal exposure to, corrosives.
◆ Presence or a high risk of renal failure, e.g. myoglobinuria, prolonged seizures.
◆ Electrolyte imbalances, diarrhoea, ileus.

Whole bowel irrigation

Consider use in poisoning by substances poorly adsorbed to activate charcoal, e.g. iron or in cases of massive ingestion where the administration of enough charcoal presents a problem. Continue administration of polyethylene glycolelectrolyte solution (Golytely) until a pure charcoal stool is passed. See page 219.

Administer antidote

Specific antidotes are available for about 5% of toxins. The antidote regime is often complex and requires detailed information from a Poison Reference Centre or a reputable handbook on poisoning. Some poisons and their antidotes are listed.

Table 37.2 Poison and antidotes

This list is not complete and the sources mentioned earlier must be consulted for guidance on indications, method, side effects and dangers of their use.

Poison	Antidote
ANILINE, NITROBENZOL, e.g. dyes or NITROBENZENE	METHYLENE BLUE
Caustic ingestion, e.g. corrosive alkalis, acids or other compounds	Milk or water per mouth
Coumarins, e.g. rat poisons	VITAMIN K1
Cyanide poisoning	Cyanide antidote kits available commercially. See current MIMS
Dystonic movements associated with phenothiazines, neuroleptics, e.g. HALOPERIDOL, METOCLOPRAMIDE	BIPERIDEN LACTATE (Akineton)
ETHYLENE GLYCOL	ETHANOL
Folic acid antagonists, e.g. METHOTREXATE	FOLINIC ACID (Leucovorin)
Heavy metal poisoning, e.g. LEAD, MERCURY	DIMERCAPROL, PENICILLAMINE
Hydrofluoric acid burns	CALCIUM GLUCONATE 10% solution for local infiltration
Indanediones, e.g. some rat poisons	VITAMIN K1
Iron poisoning	DESFERRIOXAMINE
ISONIAZID	PYRIDOXINE
METHANOL	ETHANOL
Morphines	NALOXONE HYDROCHLORIDE
Nitrates, nitrites with methaemoglobinaemia	METHYLENE BLUE
Organophosphates	ATROPINE, OBIDOXIME (Toxogonin)
PARACETAMOL	ACETYLCYSTEINE

Continue care, increase elimination of toxin, give appropriate after-care

Control body temperature

Some toxins may be associated with extreme hyperthermia, 40 °C or more. Control temperatures by sponging with tepid water and fanning.

Continue emergency measures

Continue such measures as are necessary for support or general care of the patient or are advised by Poison Reference Centre or textbook, e.g. monitoring fluid input and urine output, correcting any electrolyte or acid-base imbalance, controlling hypo- or hyperthermia, maintaining adequate nutrition, initiating further special treatment.

Special treatment regimes

These include treatment and prevention of complications, e.g. pulmonary, haematological, renal and hepatic pathology, methods to enhance elimination of the toxin, e.g. alkaline or acid diuresis, haemodialysis, haemoperfusion, appropriate diets and after-care, e.g. in chronic heavy metal poisoning, psychiatric care in intentional poisoning.

Poison Information Centres

See Appendix 5, page 688.

Recommended reading:
Dreisbach RH, Robertson WO. *Handbook of Poisoning*, 12th ed. Connecticut: Appleton & Lange, 1987.

38 PRESCRIPTIONS AND DRUG SCHEDULES

R D Gilbert

The prescribing and dispensing of medicine in the Republic of South Africa is legally controlled by the Medicines and Related Substances Control Act, 1965 (Act 101 of 1965, as amended by Act 65 of 1974).

Definition of a medical practitioner

For the purposes of the Act, a medical practitioner means a person registered as such under the Medical Act, and includes an intern registered under that Act. **Note that student interns are not included** in this definition for purposes of this Act.

Prescriptions

Every **prescription** shall be written and signed by a medical practitioner and shall state:

♦ the date of issue;
♦ the name and quantity of medicine. (For Schedule 6 and 7 drugs the quantity is to be expressed in figures as well as in words.);
♦ the name and address of the patient; and
♦ the name, qualifications and address of medical practitioner. (These may be printed on the prescription.)

Important: In paediatric prescription writing, the weight and age of the child should be included. Latin abbreviations, e.g. *t.d.s.*, *m. et n.* are **not** to be used. See Figure 38.1.

Labelling of medicines

The name of the medicine must appear on the label unless the medical practitioner considers that this would not be in the interest of the patient. In such cases he or she may endorse the prescription 'non-nomen' and initial the instruction.

Repeat prescriptions

Only unscheduled medicines and those in Schedules 1 and 2 may be repeated indefinitely. For Schedules 3-7, see Table 38.1.

Examples of medicines in the various schedules

It should be noted that the Schedule into which a medicine falls depends on its liability to misuse rather than its inherent toxicity. The Schedule(s) must be noted on every container.

Examples of the medicines in the various Schedules are given below. Note that depending on dosage form, route of administration, or the purpose for which the medicine is used, a medicine may appear in different schedules.

Schedule 1

- ♦ DAPSONE and derivatives for malaria prophylaxis.
- ♦ SODIUM CROMOGLYCATE, e.g. Lomudal.
- ♦ THEOPHYLLINE and derivatives.

Schedule 2

- ♦ Antihistamines (most).
- ♦ ATROPINE (except ophthalmic preparations).
- ♦ Barbiturates (medium-acting) and combinations within a certain dose range when used for asthma and epilepsy.
- ♦ Bronchodilators for oral use and inhalants, e.g. FENOTEROL, SALBUTAMOL, ADRENALINE, CARBOCISTEINE (Mucospect).
- ♦ MEBENDAZOLE (Vermox).
- ♦ PHENYLEPHRINE admixtures, e.g. Actifed, Dimetapp.

Schedule 3

- ♦ Anticonvulsants (except PHENOBARBITONE), e.g. SODIUM VALPROATE, PHENYTOIN SODIUM, CARBAMAZEPINE.
- ♦ ATROPINE (ophthalmic preparations).
- ♦ DIGOXIN, thyroid and derivatives, INSULIN.
- ♦ Diuretics, antihypertensives other than NITROPRUSSIDE SODIUM.
- ♦ IBUPROFEN, MEFENAMIC ACID (suspension).

Table 38.1 Conditions pertaining to the prescription of scheduled drugs in accordance with the Medical, Dental and Supplementary Health Service Professions Act (Act 56 of 1974) and the Medicines and Related Substances Control Act (Act 101 of 1965, as amended by Act 65 of 1974)

	Schedules								
	1	2	3	4	5	6	7	8	9
Prescription	Written or verbal	Written or verbal	Written or verbal	Written	Written only	Written only	Written only	—	—
Repeatable or not	Yes	Yes	Yes Max. period six months	Yes (State number of repeats and intervals)	Yes (State number of repeats and intervals)	No	No	—	—
Validity period	Not limited	Not limited	Not limited	Not limited	Not limited	Invalid after 30 days	Invalid after 30 days	—	—
Quantity	Not limited	Not limited	Not limited	Not limited	Not limited	Max. 30 days' supply	Max. 30 days' supply	Banned	Banned

	Schedules								
	1	2	3	4	5	6	7	8	9
Special instructions	—	—	—	If verbal prescription, must be followed by a written prescription within seven days	—	Quantity must be stated in words and figures	Quantity must be stated in words and figures	—	—
Keeping of registers	—	—	—	—	Keep record of all receipts for three years	Keep register for three years	Keep register for three years	—	—

Schedule 4

◆ Antibiotics and chemotherapeutic agents, e.g. SULPHO-NAMIDES, METRONIDAZOLE.
◆ Corticosteroids.
◆ FENOTEROL, SALBUTAMOL injection.
◆ METOCLOPRAMIDE, CIMETIDINE, cytotoxic agents.

Schedule 5

◆ Psychotropic agents – antidepressants, e.g. IMIPRAMINE.
◆ Tranquillizers – both major and minor, and hypnotics, e.g. CHLORPROMAZINE, DIAZEPAM, PARALDEHYDE, PHENOBARBITONE, DEXTROPROPOXYPHENE, FENFLURAMINE (Ponderax).

Schedule 6

◆ Barbiturates (medium-acting), e.g. AMYLOBARBITONE, PHENOBARBITONE, DIETHYLPROPION (Tenuate).
◆ PENTAZOCINE (Sosegon).

Schedule 7

Formerly known as habit-forming drugs (H.F.D.), e.g. COCAINE, METHYLPHENIDATE, OPIUM ALKALOIDS, TILIDINE.

Schedule 8

May be obtained only for analytical or research purposes, on permit.

Schedule 9

May be obtained only from the Director-General: Department of National Health and Population Development, for purpose of providing a medical practitioner with means to treat a particular patient, e.g. AMPHETAMINES.

Drugs in sport

In terms of International Olympic Committee regulations, drugs in the following classes are banned:

◆ Anabolic agents
◆ Diuretics

Figure 38.1 Sample prescription

Dr Peter Brown MB ChB (UCT)
101 Klipfontein Road
Rondebosch
7700

1991-7-31

John Smith (aged five years) 20 kg
7 Middle Street
MOWBRAY 7700
Tab. METHYLPHENIDATE 10 mg
30 (Thirty) tablets
One at 8 am.

P Brown

♦ Narcotics
♦ Peptide hormones and analogues (Adrenocorticotrophic Hormone (ACTH), Erythropoeitin, Human Chorionic Gonadotrophin (HCG) and Human Growth Hormone (HGH)).
♦ Stimulants

The presence of such drugs in the urine constitutes an offence, regardless of the method of administration.

The following classes of drugs are subject to certain restrictions:

♦ Alcohol
♦ Beta-blockers
♦ Local anaesthetics
♦ Marijuana

Warning

♦ Many over-the-counter cold and 'flu remedies contain banned substances.

♦ All IMIDAZOLE derivatives are acceptable for topical use, e.g. OXYMETAZOLINE. Topical vasoconstrictors, including those given with local anaesthetics, are all acceptable except EPHEDRINE.

♦ The $\beta2$ stimulants SALBUTAMOL and TERBUTALINE are permitted by inhalation only. No other $\beta2$ agonist is permitted, and oral or intravenous administration is banned.

♦ Corticosteroids given by local or intra-articular injection or by inhalation are allowed. Systemic administration is banned.

♦ The use of corticosteroids and $\beta2$ stimulants as outlined above requires prior notification by the doctor to the event organizers.

39 PROCEDURES

J D Ireland

The practice of paediatrics will always require investigations and procedures on patients. The advantages and disadvantages of invasive procedures should be considered and the investigation profile carefully planned in order to provide maximum information to the doctor with minimal emotional and physical trauma to the patient. Time spent providing information on the nature of a procedure allays parental and patient anxiety. Therefore:

♦ **plan** investigations carefully so as to obtain as much information from as few procedures as possible;
♦ **inform** parents and/or patients. Discuss indications, possible failures and risk factors where appropriate;
♦ **reassure** and support the child before, during and after the procedure; and
♦ **consider** the use of analgesia and sedation carefully, in relation to the underlying medical condition.

> ### Warning
> Do not neglect guidance and instruction on procedures to junior staff. Considerations of minimizing trauma to the patient must not impede the teaching of staff.

Restraining the patient

Restraint is necessary in almost every procedure. The age and compliance of the child are the key factors influencing the choice of method. Preparation of the patient includes optimal restraint through human holding and 'wrapping' techniques. Exposure of the procedure site, adequate lighting and the 'most comfortable' position for the 'operator', are important for

success. Because sedation takes time to work it is often therefore not administered. Adequate restraint is then more difficult,
so that haste may well result in loss of time.

Methods of restraint

◆ Wrapping the whole body and pinning it in a 'sheet'.
◆ Physical restraint: patient is held in the optimal position by
  an experienced helper e.g. nurse for lumbar puncture (LP).
◆ Splinting of limb.
◆ Restraining to the bed with arm and/or leg tie-downs.
◆ Restraint of the patient to prevent IV lines, drains etc. being
  pulled out.

Sedation, analgesia and local anaesthesia

See Chapter 3, page 29.
  It is usually safe and helpful to administer either sedation or
analgesia or both. Consider the patient's physical condition and
the underlying disease process when deciding on the form and
dosage of required medications.

Abdominal paracentesis (ascitic tap)

Empty the bladder and place the patient in a semi-sitting position with the back firmly supported. Puncture sites are in the
midline midway between the umbilicus and the pubis or in the
right or left lower quadrants a few centimetres above the
inguinal ligament. (See Figure 39.1.) Anaesthetize the skin.
Employ a needle and stylet, or 'over the needle' plastic IV
catheter, to enter the abdominal cavity. Aspirate the required
amount of fluid and withdraw. The risk of ongoing leakage of
fluid in a distended abdomen can be minimized by using a
Z-track puncture, when a subcutaneous track of 1 cm is made
with the needle before angling it inwards to enter the abdominal
cavity.

Dangers

◆ Intestinal perforation.
◆ Bladder perforation.
◆ Shock and syncope if too large a volume (>1 litre) is
  removed rapidly.
◆ Infection and peritonitis. (Ascitic fluid is an ideal culture
  medium.)

Figure 39.1 Sites for abdominal paracentesis

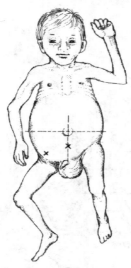

Reproduced with permission from Hughes WT and Buescher ES *Paediatric procedures* (second edition). London, WB Saunders, 1980.

Blood specimen collection

Before taking blood ensure that:

♦ you have decided on all the tests to be done on the specimen;
♦ the correct tubes are used with the correct amounts of specimen;
♦ the laboratory has been consulted and informed about 'special' tests; and
♦ the correctly labelled specimen will reach the laboratory in the required time.

Venipuncture

Common sites used are the antecubital fossa, external jugular, dorsum of hand or foot and scalp veins. Less common and more hazardous sites are the internal jugular and femoral veins. The torcular herophili (through the posterior fontanelle) is only used for critically important samples in an infant when all other sites are inaccessible.

Figure 39.2 Vascular anatomy of the neck

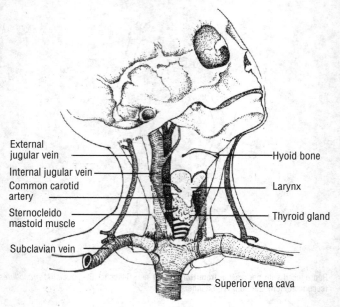

External
jugular vein

Internal jugular vein

Common carotid
artery

Sternocleido
mastoid muscle

Subclavian vein

Hyoid bone

Larynx

Thyroid gland

Superior vena cava

Reproduced with permission from Hughes WT and Buescher ES *Paediatric procedures*
(second edition). London, WB Saunders, 1980.

External jugular

Easily seen and accessible especially in the crying infant. The
vein lies superficially in the line from the angle of mandible to
mid-clavicle. (See Figure 39.2.) The restrained infant is placed
supine on a table with the head and neck suspended, partially
extended off the end of the table and turned 45°-60° from the
midline to expose the vein.

Dangers

◆ Impairment of the airway and of respiration.
◆ Damage to other structures (see 'internal jugular').
◆ Local haematoma (if not compressed after the procedure,
especially in a crying child).

Figure 39.3 Internal jugular venipuncture

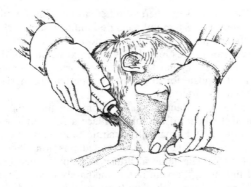

Reproduced with permission from Hughes WT and Buescher ES *Paediatric procedures* (second edition). London, WB Saunders, 1980.

Internal jugular

This vein passes on the underside of the inferior two-thirds of the sternocleidomastoid muscle and lateral to the common carotid artery. The patient is positioned as for external jugular puncture. The tip of the index finger of the operator's free hand is placed in the superior sternal notch. The needle is inserted beneath the posterior border of the sternocleidomastoid muscle at the point between its middle and lower thirds. The needle is directed at the superior sternal notch.

Advance ±4 cm beneath the muscle, maintaining suction on the syringe. If no blood is obtained, withdraw, still maintaining suction as the internal jugular may have been traversed. Sit the infant up and with a cotton wool ball maintain pressure on the puncture area for at least two to three minutes. (See Figure 39.3.)

Dangers

♦ Impairment of the airway and of respiration.
♦ Damage to the arteries, trachea, vagus and pleura with haemorrhage, pneumothorax or surgical emphysema respectively.
♦ Emotionally disturbing to the parents. They should be advised not to observe the procedure.

Femoral vein

This is only to be used when all other sites are inaccessible. The vein is found in the femoral triangle bounded superiorly by the inguinal ligament, laterally by the sartorius muscle and medially by the adductor longus muscle. In the proximal half of the triangle, the vein lies medial to the femoral artery, whereas in the distal half it is posterior to the artery. The femoral nerve in turn lies lateral to the artery.

The restrained infant is placed supine on the table with the assistant at the head of the infant. Place a forearm at each side of the infant so as to manually restrain the knees and hips in a flexed, externally rotated and abducted position. (See Figures 39.4 and 39.5.) The femoral artery is palpated just below the inguinal ligament; the vein lies immediately medial to this pulsation. The needle or scalp vein (with suction applied) is aligned with the vessel and inserted at 30° to the skin surface (i.e. angled towards the feet) until blood is obtained.

If the femoral artery is inadvertently penetrated, take the blood required quickly as the potential harm has already been done. Local pressure must be maintained for five minutes.

Figure 39.4 Anatomy of the femoral triangle

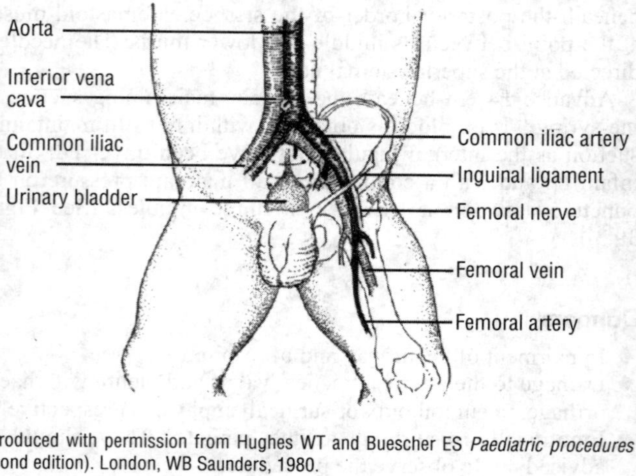

Reproduced with permission from Hughes WT and Buescher ES *Paediatric procedures* (second edition). London, WB Saunders, 1980.

Figure 39.5 Femoral venipuncture

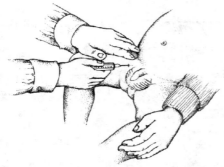

Reproduced with permission from Hughes WT and Buescher ES *Paediatric procedures* (second edition). London, WB Saunders, 1980.

Dangers

♦ Local infection, e.g. osteomyelitis of femoral head, or septic arthritis.
♦ Arterial spasm has progressed to gangrene on occasion.
♦ Haematoma: venous or arterial leakage.
♦ Arterio-venous fistulae and femoral nerve damage.
♦ Pulmonary embolus.

Posterior fontanelle (torcular herophili)

Dangerous and only warranted for critically important specimens when all other sites have been exhausted. The infant is placed in a lateral recumbent position and restrained. Hair is shaved over the area of the posterior fontanelle and this area is well cleaned. The needle is inserted in the centre of the posterior fontanelle and directed to the uppermost part of the forehead in the sagital plane. Blood is found 3-4 mm from the skin surface. Aspirate gently. (See Figure 39.6.)

Dangers

♦ Intracranial haemorrhage.
♦ Damage to brain cortex.
♦ Intracranial infection, meningitis and/or abscess.

Arterial puncture

In small infants the radial, brachial, dorsalis pedis, posterior tibial and temporal arteries may be punctured. The radial artery is

Figure 39.6 Torcular herophili

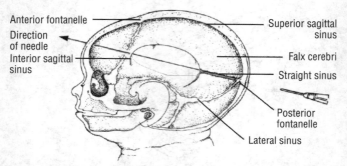

Anterior fontanelle
Direction of needle
Interior sagittal sinus
Superior sagittal sinus
Falx cerebri
Straight sinus
Posterior fontanelle
Lateral sinus

Reproduced with permission from Hughes WT and Buescher ES *Paediatric procedures* (second edition). London, WB Saunders, 1980.

preferred because of the open palmar anastomosis with the ulnar artery so that arteriospasm after puncture is unlikely to cause distal ischaemia.

Clean the site. Palpate the artery with the tips of the index and third fingers. A 25-gauge needle with a clear hub is firmly inserted between the two palpating fingers at a 45°-60° angle. The artery is pierced through both walls. Apply suction to the syringe and slowly withdraw the needle. Blood is obtained on re-entry into the lumen. After withdrawal apply firm local pressure for five minutes. Do not occlude the artery.

Cut-down technique

The best site to use is the great saphenous vein running anterior to the medial malleolus and halfway between it and the anterior tibial tendon. Other sites are the basilic vein (ulnar side) or cephalic vein (radial side) in the antecubital fossa.

Restrain, clean, drape and anaesthetize the area. Apply a tourniquet tightly enough to occlude venous return below the knee. Make a transverse incision. (See Figure 39.7.) Blunt-dissect with a curved mosquito haemostat down towards the tibia. Identify the vein and free it with blunt dissection. Place a haemostat beneath the vessel and pull through two 5,0 silk suture stays. Do not tie. The vein is held taut by the distal guide suture. Make a small V-incision with a pair of sharp-pointed scissors to a depth of about a third of the vessel's diameter. Insert a short bevelled catheter tip of suitable size into the vessel

Figure 39.7 Method for great saphenous cut-down

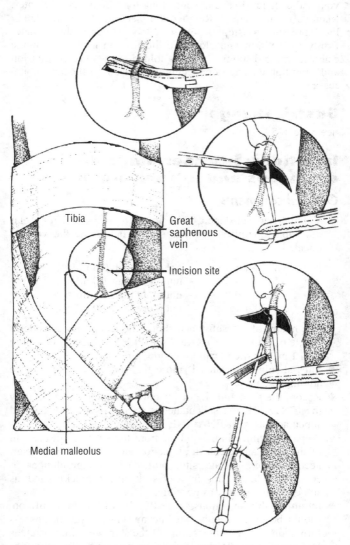

Tibia

Great saphenous vein

Incision site

Medial malleolus

Reproduced with permission from Hughes WT and Buescher ES *Paediatric procedures* (second edition). London, WB Saunders, 1980.

and advance it for 5-8 cm. Tie the proximal suture around the vein and catheter. Leave the ends long for ease of removal later. Remove the tourniquet. Remove the distal guide suture. Apply local pressure to stop oozing of blood. Anchor the catheter firmly to the skin and close the incision on each side of the catheter with 5,0 sutures. Apply a folded gauze over the incision and strap lightly. The same technique is used for the antecubital fossa.

Gastric lavage

See page 425.

Injections: intradermal, sub-cutaneous and intramuscular

General comments

◆ Volume and substance to be injected: mass and muscular development rather than age should determine the volume injected.

Less than	2,5 kg	— not more than 0,5 ml/site
	2,5-5,0 kg	— not more than 1,0 ml/site
	5,0-10,0 kg	— not more than 1,5 ml/site
	10,0 kg	— not more than 2,0 ml/site

◆ The nature of the substance should be taken into consideration, e.g. IRON DEXTRAN COMPLEX (Imferon) not more than 1 ml per site in children under three years.
◆ Sites should be rotated if more than one injection is to be administered.
◆ Record the time and site of injection. This applies especially to GENTAMICIN; subcutaneous INSULIN in diabetes and subcutaneous ADRENALINE in asthmatic patients.
◆ Prepare the injection, expel air from the syringe out of sight of the child and clean the injection site with alcohol. Insert needle at appropriate site, pull back syringe-plunger to ensure needle is not in a vessel; inject quickly and as smoothly and evenly as possible.
◆ Intramuscular injections, e.g. PENICILLIN and Imferon, should be given deeply into the muscle to prevent abscess formation. To prevent staining of the skin with drugs such as Imferon, the needle should follow a z-track through the subcutaneous tissues.

Details of injection sites

Intradermal

Figure 39.8 Intradermal injection

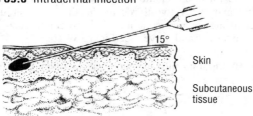

15°

Skin

Subcutaneous
tissue

Reproduced with permission from Scipien GM, *et al. Comprehensive paediatric nursing.*
McGraw-Hill, 1979.

Note angle and placement of needle. Successful injection must
raise a wheal in the skin.

Into the skin, e.g. Mantoux test for tuberculosis.

Sites: ventral surface of the forearm.

Subcutaneous

Figure 39.9 Subcutaneous injection

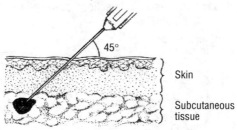

45°

Skin

Subcutaneous
tissue

Reproduced with permission from Scipien GM, *et al. Comprehensive paediatric nursing.*
McGraw-Hill, 1979.

Note angle and placement of needle.

Into the loose tissue spaces just beneath the skin, e.g.
INSULIN, ADRENALINE.

Sites: any site on limbs and trunk where loose tissue space
under the skin is obvious.

Intramuscular

Vastus lateralis area of the thigh is, in general, the only permissible site for intramuscular injections in neonates and young infants. The injection should be given at the junction of the upper third and lower two-thirds of the thigh. Never use the anteromedial area which contains vital structures such as the femoral vein, artery and nerve. See Figure 39.10.

Figure 39.10 Intramuscular injection: vastus lateralis

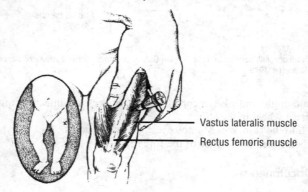

Vastus lateralis muscle
Rectus femoris muscle

Figure 39.11 Intramuscular injection: postero-lateral aspect of the gluteal area

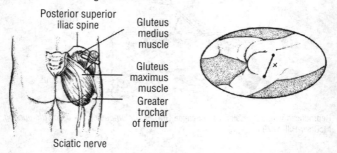

Posterior superior iliac spine
Gluteus medius muscle
Gluteus maximus muscle
Greater trochar of femur
Sciatic nerve

Reproduced with permission from Scipien GM et al *Comprehensive paediatric nursing.* McGraw-Hill, 1979.

Method: gently raise a fold of skin between thumb and forefinger and inject into apex of fold.

Figure 39.12 Intramuscular injection: mid-deltoid area

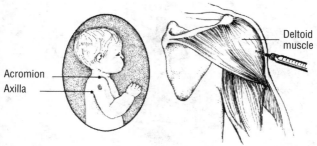

Reproduced with permission from Scipien GM et al *Comprehensive paediatric nursing*. McGraw-Hill, 1979.

The needle penetrates in a front-to-back course of the mid-lateral anterior thigh. Grasp thigh as shown to stabilize extremity and concentrate muscle mass. (See Figure 39.10.)

Postero-lateral aspect of gluteal area (upper and outer quadrant). This site is to be used only on specific written doctor's instruction and **not in a child under six years of age.** Care should be taken to avoid damage to the sciatic nerve and superior gluteal artery and vein. (See Figure 39.11.)

This is located by palpating the posterior superior iliac spine and the head of the greater trochanter. An imaginary line is drawn and the needle inserted on a straight back-to-front course lateral to the line.

The mid-deltoid area in the lateral aspect of the upper arm (Figure 39.12). This site is not generally used except for immunization against diphtheria, tetanus and pertussis. It may be used in other instances if no other site is available, e.g. in burns. The volume should never exceed 1 ml.

The injection site is determined by the acromion and the axilla as shown. Because muscle mass is limited in the mid-deltoid area, repeated injections and large quantities of medication are not recommended. Compress muscle mass prior to inserting needle.

Lumbar puncture

Proper positioning and restraint is critical for a successful tap. Neonates and small infants are often punctured in the sitting

Figure 39.13 Recumbent position for lumbar tap

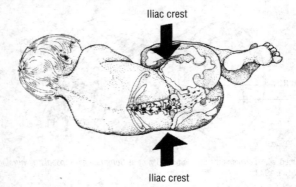

Iliac crest

Iliac crest

Reproduced with permission from Hughes WT and Buescher ES *Paediatric procedures* (second edition). London, WB Saunders, 1980.

position when the head and neck are not flexed. The lateral recumbent position is employed in older infants and children. The operator's line of vision should be on the same horizontal and vertical planes as the puncture site. The lumbar spine must be flexed, but avoid pressure flexion of the neck while attempting to flex the back. Put pressure on the shoulders rather than the head and neck. Ensure all apparatus, e.g. needles, stylets, manometers, tubes, are available.

The site of the puncture is the interspace between L3-4 or L4-5. A line joining the highest points of the two iliac crests passes just above the fourth lumbar spine. (See Figure 39.13.) After anaesthetizing skin and tissue down to the laminae, insert the short bevelled needle with stylet in the midline between L3-L4. The bevel should be in the long axis of the dura so as to part the fibres and not cut across them. Loss of resistance is felt as the needle penetrates the ligamentum flavum. The next 'pop' occurs as the needle penetrates the dura. Remove the stylet and if no fluid emerges, turn the needle through 90°. If the tap is dry, replace the stylet and advance the needle a little further. Check as before for fluid. The distance between the skin and subarachnoid space is 1,5-2,5 cm in infants; 5 cm in three to five year olds and 6-8 cm in adolescents. Pressure should be measured with a manometer in all non-crying and non-struggling patients. Normal pressure is 60-160 mm CSF.

Dangers

♦ Coning may occur immediately or after a few hours due to ongoing leakage of spinal fluid.
♦ Any indication of raised intracranial pressure, especially an altered level of consciousness, is a contra-indication to LP. Absence of papilloedema is not a reliable sign.
♦ Introduction of infection.
♦ Breakage of needle.
♦ Introduction of dermis resulting in a dermoid (non-styletted needle).
♦ Nerve or cord damage.

Nasogastric tube

Passing a nasogastric tube may be done for the following reasons:

♦ to instil a feed, electrolyte solution, or medications;
♦ to remove the gastric contents (toxin/poison);
♦ to remove amniotic fluid in neonate; or
♦ to obtain diagnostic material, e.g. for the diagnosis of tuberculosis or for post-operative decompression.

If the child is old enough, **explain** what is going to be done and do the procedure when the patient is sitting with his or her back firmly supported. Place a younger child or infant in a supine position with bodily restraint and an assistant to help.

Select the appropriate tube. Measure the length to be passed by measuring the distance from manubrium sterni to xiphisternum. Double this and add 2,5 cm if for feeding or 5 cm if for aspiration and/or drainage. Mark the tube at the selected length (Figure 39.14).

Lubricate first 3-4 cm of tube with KY jelly or water. With the head slightly flexed, pass the tube through the nostril aiming for the occiput (not vertex). If resistance is encountered, withdraw and try again. If still unsuccessful try the other side. Ask the patient to try to make swallowing motions despite gagging. Continue to pass the tube to the selected length. If severe coughing, choking or colour change occurs, withdraw immediately. Fix the tube lightly to the cheek and aspirate with a syringe. Test with litmus (blue turns pink if acid). If no fluid is aspirated, advance 3 cm and try again. If still no fluid is aspirated and you are sure the tube is in the stomach, instil 3 ml of 0,9% saline. If there is any coughing, spluttering or cyanosis, withdraw the tube

Figure 39.14 Passing a nasogastric tube

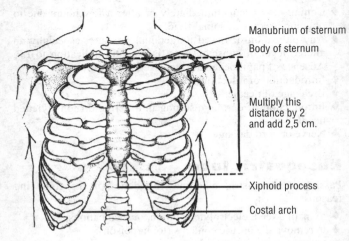

Manubrium of sternum

Body of sternum

Multiply this distance by 2 and add 2,5 cm.

Xiphoid process

Costal arch

immediately. Replace. Restrain as necessary and fix the tube firmly to the cheek using wrap-around and V-strapping. Alternatively place the bell of your stethoscope over the stomach area. Inject 5-10 ml of air rapidly down the tube. A gurgling noise on auscultation indicates that the tip of the tube is in the stomach.

Dangers

♦ Vomiting with aspiration while doing the procedure.
♦ Ulceration or infection of nasal mucosa or epistaxis.
♦ Placement of the tube in tracheobronchial tree.
♦ Otitis media or sinusitis with prolonged use.
♦ Coiling or knotting of the tube with an inability to remove it.

Pericardiocentesis (Pericardial tap)

Warning

A potentially dangerous procedure. Pericardiocentesis should ideally only be done when cardiac ultrasonography and intensive care facilities are available.

Indications

♦ Diagnostic: to determine the nature of an effusion.
♦ Therapeutic: to drain the effusion and as an emergency to relieve cardiac tamponade.

Sedate the patient (unless contra-indicated), clean and drape and use a local anaesthetic. Sit the patient with a back support at a 60° angle. Make a small incision with a scalpel blade 3-4 mm below the costal margin in the left xiphocostal angle. Insert a 10 x 7 cm gauge lock needle on a syringe through the incision perpendicularly to the skin. Advance it to a depth where the point reaches the inner (under) surface of the rib and then depress the needle hub so that the point angles upwards towards the left shoulder. Advance a further 5-10 mm and depress again so that the point is just below the inner aspect of the thoracic cage. With continuous negative pressure in the syringe advance towards the left shoulder until fluid is obtained.

The location of the needle tip may be determined during the procedure if an ECG machine or cardiac monitor or defibrillator is available. Simply attach a lead (with a crocodile clip) to the needle. The ECG may show, amongst other things, an intracardiac ECG trace, ST depression, T wave changes or arrythmias.

Once pericardial fluid has been obtained, insert a 038 guide wire (J) through the needle into the pericardial space and remove the needle. The initial incision must be sufficiently large to allow a 6,8 or 10F pigtail catheter to be inserted over the wire, which is then removed.

Check heart size and exclude a pneumopericardium (which can cause tamponade) with an AP chest X-ray.

Dangers

♦ Penetration of the heart
♦ Damage to coronary vessels
♦ Pneumothorax
♦ Pneumopericardium

Pleural drainage

Emergency drainage

Indicated when a tension pneumothorax is **suspected** on clinical grounds in a hypoxaemic or shocked child. The pleural cavity must be opened to the air as rapidly as possible. In an emergency the pneumothorax can be released with a large bore needle. **Beware of damage to the lung by the long bevel.** Opening the pleura by blunt dissection is preferred.

Make a 0,5-1 cm skin incision over the 4th or 5th intercostal space in the mid-axillary line. Dissect to the parietal pleura with a curved artery forceps. Close the forceps and, holding it 3-4 cm from the tip, push forceps through the pleura. Open the forceps to enlarge the hole and to release air. Insert a tube drain as described below.

Never use a trochar to insert an intercostal drain.

Elective drainage

This is indicated to drain air or liquids from the pleural cavity in children who are not in extremis. Sedate and use local anaesthetic. It is preferable to do the procedure under general anaesthesia in the older child who can perceive what is being done. Use the upper third of the mid-axillary line for gas or liquid. Do not enter via the pectoral muscles, as bleeding and subsequent ugly scars are common. Open the pleura by blunt dissection as described above. The use of trochars and cannulae or trochar-catheters is contra-indicated. The risk of serious and possibly lethal damage to the lung is very high in the child.

Table 39.1

Tube sizes in drainage

Neonate	10 French
Infant	10-16 French
Young child	16-18 French
Older child	18-23 French

Select a suitable tube

Use the larger sizes for pus and large air leaks. Insert the drainage tube for a distance equal to approximately one-third of the diameter of the chest. Direct the tip anteriorly for air or air and fluid, and posteriorly for fluid. Close the wound with a purse-string suture. Place one or two swabs loosely over it and retain them with thin plaster strips. Secure the tube by taping it to the abdomen to prevent traction and dislodgement. Use an underwater seal for children with spontaneous breathing. The tube should not be more than 1 cm below the water surface. Employ a Heimlich valve when a large air leak is present, especially in a ventilated patient. Alternatively fashion a valve by making a short slit at the apex of a finger stall or the finger of a rubber glove and tape it to the end of the intercostal tube. Constant suction is at times required for a large air leak during IPPV. A chronic empyema may be prevented in a pyopneumothorax with constant suction. An uncomplicated empyema or pneumothorax does not require suction. Discontinue suction whenever drainage of air or fluid ceases to prevent lung tissue from being sucked into the drainage holes and permit fluid or air to reaccumulate. Remove a pleural tube after it has ceased to drain or has become blocked. If the tube was blocked, reassess as to whether another drainage tube is required.

Subdural puncture

Place the restrained infant supine with the operator sitting facing the vertex. Shave the anterior two-thirds of the skull. An assistant should hold the head firmly. Sterilize the area and palpate the anterior fontanelle to find the puncture site at its lateral angle. Anaesthetize the area of skin. Use a 20 gauge short bevel stylet needle at right angles to the skin to enter the skull. The needle must be under complete control, but the operator's hand must be relaxed so as to move with any head movement. (See Figure 39.15.) Advance until a lack of resistance is felt. The subdural space is found 0,5 to 1,0 cm beneath the skin surface.

Figure 39.15 Site for subdural tap

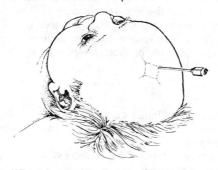

From: Hughes, WT and Buescher, ES, *Pediatric procedures* (second edition). London, WB Saunders, 1980. With permission.

Remove the stylet. Do not explore further if only a few drops of fluid are found (this is normal). Repeat on the other side using a new needle. Do not remove more than 20 ml/side. It is safer to allow it to 'drip out' than to aspirate it with a syringe.

Dangers

◆ Bleeding into the subdural space.
◆ Introduction of infection.
◆ Collapse of the patient if too much subdural fluid, i.e. >20 ml, is removed rapidly.
◆ Trauma to cortex.

Thoracentesis

Determine the site of the fluid by physical examination, percussion and X-ray. The site of the puncture is usually in the posterior axillary line at the base of the thorax. With loculated fluid the site of puncture is over the area of maximum dullness. Sedate, clean the area and use a local anaesthetic. With the restrained patient in a sitting position, enter the pleural cavity just over the superior margin of the rib to avoid the intercostal vessels which course below the inferior margin of the rib above. Hold the syringe and needle in one hand so that only a short length of needle projects beyond the fingers. Advance the needle a few millimetres at a time until a sudden lack of resistance is felt. Aspirate with the syringe to confirm that the fluid has been reached. Clamp a haemostat over the needle at the surface of the skin to prevent inadvertent further advancement of the needle. Withdraw the required volume of fluid. Withdraw the needle and apply a dressing. 'Over the needle' and 'through the needle' plastic intravenous catheter devices may also be used to diminish the risk of lacerating the lung while fluid is being withdrawn.

Dangers

◆ Pneumothorax from lung laceration.
◆ Pulmonary oedema from rapid withdrawal of too large a volume of fluid.
◆ Damage to the heart, liver, major blood vessels; air embolus.
◆ Introduction of infection.
◆ Syncope from the pleuropulmonary reflex.

Urine collection

Collection bag

Cleanse external genitalia with soap and water, dry with sterile swabs. Apply a disposable sterile plastic bag with a non-irritating adhesive over the penis or onto the perineum. Leave exposed for observation. Collect sample immediately after passing. Bag samples are often contaminated. Negative cultures exclude a urinary tract infection. This method is widely used for obtaining 'routine' specimens in the infant.

'Clean catch' with voluntary voiding

Method can be used in children over three years of age. Glans (and foreskin if present) or perineum must be thoroughly cleaned with soap and water and/or an antiseptic and dried. A midstream catch is then collected during voiding with the foreskin drawn back or labia held apart. The background sound of running water (open tap into the basin) or wetting the lower abdomen may stimulate voiding.

Bladder catheterization

Potentially hazardous and the specimen must be important enough to warrant the procedure. Single-specimen catheterization is safer than an indwelling catheter. The procedure must be done under sterile conditions with gloves, careful cleaning (see above), and with foreskin drawn back or labia held apart. A lubricated thin catheter or an F8 feeding tube is passed directly into the urethral meatus and advanced gently until a urine specimen is obtained into a sterile tube. The catheter is then carefully removed.

Suprapubic bladder aspiration

Indicated if urinalysis is urgent, the perineum excoriated or a previous culture was of doubtful significance in a child under the age of two years.

The full bladder is found intra-abdominally and is therefore accessible. Change and feed the infant. After 30 minutes check if the napkin is still dry and the bladder full. The infant is placed supine and immobilized in a frog position by an assistant. The lower abdomen is cleaned. The aspiration site is located in the midline 1-2 cm above the symphysis pubis. The needle and syringe are held 10-20° from perpendicular to the abdominal wall pointing towards the pelvis. The needle is advanced through the abdominal wall with gentle aspiration on the syringe. Bladder entry occurs after 1-2,5 cm of advancement. If no urine is obtained, attempt a second time with a further 10-15° angulation, and aiming more into the pelvis. If still dry, cease further attempts. When cleaning the abdomen, be prepared for a midstream 'catch' specimen, as urine is often voided at this stage of the proceedings.

Dangers

◆ Introduction of infection.
◆ Local haematoma.
◆ Bowel perforation and peritonitis.

40 RADIOLOGY

B J Cremin and R M Fisher

Methods of imaging

Concepts in radiology have changed radically in the last decade.
The subject has expanded beyond conventional radiology and is
now one of imaging (old radiologists never die – they just lose
their images) by many new and improved methods. This chapter
deals principally with conventional radiology, but we refer also
to ultrasound, computerized tomography, magnetic resonance
and nuclear medicine.

Ultrasound

Images are produced by the reflection of high frequency echoes
from structures with different surfaces. Real-time ultrasound is
relatively simple to use and is a dynamic study showing the
organs in motion. The picture can be frozen to produce a static
image.

   Many abdominal problems, and especially those concerning
kidney or liver pathology, are better solved with an assessment
of the images produced by ultrasound than with conventional
radiology. It is particularly useful for soft tissue lesions such as
abscesses. Ultrasound is also very useful in examining the
intracranial contents of children under one year and for cardiac
evaluation. It has also become a major imaging modality for
congenital dislocation of the hips. It has the advantage of non-
radiation, but needs a skilled operator to elicit correct findings
as sonar waves are impeded by fat or air.

Computerized tomography (CT)

The images are produced by pulsing many beams of radiation
through the head or body in a circular axial plane. The absorption of the X-ray beams is recorded digitally and a computer
reconstructs this information into an image. Sometimes pathology is better defined by an injection of contrast media. CT is

not usually the first examination of the body, though this may be so in the CNS. It is especially useful in the evaluation of the nature and extent of traumatic, inflammatory and neoplastic lesions.

Magnetic resonance imaging (MRI)

This is a relatively new field in which body protons are excited magnetically and their relaxation times estimated. As water is a main component in the body, the hydrogen proton density of various tissues is estimated and dramatic images of normal and pathological anatomy are created. It is a relatively expensive form of imaging but it is rapidly developing and gives excellent definition of soft-tissue lesions. The quality of the images for central brain lesions, white and grey matter disorders, spinal cord lesions, soft tissues, bone marrow and joint problems is unsurpassed and the images of cardiac abnormalities may soon render much present-day angiography obsolete. Its installation is expensive and it is not readily available at most children's centres. Its chief advantages are that it presents no radiation hazards, and can produce images in numerous planes.

Radiology of the different systems

Radiology can assist in the diagnosis of a great many paediatric conditions. The majority of routine problems concern the chest and abdomen. No clinician should attempt to evaluate pathology in these regions without high-quality radiographs. Under most conditions, a chest X-ray can be more useful than a stethoscope.

The chest

Various types of pneumonias and their complications can be differentiated by progress radiographs. .These are of particular importance in the diagnosis of chronic disease such as tuberculosis. In young infants, most chest infections are accompanied by bilateral over-inflation of the lungs. Inhaled foreign bodies (e.g. peanuts) must be considered when unexplained unilateral over-expansion or collapse persists. The differentiation between consolidation, masses and pleural fluid may require tomography and other radiological procedures. Barium meal studies may be used to evaluate stridor which may be caused by a vascular ring. If a child has a persistent lung infection for which no explanation can readily be found, a barium swallow may show reflux with regurgitation into the lungs. In rare instances, tracheo-bronchial fistulae may be demonstrated.

The abdomen

Serial plain radiographs of the abdomen are of great help in children with intestinal obstruction and in differentiating the causes of vomiting in infants. Erect, supine, prone and, occasionally, inverted films are taken. If the infant is gravely sick, films can be taken in the incubator by a mobile unit. In neonates, emergency barium studies may be required to exclude conditions such as malrotation of the bowel. Every infant and child with bile-stained vomiting should have either a barium meal to note duodenal configuration, or a barium enema to note the site of caecum. Other common causes of obstruction in neonates are atresias which can be diagnosed from the plain film and Hirschsprung's disease which can be suspected from the plain film and confirmed by barium enema. In typical cases a narrow transition zone is seen in the rectosigmoid region.

Another major use of barium enemas is in the infant or young child to diagnose intussusception, and hydrostatic or air reduction may obviate the need for surgery. Shock should be corrected before this is performed and the surgeon should be present to decide whether operation is necessary or not. Barium meal studies may also be used to evaluate the upper gastrointestinal tract and to exclude conditions such as hiatus hernia with reflux. Barium meal for reflux should not be requested in the first three months of life as some degree of regurgitation is usual in that period. Barium studies are no longer routinely performed for pyloric stenosis as ultrasound will demonstrate the pyloric tumour.

The renal system

Proven urinary tract infection requires radiological investigation. After the infection has been brought under control, a micturating cystogram is performed to exclude vesico-uretric reflux. In some cases stasis associated with obstruction may be shown as an antecedent cause. In cases of infection the urinary tract is also examined by ultrasound and sometimes by intravenous pyelography. Ultrasound is preferred in young infants because of their diminished excretory function.

Ultrasound is particularly useful in the renal tract where the fluid-filled structures can be readily recognized. Obstructive uropathy produces a dilated system. Hydronephrosis, dilated ureters and bladder obstruction can be readily recognized. The examinations are combined wth isotope scanning so that renal function is also assessed. Ultrasound has become the first imaging mode for renal tumours such as nephroblastomas. Differentiation from other pararenal lesions, such as neuroblastoma, is not always easy, so a combination of imaging techniques, including intravenous urography, may be used. When a nephroblastoma is diagnosed, CT is often also required to exclude lung metastisis.

The central nervous system

Skull X-rays have limited value as pathology can be better seen by other modalities and even in trauma their routine use is debatable. If there is loss of consciousness with CNS signs a CT is more appropriate. Sinus X-rays are of little value under the age of three years, and even after this age sinus opacification in children does not necessarily mean infection. The complications of sinusitis, such as orbital and brain infections, need CT for evaluation.

Ultrasound has completely changed the management of problems in the infant's head. Up to the age of six to nine months the examination is via the open frontal fontanelle. It is used mainly to diagnose and assess the causes and progress of hydrocephalus and the complications of infection and hypoxia. It is also used to assess the severity of brain haemorrhage in premature babies.

CT is used to examine the brain when the fontanelle is closed. It is particularly useful for trauma and in suspected neoplasms; in these conditions it is the main imaging modality.

In tuberculous meningitis the triad of progressive hydrocephalus, basal meningeal contrast enhancement and basal ganglia infarction may be definitive. Such findings should alert the clinician to its presence and the necessity for chest X-ray etc. to demonstrate haematogenous tuberculosis. MRI gives excellent definition of the brain and, when available, is often a superior investigation for many brain and spinal problems.

The skeletal system

Conventional radiology demonstrates congenital deformities, traumatic lesions and nutritional disorders. X-rays may also show abnormalities in diseases such as anaemia, leukaemia and haemophilia. Osteomyelitis, various forms of infection, primary bone tumours and secondary deposits all show up as areas of bone destruction. Nuclear medicine studies should be correlated in cases of infection and tumour. Marrow and neurovascular bundle involvement is best demonstrated by MRI. Radiology plays a cardinal role in non-accidental injury (NAI), which should be suspected when there are 'unusual' or unexplained fractures, frequently multiple and of different ages. A typical feature is the metaphyseal corner fracture due to twisting forces on the long bones. Skull fractures, particularly those that cross suture lines and those associated with retinal or cerebral haemorrhage may be seen. Associated abdominal and thoracic lesions are also common. (See chapter 14.)

NAI must be differentiated from minor trauma to bone weakness which causes fractures. These conditions include osteogenesis imperfecta and gross osteopenia associated with protein deficiency or scurvy; and pathological fractures seen in congenital bone syphilis. Caffey's disease with marked 'periosteal reactions', which are actually due to hyperostosis of the cortex, may also cause confusion. All these conditions can be differentiated clinically, genetically and biochemically. The presence of skull wormian bones is helpful in diagnosing osteogenesis imperfecta.

Cardiovascular system

Figure 40.1 Normal heart X-ray

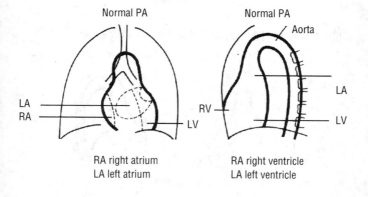

Normal PA

LA
RA

LV

RA right atrium
LA left atrium

Normal PA

Aorta

RV

LA

LV

RA right ventricle
LA left ventricle

In summary, when faced with any clinical problem, radiological imaging can usually be helpful. It is best to start with the simpler procedures and work up to the more complex and expensive methods. The radiologist will be able to advise on the best available method and will interpret the various images for you. Remember an X-ray request or a complex investigation is not like writing a prescription. If there are doubts, the radiologist should be consulted before the examination about its necessity and afterwards for the clinical interpretation of the images.

The line drawings that follow illustrate some guidelines for conventional radiological anatomy and pathology. They indicate points that one should look for in the radiograph, but since pathological appearances vary considerably, full interpretation will require the services of a radiologist.

Heart chamber enlargement

Figure 40.2 Elevated apex and anterior or substernal enlargement

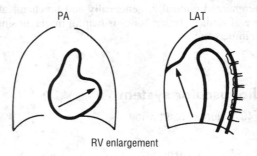

RV enlargement

Figure 40.3 Drooping apex and posterior enlargement

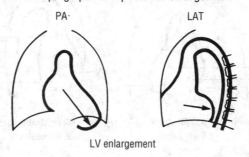

LV enlargement

Figure 40.4 Widened carina and posterior enlargement

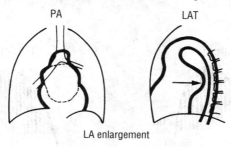

PA   LAT

LA enlargement

Respiratory system

Figure 40.5 Pleural effusion

Peripheral opacity may need lateral decubitus films.

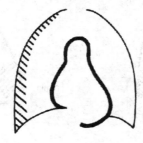

Figure 40.6 Positions of normal lobes

Consolidation may be segmental or lobar. It may also be patchy at apices and bases.

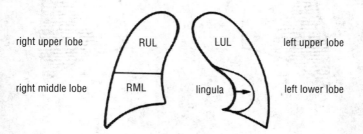

right upper lobe   RUL   LUL   left upper lobe

right middle lobe   RML   lingula   left lower lobe

Figure 40.7 Positions of normal lobes: right and left LAT

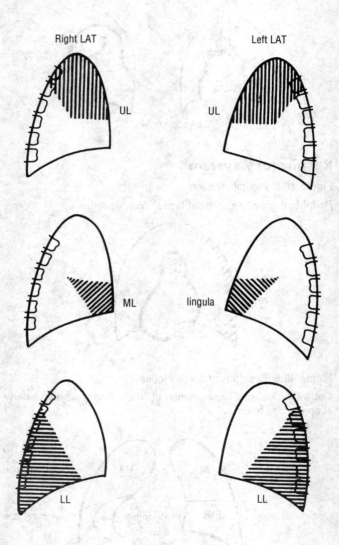

Figure 40.8 Thymus

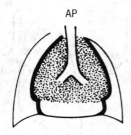

AP

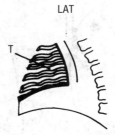

LAT

Soft paratracheal structure in middle and anterior superior mediastinum. Can be bilateral and merge with heart shadow. Many variations e.g. sail-like. Clue film is lateral chest.

Density 'T' fills in triangular space between sternum and air-filled trachea and reaches sternum in its entire vertical extent.

Figure 40.9 Saccular bronchiectasis

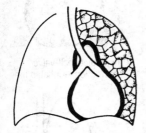

Honeycomb cystic appearance in left lung due to dilated bronchi, with fibrosis of lung and midline shift to left.

Figure 40.10 Staphylococcal pneumonia

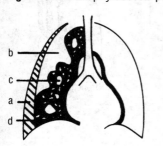

Usually unilateral.

a Empyema

b Pneumothorax

c Pneumatocoeles

d Collapsed, consolidated lung

Figure 40.11 TB chest appearances

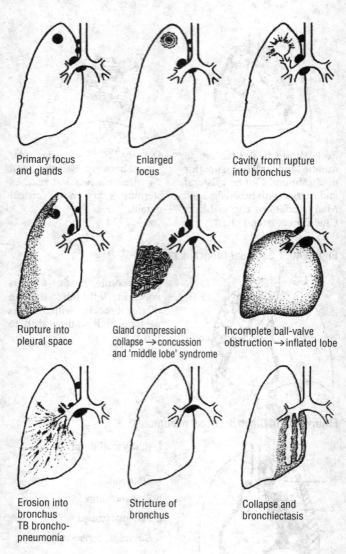

Primary focus
and glands

Enlarged
focus

Cavity from rupture
into bronchus

Rupture into
pleural space

Gland compression
collapse → concussion
and 'middle lobe' syndrome

Incomplete ball-valve
obstruction → inflated lobe

Erosion into
bronchus
TB broncho-
pneumonia

Stricture of
bronchus

Collapse and
bronchiectasis

Figure 40.12 TB chest appearances

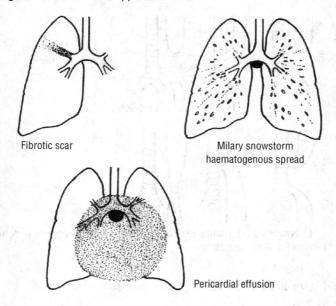

Fibrotic scar

Milary snowstorm
haematogenous spread

Pericardial effusion

Figure 40.13 Examples of foreign bodies in bronchi

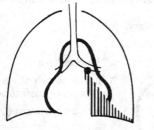

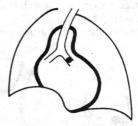

Foreign body obstructing left
lower lobe bronchus causing
collapse of lobe and compensatory emphysema of LUL.

Foreign body in left main
bronchus acting as a ball
valve causing over expansion
of whole left lung with shift
of midline structures to right
and depression of left hemi-
diaphragm.

Figure 40.14 Types of congenital oesophageal anomalies

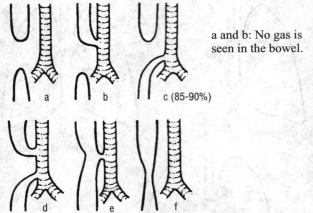

a and b: No gas is seen in the bowel.

c (85-90%)

e: H-type (1-2%) fistula may require specialized contrast techniques for demonstration.

Figure 40.15 Hypertrophic pyloric stenosis

Now diagnosed by ultrasound.

Plain film

Large distended stomach and relatively little air in rest of bowel on straight films.
Barium study – not usually necessary.

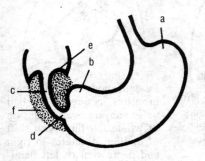

a Dilated stomach

b Tit (aborted wave of peristalsis on lesser curve

c Elongated pyloric canal

d Beak

e Mushroomed base of duodenal bulb

f Position of muscle hypertrophy

Figure 40.16 Duodenal atresia

Erect film, double bubble. No air in rest of abdomen.

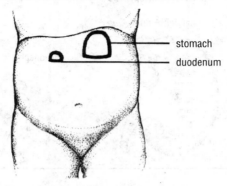

stomach
duodenum

Figure 40.17 Herniation of bowel through diaphragm

In very distressed baby at birth. Usually on left.

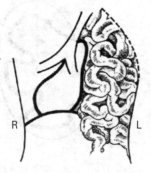

1 Heart displaced to right of midline

2 Left chest filled with loops of bowel

3 Scaphoid abdomen

Renal system

Figure 40.18 Pyelonephritis

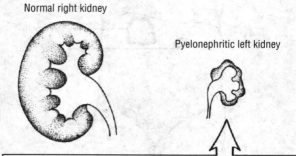

Normal right kidney

Pyelonephritic left kidney

Small kidney with decreased cortical thickness. Several cortical depressions. Clubbed calyces. Sometimes bilateral

Figure 40.19 Hydronephrosis

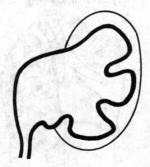

1 Large kidney
2 Thin cortex
3 Huge dilated calyces
4 Enlarged pelvis

Also well seen on ultrasound

Figure 40.20 Reflux

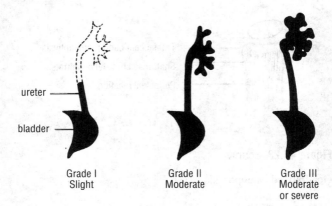

Grade I Slight	Grade II Moderate	Grade III Moderate or severe

Grades IV and V indicate more severity.

System for examining bone X-rays

1 One or multiple bones affected? (i.e. localized or generalized disease)
2 Soft tissues (often associated with bone pathology e.g. cold abscesses of TB)
3 Bone density (porotic, sclerotic, normal)
4 Periosteal reaction
5 Cortex
6 Shaft
7 Metaphysis and growth plate
8 Epiphysis and joint

Figure 40.21 Congenital syphilis

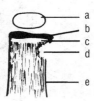

a Normal appearance of epiphysis
b Dense band
c Translucent band
d Wimbergers 'rat bite'. Sign in proximal medial metaphysis of tibia
e Periosteal reaction

Figure 40.22 Leukaemia

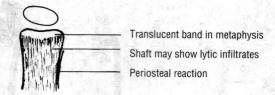

Translucent band in metaphysis

Shaft may show lytic infiltrates

Periosteal reaction

Figure 40.23 Scurvy

Generalized osteoporosis

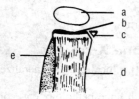

a Ring epiphysis

b Dense 'white' line of growth plate

c Small fractures (Pelkan spurs)

d Sharp pencilled cortices

e Calcified periosteal haematoma in later (healing) stages

Figure 40.24 Active rickets

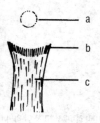

a Small, poorly defined or invisible epiphysis

b Fuzzy, cupped splayed metaphysis

c Generalized decreased bone density and loss of contrast between cortex and medulla

Localized lesions in bone

Usually in region of metaphysis.

Figure 40.25 Osteomyelitis

Lesions may take two weeks to develop but isotope scan shows lesion earlier.

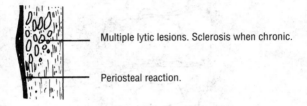

Multiple lytic lesions. Sclerosis when chronic.

Periosteal reaction.

Figure 40.26 Tuberculosis

Usually vertebrae or large bones.

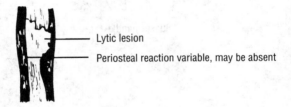

Lytic lesion

Periosteal reaction variable, may be absent

Figure 40.27 Osteogenic sarcoma

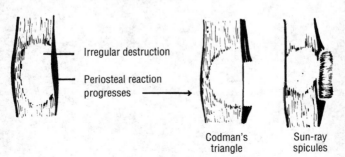

Irregular destruction

Periosteal reaction progresses →

Codman's triangle

Sun-ray spicules

Figure 40.28 Non-accidental injury

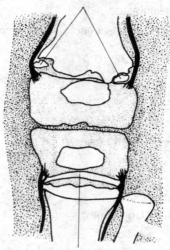

Metaphyseal fragments

Bucket-handle

Table 40.1 Suggested imaging modalities: a clinical guide

Anatomical system		Initial	Later	Remarks
Central nervous system	Brain			
	Neonate	Ultrasound		Ultrasound difficult after six to nine months as anterior fontanelle too small.
	Infant	Ultrasound	Computerized tomography	Computerized tomography best method for diagnosing tumours although magnetic resonance imaging may show them better.
	Child	Skull X-ray	Computerized tomography	Angiography and air studies now rarely used.
	Spine	X-ray	May be followed by computerized tomography	Magnetic resonance imaging best, particularly in craniocervical region.
		Myelogram	Magnetic resonance imaging superior in many cases	

Anatomical system		Initial	Later	Remarks
Respiratory system	All lesions	X-ray		Specialized studies such as bronchograms and angiograms are now less frequently used.
	Mass lesions	X-ray	Computerized tomography	
		Barium swallow		
		Tomography		
	Stridor	X-ray	May be used in mass lesions	
		High kilovoltage studies		
Cardiovascular system	All lesions	X-ray	Angiography	Doppler ultrasound now being used for flow studies
		Ultrasound		
Gastrointestinal system	GI tract Upper	X-ray	Follow through examinations for small intestine	Ultrasound now often the initial examination for all abdominal lesions. Needs user experience in order to interpret images which will otherwise be confusing.
		Barium swallow or meal		
	Lower	X-ray		
		Barium enema		
	Genito-urinary system mass	X-ray		
		Ultrasound		
		Intravenous urogram		

Anatomical system		Initial	Later	Remarks
	Infection	Ultrasound Nuclear medicine	Micturating cysto-urethrogram All cases under five years	
Skeletal system		X-ray Tomography	Isotope study for destructive, avascular or vascular lesions	Most bone lesions can be diagnosed from correlating X-rays and clinical appearances

41 RECORD KEEPING

H M Power and M D Bowie

The quality of patient care, medical research and administration depends directly on the quality of the records. Good record keeping serves to clarify thinking and improve communication. The four most common records used in paediatrics and child health care are the Road-to-Health card, the problem-orientated medical record, referral letters and their replies. Just as scientific papers are presented in a specific format, so clinical records should be structured and consistently presented. This facilitates communication between all members of the health care team, and improves the standard of care.

Road-to-Health (RTH) card

The design and layout of the RTH card has evolved in an attempt to produce a multipurpose document serving as a patient-held medical record. Perinatal data, early growth and development and immunizations are completed by nurses in neonatal services and health clinics. Medical practitioners and nursing staff often fail to use this information in detecting deviations from normal growth and missed immunizations and neglect to document further information on growth and illness. The RTH card should be inspected every time the child is in contact with health professions and a dated brief note made that records the institution or clinic, problem and management. If there is a lack of space to record such episodes, a sheet of paper can be attached to the card.

Problem-orientated medical record (POMR)

As the name implies, the POMR is a method or format of record keeping which focuses on the patient's problems. Properly used it has the advantage of being clear and concise and encourages a structured approach to patient care. Its main virtues are that it

◆ identifies and ensures attention to each of the patient's problems;
◆ forces the clinician to consider each problem on an ongoing basis and records the evidence of this;
◆ provides a logical basis of approach to clinical problems;
◆ rationalizes and reduces inappropriate investigation; and
◆ improves communication, including audit of quality of care.

The POMR has four main parts: problem list, data base, action plan, progress notes.

Problem list (Table 41.1)

This is the key and index of the POMR and is the front page of the record, although the content is derived from the other parts of the record. Active problems are current and require investigation and action. Inactive problems are part of the past history and may or may not affect the management of the patient. The problem list should be constructed and updated by the doctor in charge of the patient. This is absolutely essential for the successful use of the POMR.

Active problems

Include symptoms, signs, abnormal results of investigation, social problems, incomplete immunizations. Each problem is given a separate number. If new data establish a diagnosis, the list is amended. The original entry is not erased but linked by an arrow to the new entry which retains the orginal number (Table 41.1). If several items on the problem list become explicable in terms of one condition, then the new title should be given the number of the first listed and all the other numbers closed and not used again. However, if a complication of a single illness requires individual management it should be listed as a separate problem so that its course is more easily followed.

Inactive problems

Include past major illness, operations, and drug sensitivities for which no active care is required.

Data base

This can be divided into two parts: basic information and the current episode of illness.

Basic information

Much of the basic information need only be recorded once and this is best done on a standard form and flow charts. It is important to update the information on subsequent admissions or consultations. Basic information should include:

♦ Family history – personal details.
  ◇ Medical history of parents, siblings and relations.
  ◇ Psychosocial family history, socio-economic situation.
  ◇ Environmental influences and home circumstances.
♦ Past history
  ◇ Antenatal, natal, postnatal problems.
  ◇ Immunization.
  ◇ Growth and development — note that the RTH card is a valuable source of this information. Record on growth chart.
  ◇ Allergies and sensitivities.
  ◇ Medication history.

Current episode

In practice this will be the first part of the POMR to be recorded. This section consists of eliciting the present history and performing a physical examination in the conventional manner.

♦ History
  ◇ The reason for the consultation or admission, or any other problems, should be noted.
  ◇ Specific and systematic history relating to presenting clinical problems. Progression of problems and results of systematic enquiry.
  ◇ Dates (not the day of the week) should be recorded in the description of the presentation.
  ◇ It is important to note the concerns and expectations of the parents and, if appropriate, of the child.
♦ Physical examination
  ◇ Note the general condition of the child, examine the systems as indicated. Record growth and development.

Action plan

For every problem the initial action plan should include:

♦ Provisional diagnosis and assessment.
♦ Severity of patient's condition.

♦ Whether emergency action is required.
♦ Outline of duration, rate and degree of recovery expected.
♦ If appropriate, reasons why nothing active should be done.
♦ Diagnostic information (Dx)
  ◇ Investigations and consultations and reasons for them to be done.
♦ Therapy (Rx)
  ◇ All treatment.
♦ Monitoring (Mx)
  ◇ To monitor progress and detect any side-effects.
♦ Information (Ex)
  ◇ Information given to parent/child on the condition, investigations or management.
  ◇ The views of parents on procedures, interventions and specific therapeutic measures in chronic conditions and terminally ill patients should be recorded.
  ◇ In terminally or critically ill patients with potentially adverse outcomes, summarize or personally communicate to colleagues and staff guidelines for the management of complications of the illness.

Warning

Permission for procedures (indicated and potential) should be recorded and appropriate forms completed. See chapter 30, pages 309-12.

Progress notes

Changes in symptoms or signs, results of investigations and further action plans are recorded. These are headed by the problem number and title. Progress notes should be written in the SOAP structure.

♦ Subjective information (S)
  ◇ Information offered by child, nursing staff, parents, paramedicals or medical staff.
♦ Objective information (O)
  ◇ Changes in physical findings or results of investigations.
♦ Assessment (A)
  ◇ As in Action Plan but modified in the light of information contained in (S) and (O).

◆ Plan (P)
  ◇ Further plans prompted by the above information should be recorded and structured Dx, Rx, Mx, Ex.

Notes should be brief and concise. Flow charts are useful in most clinical situations. As further information and clarity is elicited about the listed problems, referral back to the problem list is required. Amending the list to keep it updated ensures that it is a useful ongoing statement of the patient's problems and allows for rapid assessment.

Referral letters

A letter referring a patient to a colleague should contain the following details:

◆ Letterhead (*department, institution, medical practitioner, practice number, address and telephone when applicable*)
◆ Contact information (*name and title of person making referral (not signature), time, date*)
◆ Patient information (*name, date of birth, sex, folder numbers*)
◆ Person or service to whom the referral is being made
◆ Reason for the referral
◆ Problems (*list all relevant past and present problems*)
◆ Relevant clinical information (*history, examination, special investigations, management*)

Replies to referrals for consultation

A reply to a referral letter should contain the following details:

◆ Letterhead (*department, institution, medical practitioner, practice number, address and telephone when applicable*)
◆ Contact information (*name and title of person replying (not signature), time, date*)
◆ Addressee (*person who referred the patient*)
◆ Problem under referral
◆ Other problems (*list all relevant past and present problems*)
◆ Clinical findings (*history, examination, special investigations*)
◆ Management
◆ Information given to patient and/or parents
◆ Future plans

Table 41.1 Example of a problem list

Identification (Hospital filing no.)...............
Surname: ....
First names: ....
Date of birth: ....

Problem number	ICD No*	ACTIVE PROBLEMS Include symptoms, signs and abnormal investigations not explained by another entry	Date entered	INACTIVE PROBLEMS Major past illnesses, operations, hypersensitivities. No active treatment required.	Date entered
1				Hyaline membrane disease 1983	30.10.1986
2	493.0	Recurrent wheezing attacks	30.10.1986		
		➤ Asthma	25.11.1986		
3	378.0	Squint right eye	30.10.1986		
		➤ Operation for correction	12.12.1986		
4	V03.2	No BCG immunization	30.10.1986		
		➤ BCG given	10.11.1986		
5				Right inguinal hernia repair 1983	30.10.1986

* ICD number refers to the number given from the International Classification of Disease, 9th revision, clinical modification.

42 RENAL DISEASES

J Wiggelinkhuizen

Acute post-infective glomerulonephritis

Acute glomerulonephritis (AGN) occurs seven to 21 days after a group A β-haemolytic streptococcal throat or skin infection, and occasionally follows other infections.

Clinical presentation

◆ Sudden onset of generalized oedema and/or painless macroscopic or microscopic haematuria. May present with severe fluid volume overload with hypertension, hypertensive encephalopathy and pulmonary oedema and/or oligo-anuric renal failure and/or nephrotic syndrome.
◆ Streptococcal impetigo is found in >50% of cases.
◆ Acute glomerulonephritis is uncommon before the age of two years.
◆ Clinical recovery in the vast majority of patients occurs within a few weeks, except for mild proteinuria and microhaematuria, which may persist for one to two years.
◆ Recurrences are rare, but intercurrent infection may transiently exacerbate haematuria during convalescence.

Investigations

◆ **Urinalysis:** dipstick confirmation of haematuria and proteinuria. Urine microscopy for dysmorphic red blood cells and red blood cell casts. Urine culture.
◆ **Renal function assessment:** plasma urea, creatinine, sodium, potassium, acid-base status, total protein and albumin.
◆ **Evidence of recent streptococcal infection may be looked for:** throat or impetigo swab culture, ASO and anti-DNase B titres. Reduced C3 complement.
◆ **Chest X-ray:** for pulmonary congestion, cardiomegaly, pleural effusions if clinically indicated.

Management

◆ Restrict activity until macroscopic haematuria, oedema and hypertension have resolved.
◆ Strict intake and output measurement and dipstick urinalysis on a daily basis.
◆ Monitor blood pressure and fluid balance.
◆ Restrict fluid intake to output, or less if fluid overloaded.
◆ Limit sodium intake until the fluid overload is resolved.
◆ Restrict protein intake i.e. milk, meat, eggs, fish until the plasma urea is <20 mmol/l.
◆ PENICILLIN is given orally for ten days. Long-term pro-phylaxis is not required.
◆ Manage complications: acute renal failure, hypertension and fluid overload.
  ◇ FUROSEMIDE 1-2 mg/kg/dose given orally one to three times daily is effective for fluid overload except in severe renal failure.
  ◇ Sublingual NIFEDIPINE 0,15-0,5 mg/kg/dose or HY-DRALAZINE HYDROCHLORIDE 0,1-0,3 mg/kg/dose IM/IV (Table 42.1) for hypertension over 160/110 mmHg, or if symptomatic.

Warning

Pulmonary oedema in renal failure is life-threatening and requires immediate treatment.

Emergency measures for pulmonary oedema

◆ Sit patient up in bed.
◆ Administer oxygen.
◆ Restrict fluid and sodium intake to a minimum.
◆ FUROSEMIDE 3-5 mg/kg/dose IV over five to ten minutes to induce diuresis and repeat four to six-hourly if necessary.
◆ Administer MORPHINE.
◆ Medical or surgical venesection (5 ml/kg).
◆ Intermittent positive pressure respiration (IPPR) with posi-tive end expiratory pressure (PEEP). Urgent dialysis may be required to remove fluid overload.

Refer patients with a rapidly progressive downhill course, or massive proteinuria, or if major clinical or biochemical abnor-malities persist for more than two to four weeks.

Pitfall

Hypertensive encephalopathy and pulmonary oedema in AGN may occur with only minimal peripheral oedema and mild renal failure.

Urinary tract infection

Urinary tract infection (UTI) is the presence of significant bacteriuria with >100 000 organisms per ml of a single species cultured from a fresh clean-voided urine or >1000 organisms per ml urine obtained by suprapubic bladder aspiration or catheterization. Lower bacterial counts may be significant in the presence of clinical signs and symptoms.

Significant pyuria with >5-10 pus cells per mm³ unspun urine or in a spun urine per high power field (x 400) is almost always present; if absent, invasive infection is unlikely.

Over 80% of UTI is due to *E. coli*, but infections due to Klebsiella, Pseudomonas and Enterococci spp, Proteus spp in boys, and *Staphylococcus aureus* also occur (particularly in abnormal urinary tracts). Mixed growths suggest contamination.

Clinical presentation

Infant

♦ Non-specific with fever, irritability and convulsions, diarrhoea and vomiting, failure to thrive, oedema, jaundice, anaemia and renal failure.
♦ Blood culture is positive in 30%.

Child more than two or three years old

♦ Upper tract infection (acute pyelonephritis) is likely with a fever of >38 °C, vomiting, abdominal and loin pain.
♦ Lower tract infection presents with frequency, urgency, incontinence, dysuria, haematuria (haemorrhagic cystitis), turbid foul-smelling urine.
♦ Enlarged kidney(s), a persistently full bladder, poor stream, and renal failure suggest underlying urologic abnormalities.
♦ UTI may be **asymptomatic** in recurrent infections, or be overshadowed by concomitant disease such as septicaemia or diarrhoeal disease.

Diagnosis

Dipstick urinalysis

For methods of urine collection see pages 456-8.

UTI (or other renal disease) unlikely

If blood, protein, leukocyte esterase and nitrite test strips read negative, and specific gravity and pH are appropriate for homeostasis.

UTI (or other renal disease) possible

If any of the above dipstick tests are positive. For confirmation send sample for microscopy and culture within one hour or keep overnight at 4 °C prior to culture.

Plasma creatinine, urea and electrolyte estimations, acid-base status and a blood culture are essential in the management of the severely ill child. Uncomplicated UTI in association with severe diarrhoeal disease is common in malnourished infants and young children. In others, **well-documented** UTI is often a complication of underlying congenital uropathy, commonly vesico-ureteral reflux. If so, recurrent UTI is frequent and may lead to end-stage renal failure or hypertension. Relevant imaging of the kidneys and urinary tract is thus mandatory in well-documented UTI. In the under-three year age group a prompt ultrasound scan of the abdomen and a micturating cysto-urethrogram three to four weeks later are done. In the older child initially only an ultrasound scan is done. Further investigations and their timing depend on clinical and ultrasound findings. They may include excretory urography (IVP), radionuclide studies, cystoscopy and others.

Management

♦ High fluid intake is encouraged unless in oliguric renal failure.
♦ Regular complete emptying of bladder and double micturition in vesico-ureteral reflux is advised.
♦ Treat renal failure. See pages 496-502.
♦ Antibiotic therapy (after culture specimen taken): NALI-DIXIC ACID, NITROFURANTOIN, CO-TRIMOXAZOLE, AMOXYCILLIN/CLAVULINIC ACID, oral CEPHALO-SPORIN as indicated by clinical features and antibiotic sensitivity, for five to seven days. The newer QUINOLONE

derivatives, e.g. CIPROFLOXACIN are effective but are not recommended for routine paediatric use.
◆ Septicaemic, very ill and young patients require parenteral AMINOGLYCOSIDE or CEPHALOSPORIN for seven to ten days.
◆ Exclude and surgically correct underlying uropathy if possible. Primary vesico-ureteral reflux, except when gross, resolves spontaneously in a few years, during which period recurrent UTI remains a risk.
◆ Long-term prophylaxis for three to six months or more is used for recurrent UTI with or without persisting uropathy. Give half doses of NALIDIXIC ACID, CO-TRIMOXAZOLE, NITROFURANTOIN or TRIMETHOPRIM at nighttime and rotate monthly.

Frequency – urgency – dysuria syndrome

This is seen only in girls and is due to uncoordinated bladder control. Bacterial infection cannot always be documented. Crossing the legs, squatting with the heel in the perineum and other trick manoeuvres are used to control urgency-incontinence.

Useful measures include long-term antibacterial prophylaxis, regular relaxed voiding, anticholinergics (OXYBUTININ), avoidance of constipation, showers instead of baths.

Warning

Examine the urine of any ill infant or child if the clinical diagnosis is uncertain — even if there are no leading symptoms suggestive of UTI.

Pitfalls

Primary vesico-ureteral reflux is the most common underlying uropathy, but it is not usually detected on ultrasonography. Micturating cysto-urethrography is required for diagnosis.

Bacterial resistance to AMPICILLIN, AMOXYCILLIN and CO-TRIMOXAZOLE is an increasing problem. A repeat-culture should be sterile in 48 hours. NALIDIXIC ACID and NITROFURANTOIN are inappropriate therapy for systemic infections.

Nephrotic syndrome

The nephrotic syndrome is characterized by severe proteinuria (3+ – 4+ on dipstick, >50 mg/kg/24 hours), hypoproteinaemia (albumin <25 g/l), oedema and hyperlipidaemia.

The nephrotic syndrome may occur in the course of most primary and secondary glomerular disases. Steroid-responsive minimal change nephropathy is commonest, except in black children where hepatitis B virus-associated and other forms of glomerulonephritis are more prevalent.

Clinical presentation

Gradual onset of generalized oedema with ascites and pleural effusions is characteristic of minimal change nephrotic syndrome. Macroscopic haematuria, renal failure, and/or hypertension with nephrotic syndrome is indicative of persistent or progressive glomerular disease **other** than minimal change nephropathy. Secondary infection is common.

Diagnosis

Urinalysis.

◆ Dipstick: massive (3+ – 4+) proteinuria with or without haematuria.
◆ Microscopy: granular and hyaline casts, red cells unusual in minimal change nephrotic syndrome. Send sample for culture.
◆ Quantitative 12 or 24 hour urinary protein excretion: >40 mg protein/hour/m^2.
◆ Urine protein/creatinine ratio (random early morning sample): normal <20 mg protein/mmol creatinine, ratio for nephrotic proteinuria is >200.
◆ Renal function assessment: plasma urea, creatinine, total protein and albumin, cholesterol, sodium and potassium. See page 505.
◆ Cause-directed investigations are dictated by clinical findings: hepatitis B and syphilis serology, ASO and anti-DNase B titres, total complement and C3 and C4 fractions, antinuclear factor and anti-DNA antibodies.
◆ Exclude infection.
◆ Mantoux tuberculin skin test and X-ray chest: exclude TB before administering CORTICOSTEROIDS.

Management

◆ Restricted activity does not affect course, but bed rest may promote diuresis.
◆ Dipstick urinalysis, fluid intake and output measurements daily.
◆ Restrict sodium intake. Avoid preserved, canned and packaged foodstuffs. Fluids *ad lib* unless severely oedematous.
◆ Normal to a high protein diet. Supplement protein intake if malnourished.
◆ Control of oedema: HYDROCHLOROTHIAZIDE with or without a potassium-sparing diuretic (SPIRONOLACTONE, AMILORIDE HYDROCHLORIDE or TRIAMTERENE) and/or FUROSEMIDE. Avoid diuretics if peripheral perfusion is poor. HUMAN ALBUMIN 20% infusion 5 ml/kg over one to two hours, with FUROSEMIDE 1 mg/kg IV added towards the end of the infusion, is indicated for gross oedema, hypovolaemia and in severe intercurrent infection. This may be repeated once or twice daily for three to five days.
◆ Corticosteroid therapy: for minimal change nephrotic syndrome diagnosed on clinical grounds.

   Step 1: PREDNISOLONE 2 mg/kg/24 hours (maximum 60 mg) in single or divided doses orally, until the urine is protein-free for three to five days. Alternatively for the **initial episode only,** this dosage may be given for four to six weeks.

   Step 2: PREDNISOLONE 2 mg/kg/**48 hours** in one single dose orally on alternative mornings for four weeks. The dosage is then tailed off over two to four weeks.
◆ Infection: treat vigorously. May give prophylactic PENICILLIN orally twice daily while in relapse and on high dosage PREDNISOLONE.

Relapses

◆ Relapses are treated as above. The frequency of relapses may be reduced in some cases by long-term (six to twelve months) low dosage 0,5 mg/kg PREDNISOLONE on alternate mornings. Aim at lowest possible effective dosage.
◆ Frequent relapses of steroid-responsive nephrotic syndrome with unacceptable side-effects of steroid therapy, and steroid-resistant biopsy-proven minimal change nephrotic syndrome may require immunosuppressive/cytotoxic therapy with CYCLOPHOSPHAMIDE or CYCLOSPORIN. Refer to a renal centre.

◆ Angiotensin converting enzyme inhibitors (CAPTOPRIL, ENALAPRIL) may reduce proteinuria in chronic nephrotic syndrome.

Advice

◆ Immunization: routine immunizations are best given when off all therapy or on only low dose alternative day corticosteroid therapy. Immunization against pneumococcal infection is indicated in all chronic/relapsing cases – Pneumovax 23 IM or SC 0,5 ml.
◆ Indications for renal biopsy:
  ◇ nephrotic syndrome with macrohaematuria and/or hypertension, and/or renal failure;
  ◇ suspected secondary glomerular diseases e.g. SLE;
  ◇ no response to trial corticosteroid therapy for four weeks; or
  ◇ infants under six to twelve months.
◆ Warn parents about the likelihood of relapses. Teach parents or the patient to test early morning urine with Albustix. Use a chart to record remissions and relapses, and the treatment.
◆ Over 90% of minimal change nephrotic syndromes respond to corticosteroid therapy within one to two weeks, but >90% will relapse, mostly within one to two years.

Warning

Most primary glomerular diseases, **other than minimal change** nephropathy, and most secondary nephrotic syndromes do not respond to, and may deteriorate on corticosteroid therapy. Refer to a renal centre.

Hypertension

Normal blood pressure increases with age. Hypertension is defined as a blood pressure >95th percentile for age. See pages 98-9.

A cause is found for >80% of severe childhood hypertension, usually renal or renovascular disease.

Clinical presentation

Childhood hypertension usually presents with clinical features of the primary disease or target organ involvement, i.e.

> **Warning**
>
> Measure blood pressure in **any** child who presents with neu-
> rologic, cardiovascular or renal signs and symptoms.

hypertensive encephalopathy, pulmonary oedema, congestive
heart failure, or renal disease. It may be asymptomatic or non-
specific as in adults.

Diagnosis

History and clinical examination

Look for evidence of primary disease and target organ involvement, including fundoscopy. Exclude coarctation by palpation
of femoral pulses and by measuring the blood pressure **in all
limbs.**

Baseline investigations

◆ Urinalysis.
◆ Plasma urea, creatinine, Na, K.
◆ Full blood count, smear, ESR.
◆ Ultrasound scan abdomen, kidneys and large vessels.
◆ X-ray chest.
◆ Electrocardiogram.

Referral

Further investigations oriented towards the suspected cause are
best done at a referral centre. These may include further renal
imaging, peripheral and renal vein renin activity, Tc^{99m} DTPA,
DMSA and MAG3 renal scintigraphy, renal and aorta angiography, renal biopsy, urinary and plasma catecholamines levels and
other procedures.

Management

Hypertensive emergencies

**Note: Aim at a 25% reduction in blood pressure within one
to two hours.**

Table 42.1 Management of hypertensive emergencies

Drug	Dose	Route	Comments
NIFEDIPINE (Calcium channel blocker)	0,15-0,5 mg/ kg/dose	Sublingual Oral	Puncture capsule and squeeze out under the tongue or aspirate with Mantoux syringe.
HYDRALAZINE (Direct vasodilator)	0,1-0,3mg/ kg/dose max 20 mg/ dose	IV/IM	May be repeated in 10-30 mins
LABETALOL (α and β adrenergic blocker)	1-3 mg/kg/ hour	Continuous IV infusion	Titrate to lowest dosage
SODIUM NITROPRUSSIDE (Direct vasodilator)	0,5-8,0 µg/kg/ min	Continous IV infusion. Protect from light.	Effective in minutes. Short action. Use in intensive care only Check for thiocyanate and cyanide toxicity after two to three days

Chronic hypertension

Management

The goal of therapy is the simplest regimen that controls hypertension with a minimum of side effects. Once-a-day dosage promotes better compliance. Expert advice is often required. Chronic hypertension is reduced gradually over several days to weeks to avoid ischaemic manifestations.

Step 1 PROPRANOLOL, ATENOLOL, METOPROLOL, LABETALOL, CAPTOPRIL, ENALAPRIL, HYDRALAZINE, PRAZOSIN.

Step 2 HYDROCHLOROTHIAZIDE, FUROSEMIDE, TRIAMTERENE, SPIRONOLACTONE.

Step 3 NIFEDIPINE and other calcium channel blockers.

Step 4 MINOXIDIL, CLONIDINE, METHYLDOPA.

Any drug in the Step 1 group may be used as initial mono-therapy. Dosage is gradually increased over two weeks, after which a diuretic (Step 2) is added. If control remains unsatisfactory, another drug, preferably from Step 1 or NIFEDIPINE, is added. Calcium channel blockers are increasingly used as step 1 drugs.

Mild hypertension in adolescence is best treated with diuretic therapy and non-pharmacologic measures such as weight reduction, moderate exercise, salt-restriction and avoidance of oral contraceptive pills.

Renal failure

Impairment of renal function leads to loss of normal fluid, electrolyte and acid-base homeostasis, and retention of waste products.

Aetiology
Prerenal failure

Shock, hypovolaemia and dehydration of any cause resulting in hypoperfusion of the kidneys. If not corrected, this will progress to acute tubular necrosis.

Renal failure

Glomerulonephritides. Acute tubular necrosis. Haemolytic uraemic syndrome. Septicaemia. Pyelonephritis in infants. Renovascular occlusion. Congenital renal anomalies. Acute-on-chronic failure.

Postrenal failure

Obstructive uropathy.

Clinical presentation
Acute

History and clinical features of underlying disease or precipitating cause often dominate findings. Oligo-anuria <1 ml/kg/hour (adults <400 ml/min/1,73 m^2). High output renal failure is suggestive of aminoglycoside nephrotoxicity or acute-on-chronic renal failure.

Fluid imbalance with oedema, hypertension, heart failure and pulmonary oedema is frequent. Anorexia, vomiting, pallor, urinary abnormalities, persistent metabolic acidosis, twitching, convulsions, disturbed level of consciousness. Kidneys may be enlarged.

Chronic

Chronic renal failure may present without a history of preceding disease, and with failure to thrive, chronic listlessness, short stature, polyuria, polydipsia, anaemia, 'muddy' complexion, rickets, hypertension, pruritis, anorexia, vomiting and bloody diarrhoea.

Diagnosis and assessment

Initial

♦ **Fluid-balance status:** pulse, blood pressure, capillary filling time, oedema or hydration status, jugulovenous pressure, cardiomegaly and gallop rhythm, lung bases. Record all intake and output.
♦ **Urine:** dipstick screen, microscopy, culture and sensitivity, sodium, creatinine, specific gravity or osmolality. If necessary catheterize or aspirate (infant's) bladder.
♦ **Renal function:** plasma urea, creatinine, sodium, potassium, acid-base status, calcium, inorganic phosphorus, alkaline phosphatase, proteins. Full blood count, platelets and smear. Ultrasound scan of kidneys, tract and bladder to assess kidney size, and to exclude structural abnormalities and obstructive uropathy. X-ray chest.
♦ In prerenal failure the plasma urea is raised out of proportion to the plasma creatinine, urinary sodium is <20 mmol/l, urine osmolality is >500 mOsm/kg water or specific gravity >1,020 and the fractional excretion of sodium (FENa) is <1. FENa is also low in glomerular disease. FENa is >3 in acute tubular necrosis.

$$\text{FENa} = \frac{\text{urine Na}}{\text{plasma Na}} \times \frac{\text{plasma creatinine}}{\text{urine creatinine}} \times 100$$

Ongoing investigations

Monitor plasma urea, creatinine, sodium, potassium, acid base, calcium and haemoglobin daily or more frequently.

Institute relevant investigations to evaluate cause of renal failure.

Management

Prerenal failure

◆ Correct shock or dehydration: IV fluids 20-25 ml/kg over half to one hour. If uncertain whether fluid replacement adequate give 5 ml/kg IV bolus at ten to 15 minute intervals. The fluids used depend on the circumstances: normal saline, Plasmalyte B or Ringer's lactate, half normal saline, half-strength Darrow's with 5% dextrose or Haemaccel, stabilized human serum, fresh frozen plasma or blood.

◆ Low dose DOPAMINE up to 5 µg/kg/minute IV infusion increases renal bloodflow and may have a protective effect.

◆ **Avoid** potassium-containing fluids if the risk of hyper-kalaemia exists. Add $NaHCO_3$ if necessary.
Reassess fluid balance hourly: central venous pressure measurement is the best guide to fluid balance and cardiac status.

◆ If oliguria persists **after** correction of hypoperfusion, give FUROSEMIDE 1-5 mg/kg IV slowly or MANNITOL 0,25-0,5 g/kg IV; repeat MANNITOL only if there is a good diuretic response.

Postrenal failure

Relieve any obstruction in the urinary tract.

Renal parenchymal failure

Aim at maintaining homeostasis until normal renal function is restored. In acute tubular necrosis, recovery within two to five weeks is usual.

Fluid and electrolyte balance

◆ Record daily all intake and output, weight, and monitor blood pressure and check fluid balance.

◆ Restrict fluid intake to total losses via all routes. Important: patient may be overloaded when first seen – restrict even further.

◆ Insensible loss: replace with 12 ml/kg (child) – 30 ml/kg (infant) per day as 10-20% dextrose water IV or oral glucose polymer (Caloreen) in water, cola or ginger-beer. Fever increases insensible loss.

◆ Urine output: replace with half normal saline with added 5-15% dextrose.

◆ Gastrointestinal and other losses are replaced with appropriate fluids.
◆ **Reassess** fluid balance frequently and adjust intake accordingly.
◆ FUROSEMIDE (1-10 mg/kg slowly IV) may increase the urine output (without increase in glomerular filtration) and thus facilitate fluid balance and allow a higher caloric intake.
◆ **Treatment** of pulmonary oedema: see pages 101-3.

Diet and caloric intake

◆ In acute renal failure: restrict protein intake if plasma urea >20 mmol/l. Dilute modified milk formula (low protein, low sodium) with added glucose polymer. A high carbohydrate intake >3 g/kg/day will lessen endogenous protein breakdown. Fat is poorly tolerated orally.
◆ In severe uraemia (>30-40 mmol/l): rigidly restrict protein, sodium or potassium intake. Supply all vitamins.

Note: Up to 1% weight loss daily may occur as a result of the unavoidably low caloric intake.
  Severe acute renal failure lasting for more than five to ten days may require dialysis to allow adequate oral or parenteral nutrition.

◆ In chronic renal failure: restrict protein intake to high biologic value protein 1-2 g/kg/day (meat, fish, eggs, milk). Make up calories with a high carbohydrate intake and fat. Sodium restriction is not necessary until oedema or hypertension is present.

Hyperkalaemia

The pulse may be slow and irregular.
  ECG: peaked T waves, prolonged PR interval. Progression: P wave disappears, progressive widening QRS, sine wave and cardiac arrest.
  Plasma potassium >8 mmol/l is life-threatening. Commence treatment stepwise when plasma potassium is >6,5-7,0 mmol/l. See Table 42.2.

Metabolic acidosis

◆ Correct in part with IV NaHCO$_3$ 8,4% 1-2 ml/kg if pH <7,20 or standard HCO$_3$ <12 mmol/l. Risk of fluid overload. Rapid

Table 42.2 Treatment of hyperkalaemia

Medication	Dose	Onset action	Action and duration
Step 1			
Eliminate all sources of potassium intake.			
Step 2			
Cation exchange resin (Na or Ca polystyrene sulphonate)	0,5 - 1,0 g/kg[3] by high enema or orally	Less than one hour	Removes K from body. Lasts two hours.
Step 3			
10% Calcium[1] gluconate	0,5-1,0 ml/kg IV over five to ten minutes		Neutralizes K cardiotoxic effects. Lasts 30-60 minutes.
Step 4			
8,4% Sodium bicarbonate	2-3 ml/kg IV over five to ten minutes	Less than one hour	Shifts K into cells Lasts two to four hours.
50% Dextrose water	1-2 ml/kg IV in 15-30 minutes ± Soluble insulin 1 unit for every 5 g dextrose infused may be added	Less than one hour	Shifts K into cells Lasts three to six hours. Monitor for hypoglycaemia if insulin is added.
SALBUTAMOL[2]	4 µg/kg in 5 ml water IV or 2,5-5 mg over 20 minutes by nebulization	Less than one hour	Shifts K into cells. Lasts three to four hours.
Dialysis	if above measures ineffective		

[1] IV 10% calcium gluconate preferably given under ECG control (bradycardia) is the first step in the emergency management of severe hyperkalaemia.

[2] Suspend dose 1-2 ml/kg in 5% dextrose water or sorbitol 70%. Repeat four to six-hourly until K <6-7 mmol/l.

correction may cause symptomatic hypocalcaemia – also give IV calcium gluconate but not in same line.
◆ Ongoing renal failure – repeated correction will be needed.

Hypocalcaemia

◆ 10% CALCIUM GLUCONATE 1-2 ml/kg slowly IV for significant hypocalcaemia (symptomatic or plasma calcium <1,8 mmol/l).
◆ In chronic renal failure, lower hyperphosphataemia first by giving calcium carbonate (Titralac) or aluminium hydroxide (Amphojel) to bind dietary phosphate; oral calcium Sandoz and supplemental vitamin D.

Anaemia

◆ In acute renal failure correct anaemia by slow transfusion with packed red cells 10 ml/kg. Indications: haemoglobin <6-8 g/dl, active bleeding, severe haemolysis (note the risk of hyperkalaemia and hypertension with blood transfusion in renal failure).
◆ In chronic renal failure the normochromic normocytic anaemia usually stabilizes at haemoglobin levels of about 6 g/dl and transfusion is often not indicated. Human recombinant erythropoietin is effective but expensive.

Seizures

DIAZEPAM IV (see page 411). Treat cause, e.g. hypertension, uraemic syndrome, hypoglycaemia, hypocalcaemia, hyponatraemia and conditions unrelated to renal disease.

Hypertension

See pages 494-6 for treatment.

Infection

A major hazard. Scrupulous asepsis during invasive procedures is essential. Culture suspected infection sites frequently and treat early.

Medications in renal failure

The dosage of drugs normally excreted by the kidney must be reduced. Give usual loading dose, then normal dose at longer intervals depending on severity of renal failure. Be guided by plasma levels.

Dosage modifications – check the drug package insert

None: CHLORAMPHENICOL, CLINDAMYCIN, ERYTHRO-MYCIN, FLUCLOXACILLIN, FUROSEMIDE, OXACILLIN, PENICILLIN G, DIAZEPAM, PHENYTOIN SODIUM, PREDNISOLONE, RIFAMPICIN.

Minor: AMOXYCILLIN, AMPICILLIN, CARBENICILLIN, CO-TRIMOXAZOLE, ISONIAZID, NALIDIXIC ACID, PHENOBARBITONE.

Major: CEPHALOSPORINS, DIGOXIN, AMINOGLYCO-SIDES, STREPTOMYCIN, VANCOMYCIN.

Dialysis

Indications for dialysis in acute renal failure

The decision to dialyse is based on the age and circumstances in the individual case, rather than on arbitrary biochemical criteria. Dialyse early to prevent major complications.

Guidelines for acute dialysis

◆ Oligo-anuria with plasma urea >35-50 mmol/l or plasma creatinine >400-1000 µmol/l. In the young child dialyse at lower creatinine levels.
◆ Life-threatening fluid overload unresponsive to diuretics.
◆ Clinical uraemic syndrome with disturbed level of consciousness and/or convulsions.
◆ Uncontrollable hyperkalaemia (>7 mmol/l).
◆ Uncontrollable metabolic acidosis pH <7,2.
◆ Supportive to allow total parenteral nutrition.
◆ Severe poisoning with dialysable agents.

Peritoneal dialysis

◆ Obtain consent. See page 311 for medico-legal aspects.
◆ Strict aseptic technique is essential.
◆ Ensure that the bladder is emptied by spontaneous voiding or catheterization.
◆ Sedate patient if necessary (see pages 38-9).

Technique

◆ Under local anaesthesia with 2% LIGNOCAINE make a 3 mm stab incision (no. 11 pointed blade) 2-3 cm below umbilicus in the midline through the linea alba down to the peritoneum. In small infants a site just lateral to the left lateral rectus muscle at the level of the umbilicus or left McBurney's point is preferable.

◆ Create ascites by infusing 25-50 ml/kg warmed (37 °C) dialysis fluid via a 18-20 gauge needle cannula inserted through the incision.

◆ Traverse the abdominal wall through the same incision with a paediatric peritoneal dialysis catheter with stylette in place. Once it is in the peritoneal cavity, remove the stylette and direct the catheter gently into the pouch of Douglas. Take note of the natural curve of the catheter.

◆ Ensure that all the perforations of the catheter lie well within the peritoneal cavity.

◆ Connect the Y-dialysis circuit (via blood warmer) and the drainage bag.

◆ Drain peritoneal cavity by siphonage.

◆ Complete one further exchange cycle to check that drainage is adequate. The return of the first exchange is usually incomplete as a sump is created.

◆ **Dress and secure** the dialysis catheter with strapping. A purse-string suture is not required if the incision is a snug fit around the catheter.

◆ In children >15-20 kg the dialysis fluid may be prewarmed to 37 °C, run in through the transfer line, and out through the same line once the bag has been lowered below the bed. Weigh dialysis bags before and after each exchange for fluid balance.

Fluid

1,5% or 2% dextrose Dianeal.

The addition of 10 ml (or more) 50% dextrose water per litre of dialysis fluid will increase the dextrose concentration by 0,5% and therefore the osmolality. Hyperosmolar fluid is used if the patient is fluid-overloaded. In older children, commercially available hyperosmolar 4,2% dextrose Dianeal may be used for two or three exchanges or intermittently, to remove fluid. Considerable shifts of water may result and the 4,2% strength is not used in small children.

Exchanges

Under the age of 12 months, 25-50 ml/kg via an in-line buretrol. In older children 40-50 ml/kg: use nearest 500 or 1 000 ml exchanges for convenience.

Cycles

Dialysis fluid is run in (and out) over ten to fifteen minutes and remains in the peritoneal cavity for 30-45 minutes. More rapid exchanges (shorter dwell time) will withdraw more water from the patient.

Additions to fluid

◆ HEPARIN 500-1 000 units/litre to prevent fibrin clots from blocking the catheter.
◆ 15% KCl 1-2 ml (2-4 mmol) per litre if the patient is not hyperkalaemic.
◆ GENTAMICIN 8 mg/l may be added for the first few exchanges or longer. Send dialysate sample for culture and sensitivity daily.

Note

Keep an accurate in-out fluid balance record and adjust the patient's fluid intake as needed. Do not allow retention of dialysis fluid.

Positioning the patient, gentle pressure on the abdomen, repositioning or flushing of the catheter with heparinized saline or replacement may be necessary if fluid will not run in or drain out properly. The acute peritoneal dialysis stick catheter may be left in place for five to seven days. For longer periods an acute Tenckhoff silastic catheter is placed surgically.

Complications

Include hypernatraemia, hyperglycaemia, fluid imbalance, infection (particularly with prolonged dialysis), and damage to viscera or vessels during insertion. Basal lung atelectasis is prevented by avoiding overdistention of the abdomen and physiotherapy. Small infants may require ventilatory support.

Assessment of kidney function: selected tests

Glomerular filtration function

Glomerular filtration rate

Plasma creatinine is the best simple test. The normal plasma creatinine level is proportionate to muscle mass (and therefore size of child) and the following formula is used to calculate the approximate GFR in children:

$$\text{Approximate GFR in ml/min/1,73 m}^2 = \frac{\text{Height (cm) x 38}}{\text{Plasma creatinine (μmol/l)}}$$

Creatinine clearance

Timed urine collection (24 hours) and plasma sample during collection. Measure height and weight to derive surface area from nomogram. See pages 663-4.

Calculation for creatinine clearance corrected for surface area:

$$C = \text{creatinine clearance in ml/min/1,73 m}^2 = \frac{UV}{P} \times \frac{1,73}{SA}$$

U = urine creatinine μmol/l
V = urine flow in ml/min
P = plasma creatinine μmol/l
SA = surface area in m^2

Normal values

Newborn to four weeks:	40-65 ml/min/1,73 m^2
Males over one year:	124 ±25 ml/min/1,73 m^2
Females over one year:	108 ±13 ml/min/1,73 m^2

Note: adult corrected values only reached after one year of age.

Urine concentration tests

Urine output

◆ Normal
  ◇ Infants: 3-4 ml/kg/hour.
  ◇ Adults: ±1 ml/kg/hour.
◆ Oliguria in young children: <1 ml/kg/hour.
◆ Polyuria: urine output more than twice normal.

Screening test

In the infant, blood and urine osmolality are measured after a four-hour fast. If the plasma osmolality is high in the presence of a low urine osmolality, prolonged water deprivation will result in severe dehydration and a vasopressin test is indicated instead.

Water deprivation test

Empty the bladder. Withhold all fluids for a maximum of 16 hours or until 3% of the bodyweight has been lost or the body temperature has risen to >38 °C, whichever occurs first. Measure the urine volume passed. Determine the urine and plasma osmolality at the end of the test.

Vasopressin test

Empty the bladder after breakfast.

Give aqueous Lysine Vasopressin 5 IU/m^2 SC or DDAVP (Desmopressin) 10-20 μg intranasally. No fluids are allowed for the next four hours. Collect hourly urine specimens for specific gravity or osmolality.

Normal values

◆ Specific gravity >1,025
◆ Osmolality >800 mOsmol/kg H$_2$O

43 RESPIRATORY DISORDERS

M Klein

Acute respiratory infections

After gastroenteritis, acute respiratory infections (especially pneumonia) are the leading cause of death in under-five-year-old children in South Africa. Tachypnoea, or the perception of the mother that her child is breathless, has been found to be the most reliable index of severity of acute respiratory infections (ARI).

Children below two months of age are at especially high risk, as 20-30% of all ARI deaths occur in this group. Diagnosis is complicated because severe ARI in very young children may present with symptoms such as lethargy, apnoea and hypothermia which mimic meningitis, urinary tract infection and generalized sepsis.

Air trapping

Always specify the presence or absence of air trapping when recording the physical examination because it is the most common sign of respiratory disease.

Diagnosis

♦ Inspection: a positive Hoover's sign, i.e. inspiratory retraction of both costal margins implies bilateral air trapping with depressed diaphragms.
♦ Percussion: resonance over areas of the thorax which are normally dull, i.e. reduced cardiac dullness and depressed upper border of liver.

Interpretation

Bilateral air trapping indicates diffuse peripheral airways obstruction (PAO) from conditions such as bronchiolitis, asthma, aspiration syndromes, cystic fibrosis, immotile cilia syndrome, and chronic obstructive lung disease following post-measles pneumonia. Obstruction of the larynx and trachea produces clinically apparent air trapping only when obstruction is extreme. A loud expiratory wheeze without air trapping signifies tracheal compression by tuberculous lymph nodes, aberrant vessels, or tracheal foreign body.

Unilateral pulmonary or lobar air trapping (obstructive emphysema) strongly suggests a foreign body.

Aspiration syndromes

Aspiration is a relatively common cause of recurrent cough, wheeze, pneumonia and croup in young children. Repeated aspiration may produce permanent, crippling obstructive airways disease.

Aetiology

Gastro-oesophageal reflux (GOR) is the major cause of aspiration. Laryngeal incompetence, i.e. the aspiration of fluid through the larynx while drinking, is next in importance. Tracheo-oesophageal and broncho-oesophageal fistulae are rare.

Laryngeal incompetence is most common after severe laryngeal infections (e.g. Herpes simplex croup) or trauma (intubation, burns). It generally resolves spontaneously within a few weeks or months. Laryngeal incompetence associated with velo-palatal incompetence (reflux into the nasopharynx with swallowing) suggests cleft palate, diphtheria, cerebral palsy or dysautonomia.

Diagnosis

♦ Maintain a high index of suspicion for aspiration in children below two years of age who have chronic wheezing, recurrent pneumonia or recurrent croup.

♦ A history of choking with feeds or frequent small vomits points to aspiration but is seldom obtained.

♦ Clinical and radiographic findings of aspiration are non-specific: bilateral obstructive airways disease with variable peribronchial infiltrates.

♦ The diagnosis of laryngeal incompetence is made by radiography.

♦ While GOR can be diagnosed and quantified relatively easily, it is rarely possible to prove the associated aspiration. The more severe the reflux, the more likely it is to be the cause of the respiratory disease.

Investigations

◆ **Radiography:** request 'contrast studies to exclude laryngeal incompetence, velo-palatal reflux, gastro-oesophageal reflux and tracheo-oesophageal fistula'. Standard barium swallows may miss these conditions.

◆ **Ultrasound:** in the hands of experts, competence of the gastro-oesophageal sphincter and the occurrence and severity of gastro-oesophageal reflux can be evaluated.

◆ **Isotope milk scan:** evidence of pulmonary aspiration on nuclear medicine scan with labelled feed is the only way to prove the diagnosis. However, milk scans are negative for aspiration in the majority of children who are presumed to aspirate in association with gastro-oesophageal reflux.

◆ **Sputum:** for fat-laden macrophages. A positive result is evidence of previous aspiration of milk fat. Not a sensitive test and not an index of severity.

◆ **Laryngoscopy:** under general anaesthesia with a rigid endoscope to exclude a laryngeal cleft if laryngeal incompetence is severe and symptoms date from the neonatal period. Fibre-optic laryngoscopy does not exclude a laryngeal cleft.

◆ **Oesophageal pH studies:** presently indicated only for patients being evaluated for possible anti-reflux surgery.

Management

◆ **Laryngeal incompetence:** liquids are aspirated, solids are not, and refined sugars and milk fat are damaging to the lung. Therefore, feed the child semi-solids and give water (no sugar) as the only liquid. Use milk and milk powder to make the food. Monitor weight gain weekly to ensure nutritional needs are being met. Repeat barium swallow after three months. Most cases will have resolved.

◆ **Gastro-oesophageal reflux:** GOR resolves with time, but the obstructive lung disease may be permanent. Correct GOR before irreparable damage is done. The younger the child, the more urgent the therapy. Treat surgically if a hiatus hernia is present or if there has been no improvement on medical therapy (Gaviscon and CISAPRIDE) within six weeks in a child with overt peripheral airways obstruction. Reflux in association with laryngeal incompetence is a malignant disease and requires urgent anti-reflux surgery.

Bronchiectasis

Bronchiectasis is the end of a spectrum of peripheral airway damage. Since conditions which result in permanent lung damage are rarely limited to a single lobe, bronchiectasis is usually accompanied by evidence of fairly generalized lung injury in the form of chronic obstructive (peripheral) airways disease (COPD). The COPD is often the major source of symptoms. When bronchiectasis occurs in the absence of generalized COPD, it suggests a localized airway abnormality: previous foreign body, tuberculous nodal compression, sequestration, or adenomatoid malformation.

Diagnosis

Diagnosis is clinical, not radiographic. Clubbing in association with a chronic productive cough makes the diagnosis. Symptoms attributable to bronchiectasis include: chronic productive cough, disrupted sleep, lethargy, foul breath, poor appetite, failure to thrive, and painful joints.

Warning

Poor exercise tolerance, wheeze and tachypnoea are not symptoms of bronchiectasis, but of associated COPD.

Investigation

◆ Spirometry to evaluate associated peripheral airways obstruction.
◆ Measure IgG and IgA to exclude hypogammaglobulinaemia, and as an index of severity of chronic sepsis.
◆ ECG to exclude pulmonary hypertension.
◆ Radiology: conventional chest X-rays are not reliable for the diagnosis of bronchiectasis. Thoracic CT is definitive. Bronchography with a non-water-soluble agent[1] is indicated only in children with bilateral bronchiectasis on CT in whom palliative resection is contemplated. Delayed films taken 12 to 24 hours after the bronchogram will show retained dye in the areas of lung most likely to benefit from surgical resection. See page 467.

---

[1] DIONOSIL is no longer being manufactured and alternatives are being sought.

> **Warning**
>
> There is no point in doing investigations to prove the presence of bronchiectasis unless surgical resection is indicated on clinical grounds.

Management

Surgery

Selection for operation is based on symptoms, not on the CT or bronchogram. Resection is indicated for all children with symptoms attributable to bronchiectasis unless they are tachypnoeic at rest. The objective is to reduce cough and sputum, to promote general well-being and compensatory lung growth and to reduce the risks of amyloidosis, hypertrophic pulmonary osteo-arthropathy, cerebral abscess and bacterial endocarditis (in patients with predisposing cardiac lesions). Surgery will not improve exercise tolerance, wheeze or tachypnoea. Palliative surgery may be possible in more severely affected children after further evaluation in a specialized unit.

Medical

Medical therapy aims at the control of the chronic sepsis prior to surgery and in cases where resection is not feasible. Promote drainage of sputum by postural drainage and physiotherapy, and administer bronchodilators if there is associated bronchoconstriction. Halitosis (exclude dental caries) implies anaerobic sepsis and is treated with maintenance, twice daily METRONIDAZOLE (Flagyl). Maintenance antibiotic therapy is rarely indicated. Acute exacerbations of infection are generally associated with *Haemophilus influenzae* infection.

Bronchiolitis

Acute viral bronchiolitis is a common cause of acute tachypnoea or wheezing during infancy.

Diagnosis

The following features are required for the diagnosis:

◆ age under two years, rhinitis present, air trapping present,

crackles usual, little cough or sputum, often soft wheezing, fever <38 °C axilla, no consolidation;
◆ chest X-rays (indicated if tachypnoeic) showing air trapping, no consolidation, occasionally atelectasis in the right upper lobe;
◆ neonates may present with apnoea;
◆ high fever suggests bacterial pneumonia.

Management

◆ **Oxygen** for all children requiring hospitalization. It is usually the only treatment required. Low concentrations (below 40%) correct hypoxaemia in bronchiolitis. Use a nasal catheter: oxygen at 1-2 l/min through a 6-8F feeding tube passed into nose to a depth equal to half the distance between the nose and ear lobe. Do not humidify.
◆ Evaluate and manage as for pneumonia, except that antibiotics are indicated only if consolidation or fever >38 °C are present.
◆ A test dose of IPRATROPIUM may be given by inhalation. It should only be continued (six-hourly) in those children who show objective improvement with the test dose.

THEOPHYLLINE (aqueous) 2 mg, eight-hourly, administered orally is indicated in infants with apnoea and in those under a month of age to prevent it.

◆ Steroids are of no benefit.
◆ Physiotherapy is hazardous and is contra-indicated while children are tachypnoeic. It is of questionable value in the convalescent phase unless lobar atelectasis is present.

Bronchitis

Although bronchitis does occur in childhood, it is usually an inappropriate diagnosis: most cases labelled bronchitis or wheezy bronchitis are asthma. Bronchitis is characterized by cough and relatively scanty sputum. Acute bronchitis is not distinguishable from mild bronchopneumonia. Mild bronchitis is present in all tracheotomized children but is generally only treated when the sputum becomes purulent. Chronic bronchitis is a component of airway damage in virtually all patients with chronic obstructive airways disease. Allergic tracheobronchitis is thought to be responsible for troublesome cough in some asthmatics and generally responds to inhaled CROMO-GLYCATE or steroids.

Bronchopneumonia

This is the usual form of pneumonia in childhood. See pneumonia on page 524.

Croup

Croup is the most common cause of potentially life-threatening airway obstruction in childhood. Croup, acute obstructive infraglottic laryngitis and laryngotracheobronchitis are synonymous. In croup there is inflammatory swelling of the vocal cords and the subglottic portion of the larynx.

Aetiology

Croup occurs from infection or trauma.

Infective croup is usually parainfluenza virus in generally healthy children, and Herpes simplex in children following measles. *Staphylococcus aureus, Streptococcus pneumoniae,* and *H. influenzae*, in order of frequency, are responsible for rare occurrences of primary bacterial croup. Diphtheretic croup occurs only in incompletely immunized children.

Traumatic croup follows laryngeal intubation and is avoidable: ensure that there is some air leak past the endotracheal tube when the airway pressure is raised to 15 cm water (1,5 kPa). Except in croup, an occlusively fitting tube is too large and must be removed within an hour. Following every intubation, **always record the endotracheal tube size and whether or not a leak is present**. Subsequently the leak may become sealed off by oedema or mucus but the tube need not be changed if a leak was present initially. **Tapered endotracheal tubes (e.g. Cole, Endeby) are particularly liable to damage the larynx and should be avoided.**

Diagnosis

Viral croup is by far the most common form of croup. A confident clinical diagnosis of viral croup can be made if a previously healthy child develops progressive inspiratory airway obstruction with stridor and a barking cough a day or two after the onset of an upper respiratory tract infection. A mild fever may be present (<38 °C), the child is not systemically ill, and abnormal physical findings are limited to the respiratory system. No other diagnosis need be entertained in a child with a typical history and physical findings.

Features which suggest a different diagnosis are: dramatic onset of severe obstruction (foreign body); incomplete immunization (diphtheria); dysphagia or the patient prefers a sitting position (epiglottitis, retropharyngeal abscess); toxic with erythematous rash (staphylococcal croup); or aphonia in a black child with a previously hoarse voice (laryngeal papillomatosis).

Recurrent croup in an infant is suggestive of an associated congenital subglottic stenosis or gastro-oesophageal reflux. In older atopic children, recurrent croup often occurs as short-lived attacks of so-called spasmodic croup which generally respond dramatically to inhaled ADRENALINE.

Investigations

◆ Radiographs of the larynx are indicated only if there is serious doubt concerning the diagnosis.
◆ Check oxygen saturation in air by pulse oximetry. Measure acid-base and blood gas balance prior to intubation to exclude unsuspected metabolic acidosis from dehydration which, by stimulating respiration, increases the apparent severity of croup. Blood gases are not a reliable indicator of the need for airway intervention.

Assessment of severity

The degree of airway obstruction is graded according to Table 43.1.

Table 43.1 Severity of airway obstruction in croup

Severity	Inspiratory obstruction	Expiratory obstruction	Palpable pulsus pardoxus
Grade 1	+		
Grade 2	+	passive	
Grade 3	+	active	+
Grade 4	marked retractions, apathy, cyanosis		

Signs of inspiratory obstruction are: inspiratory stridor, prolongation of inspiration, retractions and tracheal tug. Prolonged expiration is the major sign of expiratory laryngeal obstruction. 'Active' expiratory obstruction implies visible or palpable contraction of abdominal muscles. 'Passive' obstruction: prolonged expiration without apparent abdominal muscle contraction. Although the vocal cords are invariably swollen in viral croup, the cry is often surprisingly well preserved. Pulsus paradoxus is present when the pulse becomes weaker or disappears with inspiration. Use only a light touch to feel the pulse, or the paradoxus will not be detected.

> ### Warning
> (a) the grading is applicable only to croup, not to other causes of airway obstruction, and (b) it is the severity of airway obstruction which is graded, not the severity of stridor. Stridor becomes softer as the airway obstruction becomes more severe.

Management

Remove the cause

♦ Antibiotics are indicated in diphtheria and when bacterial croup (*S. aureus, H. influenzae and pneumococci*) is suspected: fever >38 °C, purulent sputum, pneumonia. Treat all children with post-measles croup for Herpes simplex virus infection with intravenous ACYCLOVIR and substitute oral ACYCLOVIR a day after fever subsides to complete seven days of therapy.

Do not make matters worse

♦ Crying and hyperventilation with fever and metabolic acidosis increase the oedema. Keep the child comfortable and happy. Continue feeding orally. Encourage parents to remain with the child. Avoid painful procedures. Prescribe PARACETAMOL if febrile.
♦ Sedate the child with CHLORAL HYDRATE (50 mg/kg/dose) or TRICLOFOS (50 mg/kg/dose) only if he or she cannot be consoled in any other way. Sedated children require tube feeding to maintain hydration.

Steroids

Steroids are beneficial in viral croup. Give a stat dose to children with viral croup grade 1 or 2 if there has been no measles within the past month, fever <38 °C and no evidence of oral herpes. Use a single dose of PREDNISONE or PREDNISOLONE 2 mg/kg oral or DEXAMETHASONE 0,5 mg/kg IM or IV or METHYLPREDNISOLONE 2 mg/kg IM or IV. Repeat after 24 hours if no improvement.

Relieve the obstruction

Management is tailored according to the severity of the obstruction.

Grade 1 obstruction: Observe at home if conditions are favourable and the obstruction does not appear to be getting worse. Steroids may be beneficial. A misted room (not tent) may have a soothing effect.

Grade 2 obstruction: Hospitalize. Give steroids as above and nebulized ADRENALINE inhalations by mask. (Mix 1 ml ADRENALINE 1:1 000 (1 mg) with 1 ml saline. Nebulize the entire volume with oxygen. Repeat every 15 minutes or more frequently until improved. Continue every 30 minutes until expiratory obstruction has been virtually abolished. Caution: observe the child carefully for deterioration and be prepared to provide an artificial airway.) Keep the child happy. Feed. Sedate if the child is fretful and cries when nebulized.

Grade 3 obstruction: give steroid and ADRENALINE inhalations. Monitor oxygen saturation. If obstruction is not relieved within two hours, pass endotracheal tube (ETT) under general anaesthesia or do a tracheostomy. Use the smallest ETT that permits aspiration of secretions and comfortable breathing. Approximate ETT sizes for normal children are given on page 8.

Table 43.2 Appropriate endotracheal tube sizes for croup

Age	ETT size
Birth to six months	2,5 to 3,0 mm
Six months to 18 months	3,0 mm
Eighteen months to three years	3,5 mm
Three years to five years	4,0 mm
Over five years	4,5 mm

The choice between ETT and tracheostomy depends on local circumstances. ETT's block and become dislodged more readily. Tracheostomy is safer but carries greater morbidity. Tracheostomies are always done under general anaesthesia with an ETT *in situ*. It is always possible to insert a 2,5 or 3,0 mm ETT in croup, no matter how severe. Do not warm the tube as it may become too soft to pass the obstruction.

Grade 4 obstruction: give 100% oxygen and nebulized ADRENALINE continuously if available. Emergency intubation may be required for patients with grade 4 obstruction, although it is preferable to perform intubation under anaesthesia when circumstances permit.

Effusion and empyema

The primary classification of pleural effusion is into septic and aseptic groups.

Septic (Pyogenic): *S. aureus, S. pneumoniae, H. influenzae.*

Aseptic: partially treated septic, tuberculous, post-traumatic (e.g. surgery), blunt or penetrating trauma, malignant (e.g. lymphoma), fungal (e.g. actinomyces), viral, mycoplasmal, amoebic, nephrotic syndrome and acute glomerulonephritis.

Aseptic effusion

Diagnosis

The aetiology of aseptic effusions is often evident from the history and associated findings on physical examination. Diagnostic pleural aspiration is indicated when the diagnosis is not apparent. The appearance of the fluid should be noted (serous, haemorrhagic, chylous) and it should be sent for chemistry (protein, adenine deaminase), cytology, and culture for mycobacteria and unusual pathogens.

Management

Management of aseptic effusions is that of the underlying disorder. Repeated needle aspiration is generally sufficient for relief of symptoms related to pulmonary compression. Effusions following blunt chest trauma (associated pulmonary contusion) and chylous effusions are generally managed with intercostal tube drainage. See pages 453-455.

Septic effusion: empyema

Staphylococcus is the most frequent cause, followed by pneumococcal and *H. influenzae* infection.

Diagnosis

Effusions in children who are acutely ill and febrile must be regarded as septic. **Diagnostic needle aspiration of the pleura is not recommended.** In such cases it is often misleading: coagulated exudate may block the needle, producing a falsely dry tap, or only thin supernatant is obtained, creating the impression that no pus is present. In toxically ill children, proceed to immediate intercostal tube drainage (see page 453) and submit the fluid for Gram's stain, Ziehl-Neelsen (if tuberculosis is suspect), and culture.

Clinical and radiological features

Clinical

A spontaneous pneumothorax in a febrile child who was previously well is virtually diagnostic of staphylococcal pyopneumothorax. Pneumothorax rarely occurs with *S. pneumoniae* or *H. influenzae* effusions.

Radiography

A pneumothorax is typical of staphylococcal pleuro-pulmonary sepsis. A multicystic appearance is common, due to intrapleural fibrin strands. True pneumatocoeles are relatively rare, there are seldom more than two per lung, are confined anatomically within lobar boundaries, and develop slowly over several days. See page 465.

Warning

Children who remain ill after two days of adequate antibiotic therapy (see 'pneumonia') and attempted intercostal drainage in the ward must be referred for formal drainage and pleural toilet under general anaesthesia by a thoracic surgeon.

Management

It is just as important to remove the pleural pus by adequate intercostal drainage as it is to administer antibiotics. See page 453.

Epiglottitis

Epiglottitis is a condition of children and young adults due to *H. influenzae* type B infection.

Diagnosis

◆ Epiglottitis is characterized by a very sore throat, dysphagia, toxaemia, and rapidly progressive airway obstruction. Total airway obstruction is imminent by the time stridor appears.
◆ The child's appearance is most deceptive. The child does not appear to be in grave danger because the airway obstruction is masked by measures the child adopts to protect its airway: the child sits, the head is kept still and jaw pushed slightly forward, there is reluctance to open the mouth wide, breathing is shallow with slow deliberate inspirations. The child will also be reluctant to speak (speech is soft), and reluctant to swallow and may drool.
◆ **The airway may occlude acutely if these protective mechanisms are interfered with,** as when the child is provoked to cry or if any attempt is made to change its posture, e.g. to take radiographs. Inspect the throat only if the patient voluntarily opens its mouth. Make no attempt to see the epiglottis: the patient may choke on the spatula and arrest. Peritonsillar and retropharyngeal abscess may mimic supraglottitis. It is not necessary to differentiate between them since all require urgent therapy in the operating theatre.

Investigations

Lateral radiographs of the pharynx show the swollen epiglottis and aryepiglottic folds. Because radiography is dangerous, laryngeal X-rays are justified only:

◆ if there is real doubt regarding the diagnosis and if someone competent is available to read the X-rays; and
◆ if a doctor with skill and equipment for immediate intubation accompanies the patient. **Do not forcibly reposition the child or attempt to hold it down for X-rays or procedures.**

Intravenous drip and blood sampling (blood culture, blood count) must be delayed till after the airway is secured.

Management

Upon making a clinical diagnosis of supraglottitis, take the patient directly to the operating theatre for examination under general anaesthesia. Do so irrespective of the apparent degree of airway obstruction, because total obstruction may occur suddenly and quite unpredictably.

If epiglottitis is confirmed on endoscopy, insert an endotracheal tube of the usual size for the patient's age, taking care to ensure that a leak is present when airway pressure is raised 15-20 cm water (1,5-2,0 kPa) see page 8 and Table 43.2. Do not try to see the vocal cords when intubating, since it is not possible. Pass the bevel of the endotracheal tube along the posterior groove of the swollen epiglottis and it will slide easily into the larynx. A blood culture and blood count can now be taken and intravenous CHLORAMPHENICOL commenced. Substitute AMPICILLIN if the blood culture is sterile or grows sensitive organisms. See Appendix 1. Attempt extubation after the fever and sore throat have subsided (48-72 hours later). Give daily oral steroid (PREDNISOLONE 2 mg/kg or equivalent) as a single daily dose until the tube is out.

Foreign bodies (FB)

Laryngeal foreign bodies

Rare. Usually presents with acute onset of stridor and airway obstruction following a choking spell. Rarely confused with croup. Laryngeal foreign bodies are generally sharp objects (e.g. fish bones) which are small and seldom seen on radiographs. Removal is by laryngoscopy.

Tracheobronchial foreign bodies

Common. Usually smooth objects such as peanuts which are able to slip through the larynx. Rarely radiographically visible.

Diagnosis

History

A choking spell followed by persistent cough, wheeze or respiratory distress is diagnostic of a tracheobronchial foreign body. However, a typical history is not always obtainable.

Clinical

Soft breath sounds over a lobe or lung which is resonant to percussion or shows radiographic evidence of obstructive lobar or pulmonary emphysema should be regarded as evidence of a foreign body until the diagnosis is excluded by bronchoscopy.

Management

Endoscopic removal under general anaesthesia.

Laryngomalacia

Usual cause of stridor that begins within a few weeks of birth. Laryngeal cartilage is normal. The soft tissues of the larynx are hypotonic and bulky and prolapse into the laryngeal lumen with inspiration.

Diagnosis

Clinical signs are typical: onset of inspiratory stridor during first two weeks of life, inspiratory obstruction which varies from breath to breath, no expiratory obstruction, and a normal voice. Suspect vocal cord paralysis if the voice is soft.

Investigations

Fibre-optic laryngoscopy when available, otherwise a lateral neck X-ray to exclude a supraglottic cyst or mass. Formal laryngoscopy under general anaesthesia is not warranted unless the obstruction is sufficiently severe to warrant surgery or tracheostomy.

Management

Reassurance is sufficient in the vast majority of cases. Children generally outgrow laryngomalacia within two years. Laser excision of excessive supraglottic tissue is indicated if the child fails to thrive, has marked retractions or chest deformity, or has apnoeic spells or frank hypercapnoeic respiratory failure. Tracheostomy is rarely required.

Laryngotracheobronchitis (LTB)

See 'Croup' on page 513.

Near-drowning

Near-drowning refers to initial recovery after immersion. Victims of near-drowning may subsequently succumb to pulmonary oedema and hypoxaemia, cerebral oedema, or infection. The late pulmonary complications are often referred to as secondary drowning.

Treatment at the scene

The quality of initial resuscitation at the scene is the essential factor that determines the outcome in near-drowning. (See page 1 for cardiopulmonary resuscitation (CPR).) Do not discontinue resuscitation even if the situation appears hopeless. Do not rush the victim to hospital until everything possible has been done to resuscitate the victim. Continue active CPR during transport using 100% oxygen if available. Hypothermia may be present. Dry and cover the victim to avoid further cooling. Victims who are not breathing on arrival at hospital will probably die, unless the cause is hypothermia.

Hospital admission criteria

A decision to terminate CPR should only be taken after full assessment in hospital. Victims who have suffered any disturbance in their level of consciousness, who have been confused or who have any respiratory symptoms must be admitted to hospital for at least 12 hours. They are at risk for secondary drowning and cerebral oedema. If possible, administer oxygen en route by nasal prongs or facemask, even when there is no clinical evidence of hypoxaemia.

Hospital care

Hypoxaemia and post-hypoxic cerebral oedema are the major causes of morbidity and death.

◆ Hypoxaemia during the first six hours is due to pulmonary oedema, fluid overload, or aspirated chemicals or particulate matter. Subsequent hypoxaemia is usually secondary to infection. Continue oxygen therapy (and IPPV if in progress) until chest X-ray and blood gas results are available.
◆ Cerebral oedema is a late (six to 12 hours) consequence of cerebral ischaemia. See pages 333-4.

General measures and investigations

◆ Drain the stomach by nasogastric tube.
◆ Do blood gases, blood count and serum electrolytes.
◆ Culture gastric aspirate, blood cultures and tracheal or nasopharyngeal aspirates.

Hypervolaemia and hypovolaemia

Hypervolaemia and pulmonary oedema are common. Associated water intoxication may precipitate convulsions.

◆ Give FUROSEMIDE 0,5 mg/kg if there is clinical suspicion of pulmonary oedema on arrival.
◆ Blood volume expansion may be required following sea-water aspiration. Insert a central venous pressure line and catheterize the bladder to monitor fluid therapy in patients who require IPPV or whose hypoxaemia has not improved following the diuretic.

Medications

Because they may have aspirated, oral antibiotics are usually prescribed for patients who have lost consciousness. Steroids are indicated only when the victim is known to have vomited and aspirated gastric content. Steroids do not prevent post-hypoxic cerebral oedema and may mask the signs of infection.

Discharge criteria

Patients may be discharged after a minimum 12-hour period of observation if they are fully conscious, afebrile, have normal white blood counts, normal chests on clinical and X-ray examination and normal acid-base and blood gases in air.

Follow-up examination

The effects of infection with unusual pathogens may appear up to a month after discharge. All children who have been sent home before culture results are known should be examined again within two days for clinical evidence of pneumonia. Advise parents to report any unexplained fever, tachypnoea or chest pain developing during the ensuing month.

Oropharyngeal obstruction (OPO)

See 'Snoring', page 526.

Pneumonia

Pneumonia is the leading cause of death from acute respiratory infections, killing up to five million under-five year olds annually in developing countries.

Diagnosis

Bronchopneumonia is the usual form in young children. Lobar pneumonia becomes more common with increasing age. Bronchopneumonia may be difficult to distinguish clinically from acute bronchiolitis: fever tends to be higher in bronchopneumonia and crackles are less prominent. Typically bronchopneumonia manifests on chest radiographs with peribronchial infiltrates clustered around the hila (so called para-hilar infiltrates), some air trapping, and varying degrees of focal parenchymal consolidation.

Investigations

All cases

Chest X-ray routinely.

Hospital admission

Blood culture and nasopharyngeal aspirate prior to commencement of antibiotic therapy. Measure haemoglobin concentration. Record oxygen saturation in air by pulse oximeter **or** measure arterial blood gases.

Management

Antibiotics

Viral bronchopneumonia cannot be distinguished from bacterial bronchopneumonia clinically or radiographically. The more ill the child, the more likely is a bacterial infection. Antibiotics should be used for all acutely ill children with bronchopneumonia: fever >38 °C, persistent tachycardia >140 per minute, alar flare, marked retractions.

The clinical setting determines the choice of antibiotic for initial therapy of pneumonia (see page 584). It may require modification in the light of bacterial culture. Therapy should be reviewed if there is no clear improvement within 36 hours.

Antibiotics should be discontinued as soon as the child is asymptomatic (usually within five days) except for staphylococcal pneumonia which is treated from three to six weeks.

Oxygenation

Death in pneumonia occurs from hypoxaemia. All children requiring hospital admission with pneumonia need oxygen by nasal catheter (see page 512) or head box. Hypoxaemia cannot be judged clinically. Failure to monitor oxygenation may result in 'unexpected' death or respiratory arrest.

If haemoglobin <8 g/dl, transfuse with packed cells. Maintain haemoglobin above 10 g/dl in children who require >35% to achieve haemoglobin saturation >95%.

Fluid therapy

The aim is to maintain normal hydration and nutrition. Feed with milk at the usual recommended volume for age, preferably as three-hourly feeding to avoid gastric distension.

Because of the low solute content, intravenous fluid requirements are much less than those for milk. Fully correct fluid deficits. No more than 50-60 ml/kg/day of intravenous fluid should be given for maintenance to children with pneumonia. The use of a greater volume will produce water overload and may cause pulmonary oedema. Only give solutions containing bicarbonate or lactate if buffer is specifically indicated.

Pneumothorax and pyopneumothorax

Spontaneous pneumothorax without apparent underlying pulmonary pathology is encountered only in the first week of life. At all other times a definite cause is present: cardio-pulmonary resuscitation, ventilator barotrauma and acute severe asthma. A pneumothorax without definite cause in a febrile child implies almost certain staphylococcal infection and associated empyema. See Empyema (page 518) and Pleural effusion (page 517).

Diagnosis

The effects of a pneumothorax depend on the condition of the underlying lung and, only secondly, on the volume of the

pneumothorax. A small pneumothorax in a patient with pneumonia can have severe consequences. The term 'tension
pneumothorax' is used to indicate that the pneumothorax is producing marked symptoms. The diagnosis of tension pneumothorax is therefore clinical and not radiographic: unilaterally
reduced breath sounds, resonance to percussion and evidence of
tamponade such as hypotension or hypoxaemia. Lesser degrees
of pneumothorax are detectable only by radiography, or by
transillumination in low birthweight neonates.

Investigation

Diagnostic needling of the pleura for pneumothorax is unwar-
ranted, since lung puncture is unavoidable. If there was no
pneumothorax before, there will almost certainly be one
afterward.

If the child is severely distressed and a pneumothorax is suspected the pleura should be drained as described on page 453. If
the child is not severely distressed, the pneumothorax should be
confirmed by X-ray before drainage.

Management

Therapy depends on the cause and effects. Patients with presumed staphylococcal infection (see above) should have an
intercostal drain inserted immediately. Moderately ill children
can be given 100% oxygen to promote absorption of the pneumothorax and be observed, or the pneumothorax can be treated
by needle aspiration, and an intercostal drain inserted if it
recurs. See page 453.

Snoring

It is abnormal for a child to snore regularly. All such children
require treatment. Routinely enquire about snoring when taking
the history because parents will rarely volunteer the
information.

Snoring is a symptom of oropharyngeal airway obstruction
(OPO) and occurs typically during sleep when the oropharyngeal muscles relax. However, in severe OPO, the child may
snore even when awake. In small infants, snoring may be high-
pitched and can be confused with stridor.

Children are predisposed to OPO because of the small size of their oropharyngeal airway. Severe OPO with acute respiratory failure may be precipitated by a simple cold.

Adverse effects of OPO are listed in Table 43.3. Children under two years of age are most severely affected. Ill effects may become irreversible if therapy is delayed. OPO may cause death.

Table 43.3 Adverse effects of OPO

Effects	Symptoms
Fragmented sleep	The most common but subtle and non-specific: irritability, learning problems, enuresis, and developmental delay.
Asphyxia	Acute respiratory failure, pulmonary hypertension, systemic hypertension, cardiac failure. Rarely polycythaemia.
Increased working of breathing	Failure to thrive, chest deformity.

Investigations

Lateral X-ray of the postnasal space to see if the adenoid is present — not whether it is enlarged! Blood count to detect polycythaemia, ECG to detect cor pulmonale.

Management

Chronic OPO, i.e. habitual snoring

OXYMETAZOLINE (Drixine, Iliadin) nose drops at bed time and other measures to control allergic rhinitis. See page 23. Adenoidectomy if these measures fail, even if the adenoid appears normal or small. Over 90% of children with chronic OPO will be cured by adenoidectomy. Failure to respond suggests that the adenoidectomy was incomplete.

Acute life-threatening OPO

Endotracheal intubation, but continuous insufflation of the

pharynx (CIP) is simpler and safe: warm humidified air is flowed through a 2,5 mm or 3,0 mm endotracheal tube secured in place with the tip midway between the margin of the soft palate and epiglottis. Use the lowest flow rate that keeps the child comfortable during sleep (3-6 l/min). Oxygen supplementation will only be required if there is an associated pneumonia.

Severe OPO unresponsive to the above measures necessitates tracheostomy.

Stridor

Stridor is a symptom, not a diagnosis.

Inspiratory stridor

The usual causes are laryngomalacia and croup. In epiglottitis, stridor is soft and may have a low-pitched gurgling quality.

Expiratory stridor

This implies obstruction of the intrathoracic trachea or main bronchi. Vascular rings and airway compression by large tuberculous lymph nodes are the main causes.

Table 43.4 Differential diagnosis of wheezing

Air trapping	Site of obstruction	Causes
Bilateral	Peripheral small	Less than two years old: bronchiolitis, bronchopneumonia, aspiration syndromes, asthma uncommon. More than two years old: asthma usual, post-infective (measles, adenovirus) or post-GOR, obstructive airways disease, cystic fibrosis.
Unilateral	Main bronchi	Foreign body, e.g. peanut, TB, lymph nodes.
Lobar	Lobar bronchi	Foreign body, congenital lobar emphysema.
None	Tracheal	Extrinsic compression: vascular ring, TB nodes. Rare: tracheo-oesophageal fistula, foreign body, croup.

Tachypnoea

Transient increases in respiratory rate are common in normal children. Tachypnoea is defined as a respiratory rate persistently (observations repeated 30-60 minutes apart) above the upper limit for the child's age. See page 684.

Wheezing

Expiratory wheezing implies intrathoracic airway obstruction. Soft wheezing is heard only with a stethoscope, loud wheezing is heard without one.

Differential diagnosis

The differential diagnosis of wheezing is much broader in children than adults. It is helpful to approach it according to whether or not air trapping is associated. (See Table 43.4.)

Diagnose asthma in every child with recurrent wheeze, dyspnoea, or cough which responds to a bronchodilator. By response one means a reduction in airway obstruction within 5-10 minutes of the administration of an inhaled (or parenteral) bronchodilator. Failure to make an explicit diagnosis of asthma results in inadequate or inappropriate therapy and increased morbidity from the disease.

By perpetuating airway hyper-responsiveness, allergy plays an integral role in childhood asthma. However, proof of allergy is not required for the diagnosis of asthma, nor is identification of specific allergens helpful in the management of most asthmatics. Passive smoking is a cause of increased severity of asthma and parents of asthmatics must be strongly counselled against having anyone smoke in the child's presence.

Although asthma may occur in children below two years of age, it is not the most common cause of chronic or recurrent peripheral airways obstruction at this age. Other causes of peripheral airways obstruction, particularly gastro-esophageal reflux, should be excluded before diagnosing asthma in a child below two years. See Table 43.4.

44 SKIN DISEASES

N Saxe

Candida infection
Monilia (thrush) of the mouth
Appearance

A white cheesy membrane which is easily scraped off the oral mucosa.

Treatment

MICONAZOLE (Daktarin) oral gel four times daily or NYSTATIN suspension:

♦ Infants 2 ml (200 000 units) four times daily for one to two weeks. Half the dose is placed on each side of the mouth and is then swallowed.
♦ Older children 5 ml (500 000 units) four times daily. Liquid swished around in the mouth for five minutes before swallowing.

Monilia of the skin
Appearance

Beefy red scalded skin with satellite pustules.

Treatment

NYSTATIN ointment or VIOFORM 2% and steroid ointment 10% in zinc cream or equal parts of Mycostatin, steroid cream and zinc cream or newer broad-spectrum antifungal preparations (see 'Ringworm', page 536).

Eczema (or dermatitis)

The eczematous pattern is the most common condition encountered in a paediatric dermatology clinic. Causes include atopic eczema, seborrhoeic dermatitis and nummular eczema.

Appearance

Eczema may be acute with erythema, scaling and/or vesicles, or chronic with thickening pigmentation and increased skin markings (lichenification).

Atopic eczema is very itchy and the child is usually severely distressed. The lesions begin on the face, spread to the flexor surfaces and become generalized. The skin is often very dry. Asthma, hay fever and allergies may be associated. Seborrhoeic dermatitis occurs in infants aged one to three months; there is greasy scale in the scalp and red moist scaling in the flexures.

Nummular eczema manifests as well-rounded patches of eczema, often on the legs, and may be associated with atopic dermatitis.

Topical treatment

This is the same for all eczemas. Tar and/or steroids are the best. In the acute, wet 'weeping stage' use a cream or lotion. In the dry, scaly or lichenified stage use ointment. Use the weakest topical steroid that will control the eczema, e.g.

◆ HYDROCORTISONE 1% in HEB; or
◆ 10% of steroid (potent group) ointment in HEB; or
◆ solution of coal tar 5% (LPC) in **emulsifying ointment** B.P. (HEB).

Very rarely a stronger (i.e. fluorinated) steroid, e.g. Synalar, Betnovate, Celestoderm V or Cortoderm, etc., may be required for a week or two. When improvement occurs, change to a weaker maintenance steroid. In infected eczema use potassium permanganate soaks, and VIOFORM 2% and steroid 10% in HEB to the body and VIOFORM 2% and HYDRO-CORTISONE 1% in HEB to the face. With severe infection Betadine cream under occlusive dressings is indicated for up to a week.

Special precautions

◆ Avoid potent steroids in children, particularly on the face. Try to adhere to HYDROCORTISONE 1% in HEB.
◆ Attempt to change treatment to a tar preparation.

Topical steroid preparations with mild potency, i.e. HYDRO-CORTISONE (base + acetate) 0,1-2,5%, include Mylocort, Procutan, Cutaderm and Dilucort.

General measures

If the eczema is infected, i.e. pustular or crusted, use a systemic antibiotic, such as PENICILLIN, FLUCLOXACILLIN or ERYTHROMYCIN.

Special measures

Avoid soap and wool next to skin. Showers are preferable to baths. Antihistamine, e.g. HYDROXYZINE (Aterax) or TRI-MEPRAZINE (Vallergan) for itch or sedation. Teach stress management and institute family therapy. Apply AQUEOUS CREAM (UEA) or CETAMACROGOL cream to lubricate dry skin or to use in place of soap.

Haemangioma and vascular lesions

See page 551.

Ichthyosis

Appearance

Dry skin with scaling. Inheritance influences the type of ichthyosis.

Treatment

Topical therapy with AQUEOUS CREAM (UEA) or CETA-MACROGOL cream or 10% UREA in Vaseline. Refer severe types for further investigation.

Impetigo

Appearance

Honey-coloured crusts due to superficial streptococcal or staphylococcal infection of the skin. It may be primary or may supervene on other dermatoses, i.e. infected eczema may become crusted or impetigenized.

Treatment

◆ 2% VIOFORM in zinc cream to the skin and local hygiene. VIOFORM 3% in Eucerine or Betadine shampoo or Beta-dine cream to the scalp.
◆ If extensive: ERYTHROMYCIN or PENICILLIN orally.

Pitfall

If impetigo or eczema is on the face or the neck, tinea capitis or pediculosis of the scalp should be excluded.

Moles and pigmented naevi

See page 555.

Molluscum contagiosum

Appearance

Multiple flesh-coloured dome-shaped umbilicated papules. It is caused by pox virus.

Treatment

Apply a light application of liquid nitrogen. If the latter proves unsuccessful perform a gentle curettage or apply a pointed orange stick/cotton-tipped swab dipped in PHENOL 1% or 30-50% trichloracetic acid for a few seconds until the lesion turns white, or apply Duofilm (lactic acid 1 part, salicylic acid 1 part, collodion 3 parts).

Papular urticaria

Papular urticaria is very common. It is due to an insect bite allergy which causes recurrent itchy eruptions.

Appearance

The eruption is polymorphous and includes itchy papules with central excoriation, vesicles, impetigo and often bullae which may be large on the palms and soles. Older lesions on the trunk are pigmented or hypopigmented. The typical history is of improvement followed by recurrence.

Treatment

It is important to inform the mother that the eruption will recur possibly for years until the child develops an immunity to insect bites. Treatment is symptomatic. LOTION CALAMINE with menthol 0,25% and phenol 0,5% is applied to the eruption. It may be necessary to use HYDROCORTISONE 1% in HEB. HYDROXYZINE (Aterax) or TRIMEPRAZINE (Vallergan) given at night for sleep may be helpful.

Pediculosis

Louse infestation

Appearance

The patient presents with pruritus and crusted excoriations. These most often occur in the scalp, where the nits are attached to the hairs. Their presence may be confirmed by the examination of hair under a microscope.

Treatment

◆ Examine others in the household. Treat infected members with GAMMA BENZENE HEXACHLORIDE 1% (Lindane or Quellada lotion or shampoo) or BENZYL BENZOATE. Apply Lindane shampoo to the scalp for five minutes. Wash the Lindane out thoroughly. Repeat the treatment after seven to ten days.

◆ Children over two years: saturate the hair and scalp with a PERMETHRIN 1% cream rinse as a single treatment. Leave for ten minutes. Rinse with water. PERMETHRIN should not be used by nursing mothers.

Removal of nits

◆ Hair: soak the hair with 3-5% acetic acid solution and cover with a towel saturated with the same solution. The nits are combed from the hair with a fine-tooth comb.

◆ Eyelashes: apply Vaseline to the eyelashes twice daily for eight days. This is followed by mechanical removal of remaining nits.

Pityriasis rosea

Appearance

A widespread rash on the trunk with collarette of scale a few days after the herald patch.

Treatment

No specific therapy. Use HYDROCORTISONE 1% if an itch is present. Reassure parents that it is self-limiting, lasting about six weeks.

Pitfall

The herald patch is often mistaken for *tinea corporis.*

Pityriasis sicca alba

Appearance

Depigmented scaly white patches on the faces of young children.

Diagnosis

The diagnosis of *tinea versicolor* can be excluded by examining scale with KOH under a microscope.

Treatment

Mild emollient, e.g. UEA or HYDROCORTISONE 1% in HEB if severe or LPC 5% in HEB.

Pitfall

Pityriasis sicca alba is often mistaken for fungal infection, i.e. *tinea versicolor*. The latter is usually on the trunk and occurs largely in adults. Treatment with Whitfield's ointment will aggravate pityriasis sicca alba.

Psoriasis

Appearance

Erythematous lesions with silvery scale. The onset occurs at any age.

Treatment

◆ Use 5% crude coal tar in HEB or 5% LPC in HEB, or DITHRANOL: **expert supervision, clear detailed instructions and understanding are required.** Warn the patient that DITHRANOL can burn and stain the skin temporarily. DITHRANOL 0,5% in salicylic acid ointment 5% in yellow Vaseline is applied for half an hour only, then washed or showered off immediately.
◆ **Scalp:** apply salicylic acid ointment 2%, precipitated SULPHUR 2% in UEA to the scalp at night initially.
◆ **If no response:** apply DITHRANOL 0,5% in LYGOL solution (salicylic acid 3%, ppt sulphur 5% in HEB) for half an hour to scalp. Use Teepol shampoo to remove the DITHRANOL. Give precise and careful instructions about burning and care of the eyes to the patient.

Alternative treatment

Tar shampoo. Leave the lathered shampoo for half an hour under a shower cap followed by a rinse with water.

Severe lesions: special psoriasis scalp lotion at night.

Ringworm

I.e. *tinea* of the body (*corporis*), *tinea* of the scalp (*capitis*).

Appearance

A 'ringworm' is a dermatophyte fungal infection which produces an eczematous-type reaction with the clinical appearance of an annular 'ring' lesion, i.e. the inflammation is accentuated on the circumference where it is red and scaly or pustular. The diagnosis is made by the microscopic examination on a slide of a scale scraped from the edge of the lesion. A drop of potassium hydroxide 10-30% is added and the slide is warmed. The presence of fungal hyphae under the microscope or laboratory culture of the dermatophyte confirms the diagnosis.

Treatment

Tinea of the body

Topical therapy with Whitfield's ointment or colourless Castellani's paint for two to four weeks is usually adequate unless the lesion is very extensive or resistant. Newer preparations such as CLOTRIMAZOLE 1% cream (Canesten) or MICONAZOLE 2% cream (Daktarin), KETOCONAZOLE (Nizcreme) or ECONAZOLE (Pevaryl) are all equally effective, but they are more expensive than older treatments.

Tinea of the scalp

Topical therapy is of no value. Requires oral GRISEOFULVIN for six weeks. Instruct the patient to crush tablets and take with food or milk.

For children over two years ultra-microsize GRISEOFULVIN 10 mg/kg/day. Standard dosages are as follows:

♦ Two year old child: 125 mg (one tablet) daily.
♦ Five year old child: two tablets daily.
♦ Seven year old child: three tablets daily.
♦ Ten year old child: adult dose – four tablets a day for six weeks in divided doses.

Pitfall

Topical therapy is of no value in tinea of the scalp.

Scabies

Appearance

Patients present with a generalized itch. Look for burrows on the hands, between the fingers and on the genital area. Itchy papules on the faces of young infants occur occasionally but such lesions are usually confined to the trunk. The diagnosis is confirmed by finding the burrow and the mite.

Treatment

The whole family and everyone in the household must be treated simultaneously. Give written instructions. Apply Lindane (or Quellada) lotion (GAMMA BENZENE HEXACHLORIDE 1%) to the entire body below the neck. Do not soak in a hot bath prior to the application as this may cause absorption. Reapply if the hands need to be washed.

An application of the lotion is left on for 12-24 hours and washed off thoroughly. The lotion should be kept away from the eyes and mucous membranes. A second application is appropriate only when there is failure to comply, re-infestation or resistance. 10% of the Lindane applied to the skin can be recovered in the urine. Clinical central nervous system toxicity has occurred only with misuse related to abuse, overuse or failure of the patient to comprehend warning instructions.

Scabicides other than Lindane are preferred for infants, young children, pregnant or nursing women. In young infants apply sulphur 2,5% ointment three times daily for three days. Tetmosol soap is used in institutions in addition to the definitive treatment. BENZYL BENZOATE may alternatively be applied for 24 hours. It is cheaper but burns. Patients often wash it off and fail to carry out instructions properly. PERMETHRIN with 70-80% ovicidal activity has no reported adverse properties. Apply the cream rinse for ten minutes and then rinse it off with water.

Sunscreens

Long-term damage by excessive exposure to ultraviolet light may cause skin cancer, including melanoma. Fair-skinned children in particular should be advised to use sunscreens with a sun protection factor of 15 or more from early childhood. Sunbathing and sun exposure should be avoided from infancy and the use of protective clothing and hats is advisable.

Urticaria

Appearance

Lesions vary from erythema with little oedema to elevated, intensely itching, massive wheals with giant pseudopods.

Treatment

Cure depends on the identification and elimination of the aetiologic factor whenever possible. Symptomatic treatment consists of treatment with antihistamine for up to one month to prevent the development of chronic urticaria. The treatment of choice for the latter is HYDROXYZINE (Aterax).

Acute or severe urticaria and anaphylactic reaction and angioedema: see page 27.

Warts (Verruca vulgaris)

Extremely common and caused by a virus.

Appearance

Raised papules with a rough or digitate surface. They commonly measure from 3 to 10 mm in diameter.

Treatment

Instruct the patient carefully. Soak the wart(s) in hot water. Scrub with nailbrush. Apply wart paint and cover with plaster directly. Wart paint: salicylic acid 1 part, lactic acid 1 part, collodion 3 parts (available as Duofilm).

Warts may be pared after a few weeks. This method is particularly useful in plantar warts.

Note

Freezing with LIQUID NITROGEN is possible but is painful and not feasible when there are a large number of warts.

45 SURGERY

S Cywes, H Rode, A J W Millar and R A Brown

Newborn infants
Indications for surgery

Congenital abnormalities which if untreated are incompatible with life: diaphragmatic hernia; omphalocoele or gastroschisis; oesophageal atresia and trachea-oesophageal fistula (TOF); intestinal obstruction; anorectal malformations.

Contra-indications to surgery

Severe multiple congenital anomalies, some uncorrectable and incompatible with life.

Clinical presentation

Respiratory distress, gastrointestinal obstruction or obvious surface defects.

Factors influencing survival

♦ Uncontrollable: multiple congenital anomalies and prematurity.
♦ Controllable:
   ◇ **early diagnosis** by antenatal ultrasound and recognition during the perinatal period of the significance of symptoms;
   ◇ **prompt referral** to a specialist centre;
   ◇ **meticulous** peri-operative care;
   ◇ **correct timing of appropriate** surgery.

Diaphragmatic hernia (congenital)

Usually a posterolateral defect on the left side (15% right-sided).

Clinical presentation

♦ Antenatal diagnosis: ultrasound.

◆ Postnatal diagnosis: respiratory distress, apparent dextrocardia, bowel sounds in the chest and scaphoid abdomen.

Diagnosis

Chest X-ray confirms the diagnosis showing the deviated mediastinum and air-filled bowel in the hemithorax. See page 460.

Differential diagnosis: large pneumothorax, cystic adenomatoid malformation, eventration of the diaphragm and air-filled duplication cyst.

Management

◆ Nasogastric decompression.
◆ Respiratory support with oxygen and ventilation with paralysis if necessary.
◆ Stabilize before surgery over a matter of hours or days.
◆ Anticipate the formation of a pneumothorax.

Exomphalos (unruptured)

Clinical presentation

◆ Minor: abdominal wall defect <4 cm with bowel contained within a sac of peritoneum and amnion.
◆ Major: abdominal wall defect >4 cm with bowel and liver contained within the sac.

Management

◆ Transport: decompress the stomach with a nasogastric tube. Cover the exomphalos with plastic to prevent heat and fluid loss.
◆ Attempt a primary repair in most.
◆ Where there is a large defect in a small or unfit baby, paint the sac with 1% aqueous MERCUROCHROME. Delay repair if necessary for months.

Warning

◆ Exclude hypoglycaemia which may last for several weeks in a patient with the Beckwith-Wiedeman syndrome characterized by macroglossia, exomphalos or umbilical hernia and gigantism.
◆ Mercurial poisoning may result from the excessive use of MERCUROCHROME.

Gastroschisis and ruptured exomphalos

Clinical presentation

Gastroschisis: eviscerated bowel through a small defect to the right of the umbilicus. The bowel is thickened and oedematous.

Ruptured exomphalos: a larger central defect in the abdominal wall and evidence of the ruptured membranes which occur at delivery. Liver may be present outside the abdominal wall.

Management

♦ Cover with a plastic film or place the lower half of the baby in a plastic bag. Control heat and fluid loss, particularly during transport. Prevent infection.
♦ Attempt primary closure. Beware of impairment of respiration and venous return. Failure of primary closure requires the placement of a silastic silo. The bowel should be reduced and the abdominal wall defect repaired within ten days, before local sepsis develops.

Intestinal obstruction

High

Duodenal atresia or stenosis.
Malrotation with volvulus.
Proximal small bowel atresia.

Low

Distal small bowel or colonic atresia.
Meconium ileus.
Hirschsprung's disease.
Meconium plug syndrome.
Ano-rectal malformation.

Clinical presentation

♦ **Bile-stained** vomiting or **persistent** non-bile-stained vomiting.
♦ High obstruction: polyhydramnios and emphasis on vomiting.
♦ Low obstruction: emphasis on distension and failure to establish normal stooling. (Normally a large meconium stool is passed on day 1).

Diagnosis

Request an abdominal X-ray (AXR) in all patients and Barium (Ba) meal in those patients with bilious vomiting or incomplete proximal obstruction.

◆ **Duodenal atresia:** vomiting from birth. Stomach and duodenal fluid levels (double bubble), no gas distally unless there is a stenosis on AXR. See page 461.

◆ **Malrotation:** history of normal feeding then a **bile-stained vomit** or intermittent episodes of bile-stained vomiting. **There may be no other clinical evidence.** AXR shows evidence of high small bowel obstruction in 80% of cases but may be normal in 20%. Barium meal (Ba meal) is diagnostic showing malrotation and obstruction in the distal duodenum.

◆ **Proximal small bowel:** AXR usually diagnostic with several loops of distended bowel with fluid levels.

◆ **Distal small bowel:** distension marked and AXR shows many fluid levels. Prone film demonstrates the absence of gas in the distal bowel. Ba enema confirms the level of obstruction and patency of the colon (a second colonic atresia is present in 5% of small bowel atresias).

◆ **Meconium ileus:** family history of cystic fibrosis. Abdomen distended from birth. Minimal vomiting. Palpable loops of bowel. AXR has ground-glass appearance with dilated bowel, but few fluid levels. Ba enema: micro-colon.

◆ **Hirschsprung's disease:** suspect in an infant with bowel dysfunction where the continuity of intestinal tract is evident. Explosive decompression on rectal examination. Ba enema: transition zone between dilated proximal innervated and distal narrow aganglionic bowel. Suction rectal biopsy shows, on histology, absent ganglia with increased parasympathetic nerve fibres in the muscularis mucosa on the acetyl cholinesterase stain.

◆ **Meconium plug syndrome:** the diagnosis is by exclusion of Hirschsprung's disease, cystic fibrosis, hypothyroidism, the infant of a diabetic mother, medication in pregnancy or during labour affecting peristalsis, prematurity, and sepsis. Identify by Ba enema.

◆ **Ano-rectal obstruction:** evident on inspection. If in doubt, probe gently with a firm catheter.

◆ **Ano-rectal anomaly:** diagnosis **clinical.** Look at the perineum. Is the bladder palpable? Are the sacrum and coccyx normal?

Translevator (low)

◆ Male: anal pit, midline raphe or 'handle bar' across anal pit, meconium on perineum via ano-cutaneous fistula.
◆ Female: anus/fistula in vestibule separate from vaginal orifice. Direction on probing is posterior under skin of perineum.

Supra levator (high and intermediate)

◆ Male: meconium in urine via recto-urethral fistula.
◆ Female: anus/fistula not seen to be separate from vaginal orifice. Direction on probing is axial.

Lateral invertogram AXR. May need to wait 24 hours. Rectal gas shadow in relation to ischium: below inferior tip = low; higher than this or gas in bladder = high.

> ### Warning
> Meconium evident on a nappy does **not** exclude an anorectal malformation.

Management

General

Resuscitate, rehydrate and perform a surgical correction of the anomaly.

Special

◆ **Hirschsprung's disease:** decompress the bowel obstruction with rectal washouts before creating a colostomy proximal to the aganglionic bowel. Definitive correction by pull-through is performed as a second stage procedure six to nine months later.
◆ **Meconium plug syndrome:** treat with a half-strength GAS-TROGRAFIN enema. Laparotomy and the creation of a stoma proximal to the obstruction is performed if there is clinical deterioration or failure of decompression. Biopsy the distal bowel to exclude Hirschsprung's.
◆ **Meconium ileus:** uncomplicated, i.e. there is no evidence of meconium peritonitis or volvulus. Treat with a half-strength

GASTROGRAFIN enema. Complicated, delayed presentation, or unsuccessful enema requires laparotomy.
♦ **Ano-rectal anomaly:** low anomalies: cut back anoplasty. If in doubt, colostomy. High or intermediate: colostomy (proximal sigmoid) or transverse. Exclude other system anomalies, e.g. of the urinary tract by ultrasound and a micturating cysto-urethrogram (MCUG). An ano-rectoplasty is performed at between three and nine months of age.

Oesophageal atresia

Clinical presentation

♦ Polyhydramnios
♦ Frothy oral mucus
♦ Immediate regurgitation of feeds.

Diagnosis

Failure to pass a firm nasogastric tube (No. 12 Fr). Chest X-ray shows the nasogastric tube in the upper pouch. If a thin tube has been passed for feeding, the tube will be seen coiled in the upper pouch. See page 460.

Management

♦ Keep upper pouch empty by continuous aspiration, preferably with a Replogle tube.
♦ Place the infant in a 45° head-up position to prevent reflux via a tracheo-oesophageal fistula (TOF).
♦ Examine for, assess and manage other congenital abnormalities.
♦ Treat pneumonia if present (see page 524).
♦ Extrapleural thoracotomy, closure of the TOF and primary repair of oesophagus. Stage the repair and feed via a gastrostomy if the gap is wide or in the presence of a major life-threatening anomaly.

Cleft lip and palate

A common congenital anomaly in which the lip and/or the palate is cleft along the lines of embryological fusion. There is a family history in 20% of cases. Cleft lip and cleft lip and palate are genetically distinct from isolated cleft palate.

Clinical presentation

Approximately 50% of patients present as cleft lip and palate, 25% isolated cleft lip, and 25% isolated cleft palate. Associated anomalies are found in 20%. Only the uvula may be cleft or grooved (submucous cleft palate), which may cause early otitis media.

Management

◆ **Cleft lip:** breast feeding should be encouraged but, if not possible, use expressed breast milk. Refer to plastic surgeon for reassurance of parents and arrangement of surgery between three and six months. In a few cases, surgery can be done a few days after birth.

◆ **Cleft palate:** encourage breast-feeding and in general avoid using nasogastric feeding unless too weak to feed normally. An adapted teat may be required for wide cleft or Pierre Robin syndrome.

◆ **Cleft lip and palate:** feed the baby with expressed breast milk via a nasogastric tube. Refer to orthodontist for a special feeding plate and to a plastic surgeon for parent counselling and arrangement for surgical correction at three to six months. At the Red Cross War Memorial Children's Hospital, the lip and the palate are repaired in a single operation where possible.

Early surgery minimizes the risk of middle ear infection. In bilateral clefts or very wide clefts of the palate, the repair may have to be accomplished in stages and may be delayed until sufficient tissue has developed.

Post-operative management

The babies stay in hospital for three days post-operatively and are fed with a teaspoon for about ten days. During that time the arms should be restrained so that the baby cannot push a finger through the repaired tissues.

Regular follow up at OPD clinic. Further surgery may be necessary for revision of the lip and nose before school; or secondary surgery of the palate for fistula or nasal speech; bone graft of the alveolus at about nine to 11 years; and final cosmetic correction of the nose at about 16 years.

Specific surgical conditions
Abscess
Extremely common.

Clinical presentation
Pus under pressure leads to pain, swelling, loss of function and toxaemia. All soft tissue and lymph node drainage areas are affected.

Management
Surgical drainage. Treat with antibiotics. See Appendix 1.

Special sites
◆ **Breast:** complication of neonatal hyperplasia.
Management: avoid manipulation or massage. Peripheral dependent incision and drainage. Administer broad spectrum antibiotics, as necrotizing fasciitis and breast bud damage may occur.
◆ **Abdominal wall:** deeply placed intramuscular abscess. May mimic intra-abdominal pathology, i.e. RUQ — liver abscess; RLQ — appendix abscess; flank — perirenal abscess.
◆ **Pyogenic psoas abscess:** common in boys. Pain, fever and fixed flexion of the hip with lack of gastrointestinal symptoms. Walks with a limp. Mass palpable in iliac fossa. Confirm diagnosis by ultrasound.
Management: via an extraperitoneal approach, pus is located in pale oedematous muscle with needle aspiration prior to incision and drainage.
◆ **Liver abscess:** fever and RUQ pain with tender hepatomegaly. Pyogenic abscess is three times more common than amoebic abscess. Confirm diagnosis with ultrasound and the complement fixation test.
Treat with antibiotics. See Appendix 1. See page 592.
Surgical drainage: if signs and symptoms persist beyond two days of medical treatment or worsen. Most left-lobed abscesses require surgery, which is necessary in 60-70% of cases overall.
◆ **Suppurative adenitis of the deep external iliac nodes:** the presentation and treatment are similar to psoas abscess. Healing septic skin lesion is evident on the leg of the affected side.

Anal fissure

(See 'Constipation', page 218.)

This is the most common cause of fresh rectal bleeding. Identify by inspection. May require examination under anaesthetic, anal stretch and removal of faecaloma.

Appendicitis

Clinical presentation

Anorexia, nausea, vomiting, abdominal pain, disturbance of stooling pattern. Localized signs of inflammation in RIF, right flank or pelvis. Evidence of a systemic response with pyrexia, tachycardia, raised WBC.

A urinary tract infection and renal colic must be excluded and, in girls with high fever and a vaginal discharge, a primary peritonitis.

AXR: localized ileus, faecolith, scoliosis concave to right and blurring of soft tissue definition.

Management

◆ Full resuscitation prior to appendicectomy is important.
◆ Prophylactic antibiotics: PENICILLIN, Gram-negative cover + METRONIDAZOLE (Flagyl) to prevent wound infection. See page 646.

Ascariasis

See page 294.

Clinical presentation

Age four to ten years.

Heavy infestation leads to bolus obstruction ('worm colic') with colic, vomiting and palpable masses. AXR: whorls of worms and signs of partial obstruction.

Management

◆ Treat with bed rest, IVF, nasogastric tube, analgesia, antispasmodics, e.g. HYOSCINE BUTYLBROMIDE (Buscopan).
◆ 95% resolve within 24 hours.
◆ A vermifuge is only administered when asymptomatic.
◆ Beware of complications, viz impaction necrosis producing a

tender mass – or volvulus – a tender mass with shock. In these cases, management requires laparotomy.

Complications

◆ **Biliary ascariasis:** presents with biliary colic. Worms may enter the liver with heavy intestinal infestation.
The majority (95%) resolve on conservative treatment (see page 293). Monitor with ultrasound.
Complications: cholangitis, liver abscess, biliary strictures. Identify worms with endoscopic retrograde cholangio-pancreatography (ERCP) and extract endoscopically if symptoms fail to resolve, or worms still present after more than four weeks. Surgical exploration if ERCP unavailable or fails.
◆ **Pancreatitis:** generalized pain with raised serum amylase. Treatment: resuscitation and supportive therapy.
◆ **Intussusception:** treat as described (see page 554).
◆ **Appendicitis:** treat as described (see page 557).

Biliary atresia and neonatal cholestasis

See page 360.

Clinical presentation

Pale stools, dark urine and clinical jaundice after the first two weeks of life must be considered pathological until proven otherwise by investigation that shows patency of the extrahepatic biliary tree. See page 356.

Diagnosis

The neonatal hepatitis syndrome is often impossible to differentiate from biliary atresia before operative cholangiogram. Delay in diagnosis of biliary atresia leads to progressive biliary cirrhosis and a rapidly decreasing chance of obtaining bile flow through a Kasai (porto-enterostomy) procedure.

Plan of investigation

◆ Stool observation (the bakkie test, see page 658) shows acholic stools over a period of one week.
◆ Haematology and liver function tests that demonstrate evidence of cholestatic jaundice.
◆ Ultrasound and radio-isotope imaging.

♦ Screening tests to exclude infection (TORCH), metabolic and genetic disorders.
♦ Refer to surgeons early for open liver biopsy and cholangiography.

Branchial arch and cleft remnants

Cysts which may become infected. Fistulae or sinuses. Cartilaginous skin tags.

♦ **Pre-auricular skin tag:** requires cosmetic excision.
♦ **Pre-auricular sinus:** leave. Treat with antibiotics if infected. Follow with total excision of the fistulous track in quiescent phase.
♦ **First branchial arch cyst and first branchial arch fistula:** opens under angle of the jaw below and extends to external auditory canal above. Excise carefully as the fistula lies close to the facial nerve.
♦ **Branchial cyst:** presents late in childhood as a lateral cystic swelling in the anterior triangle of the neck. Excise when diagnosed.
♦ **Second arch fistula:** opens along the lower anterior border of the sternomastoid and extends to the tonsillar fossa through the carotid bifurcation. 15% bilateral. Mucous discharge. Excise before three years of age if possible. Its course through the neck is horizontal at this age.

Cervical lymphadenopathy

Aetiology

♦ Reactive hyperplasia: viral.
♦ Acute suppurative lymphadenitis: coccal or haemophilus infection.
♦ Chronic adenitis: *Mycobacterium-avium-intracellulare-scrofulaceum complex* (MAIS): subacute course, unilateral, negative Mantoux, not responsive to anti-TB therapy, requires excision for a cure.
♦ Tuberculosis: chronic course and often associated with pulmonary infection. Responds to anti-TB therapy. See page 566.
♦ Neoplasia.

  ◇ Primary: Hodgkins/non-Hodgkins lymphoma.
  ◇ Secondary: less common in children.

Management

◆ Exclude generalized systemic, regional and local disease.
◆ FBC, ESR, CXR, and Mantoux test.
◆ Treat acute infections with antibiotics. See Appendix 1.
◆ Indications for excision biopsy: clinically suspicious, e.g. long history, >2,5 cm diameter, firm, hard, matted or failure to respond to antibiotics in two weeks.

Circumcision

The only medical indication is phimosis caused by recurrent episodes of balanoposthitis.

Adherence of the inner foreskin is a normal phenomenon (15-20% are still adherent by five years, <1% at 12 years).

Management

◆ Absolute contra-indication: hypospadias or ammoniacal dermatitis.
◆ Delay till out of nappies if not done as a neonate.
◆ Do not attempt forcible retraction.
◆ Mild degrees of phimosis respond to 1% HYDROCORTI-SONE cream applied locally for ten days.
◆ Complications: bleeding, infection, coronal fistula, too much skin removed, meatal ulceration and stenosis. Plastibell circumcisions done as outpatient procedures have a higher incidence of complications.

Cystic hygroma

Clinical presentation

Multiple fluid-filled endothelial-lined cysts. Usually evident from birth in cervicofacial region. Multiple cysts often surround vital structures in the neck.

Management

◆ Do **not** aspirate.
◆ Early referral.
◆ Infection may be lethal with gross tissue oedema obstruction of the airway.
◆ Spontaneous resolution unlikely.
◆ Careful surgical excision, which may be done in stages.

Ear deformities

Can be corrected at any time after nine months, but preferably before school-going age. (See page 192.)

Ectopia vesicae (bladder exstrophy)

Clinical presentation

The anterior abdominal wall below the umbilicus is deficient and the bladder lies open and exposed. The anus is anteriorly placed. There is epispadias or a bifid clitoris and wide separation of the symphysis pubis. Associated exomphalos is common.

Management

Early closure is advocated and immediate referral to a specialist centre is imperative.

Fused labia

Clinical presentation

Often referred to as absent vagina, or with wetting problems. Delicate incomplete fusion of labia minora in midline.

Management

Treat with local application of oestrogen cream. If this fails, separate under sedation or general anaesthetic. Apply cream locally to prevent recurrence.

Haemangioma and vascular malformations

Clinical presentation

♦ **'Stork bites':** small pink or red marks (macular stains) on the forehead and eyelids. Most fade in the first six months.
♦ **'Strawberry naevus'** (capillary haemangioma): raised bright red lesion. May increase in size in first months of life but will resolve completely. Best left alone.
♦ **Mixed haemangioma (capillary cavernous):** there may be extensive proliferation in the first months of life. Systemic complications such as thrombocytopenia or cardiac failure are common. Local interference with vital functions (airway, eye) may warrant intervention.

◆ **Cavernous haemangioma:** soft, puffy, usually well-circumscribed lesion which is often found deep in soft tissue or muscle. Excision is usually required for diagnosis and cure.
◆ **Vascular malformation** (Port Wine stain): present at birth. Grows commensurately without involution.

Management

◆ **Haemangiomas**
Essentially observation in the majority.
Small lesions causing trouble (bleeding, infected or traumatized): local steroid injections or local excision.
Large lesions with rapid growth: PREDNISOLONE 4-8 mg/kg/day for three weeks. Discontinue if there is no response. If there is a good response, continue for three months and gradually tail off over four to six weeks.
Prognosis: most will undergo considerable spontaneous involution which is complete by about seven years of age.
◆ **Malformations (Port Wine stain)**
Pulsed dye flash lamp laser therapy may result in good cosmetic result.

Hernia

Hydrocoeles

Present at birth due to a thinly patent processus vaginalis and entrapment of fluid within the tunica vaginalis testis. Diagnosis is confirmed by the ability to 'get above it' and with transillumination. Resolution is usually spontaneous.

Herniotomy is indicated:

◆ when the hydrocoele is huge and tense;
◆ when it persists beyond 12 months of age;
◆ if the hydrocoele develops later in childhood or is associated with an abnormal testis.

Fluid hernia

This implies a wider patency of the processus vaginalis with fluctuation in size. Elective herniotomy is indicated as bowel-containing hernias commonly develop and spontaneous resolution is unlikely.

Inguinal hernia

◆ All inguinal hernias at any age require surgical treatment without delay.
◆ The younger the patient, the greater the incidence of complications, viz. irreducibility, obstruction, strangulation and gonadal ischaemia.
◆ Irreducible hernias with evidence of strangulation (local oedema being the first sign) require immediate surgery after resuscitation.
◆ Irreducible hernias without evidence of strangulation. A single attempt at gentle manual reduction can be made after sedation. If successful: repair after 24-48 hours. If unsuccessful: immediate operation.

Warning

In females a gonad may be found in the hernial sac. This should be examined and biopsied at surgery to exclude androgen insensitivity (testicular feminizing syndrome). Chromosomal sexing should be done prior to surgery if the hernias are bilateral and contain gonads. The passage of a thin probe into the vagina, confirming its presence and length >3 cms, also confirms female sex.

Para-umbilical and supra-umbilical hernias

Do not regress, frequently strangulate, and should be repaired.

Umbilical hernias

These tend to regress spontaneously and rarely strangulate. Repair at five years of age if there are no signs of closure.

Complications may occur in association with pica (sand-eating) as the intestinal contents are putty-like and become entrapped in the hernia. They usually reduce on bed rest and sedation. Treatment of iron deficiency and elective repair are indicated.

Hypospadias and chordee

Meatal obstruction does not occur and circumcision is contra-indicated. May be corrected surgically from the age of one year and should be completed before school-going age.

Intersex
Clinical presentation

It is difficult to determine the correct gender from the appearance of abnormal external genitalia. Practical issues related to phallic size may direct one to female gender of rearing regardless of chromosome genotype. This decision should be made as soon as possible after birth.

Refer for immediate evaluation:

◆ any infant with abnormal or ambiguous genitalia;
◆ a 'boy' with hypospadias and undescended testes;
◆ a 'boy' with perineo-scrotal hypospadias;
◆ boys with bilaterally impalpable testes;
◆ girls with bilateral gonad-containing inguinal hernias.

Intussusception
Clinical presentation

This typically presents as a sudden onset of colic with vomiting in a previously healthy infant of less than two years of age. Bloody stools and evidence of obstruction occur later. An abdominal mass may be more easily palpable by rectal examination. Delay in diagnosis leads to significant morbidity and even mortality. Diagnosis is excluded by contrast enema as most arise from lymphoid hyperplasia in the ileo-caecal region. If it occurs in a child older than two years, think of lead-point pathology, e.g. Meckel's diverticulum, hamartoma, duplication cyst or lymphoma.

Management

◆ Uncomplicated cases with early diagnosis: hydrostatic barium enema or pneumatic reduction after resuscitation by restoration of circulating blood volume (use colloid 10-20 ml/kg) and adequate sedation (1 mg/kg PETHIDINE IM). Success rate ±60%.
◆ Contra-indications to attempted reduction are: tender mass, peritonitis, generally poor condition, more than 36 hours of symptoms, established small bowel obstruction with distension and multiple fluid levels on AXR. These patients are managed by laparotomy after full resuscitation. Manual reduction may still be successful but if this fails, bowel resection.

Lymphangioma

These hamartomas contain a mix of mesodermal elements (angiomatous, lymphatic and other soft tissues). A wide field of abnormality may be present with associated bony deformity. Infections are common and may be indolent.

Management

Treatment is directed at the control of infection.

Staged conservative excision is indicated on cosmetic grounds from the age of three months or because of interference with function.

Macroglossia (enlarged tongue)

May be encountered with: Beckwith-Wiedeman syndrome; Down's syndrome; hypothyroidism; lymphangiomatous, haemangiomatous or neurofibromatous involvement.

Management is by partial glossectomy if the tongue cannot be comfortably accommodated in the mouth. Beware of severe post-operative oedema and airway obstruction.

Meatal stenosis

A pinhole meatus with a thin stream on micturition, which usually results from inappropriately-timed circumcision and a healed meatal ulcer. Management is by a generous meatotomy.

Moles or pigmented naevi

Most are innocent junctional or compound naevi. Deeply pigmented large naevi (giant hairy naevi) require excision with skin grafting if necessary. Those that need to be completely excised to exclude malignancy include those subject to repeated trauma, sudden change in size or colour, or where itching, halo formation and ulceration occur. Malignant melanoma is very uncommon.

Parotid enlargement

Aetiology

Inflammatory causes

◆ Parotitis
  ◇ Viral, e.g. mumps.

◇ Acute suppurative: often associated with trauma to the meatus of the parotid duct during teething or sucking. Commonly seen in AIDS. Treat with antibiotics. See Appendix 1.

◆ **Recurrent parotitis of childhood:** unilateral mild symptoms, four to ten years of age, and due to rupture of acini and chemical inflammation (sialectasis). Spontaneous resolution at puberty.

Other causes

Lymph node enlargement within the gland capsule, e.g. pyogenic, TB, lymphoma. Also auto-immune disease, starvation, mesodermal malformation, haemangioma, first branchial arch cyst and tumour.

Management

Identify the cause by biopsy if necessary. Take a conservative approach to hamartoma or haemangioma because of the danger of facial nerve damage. Refer tumours to a specialist centre.

Pyloric stenosis

Clinical presentation

The incidence in the first six weeks of life is one in 500 infants. Male to female ratio is 4:1. Persistent non-bile-stained forceful vomiting develops after some weeks of normal feeding. Constipation or green mucoid 'hunger' stools.

Complications

◆ Haematemesis: due to gastritis, Mallory-Weis tear or oesophagitis.
◆ Metabolic: jaundice, dehydration, hyponatraemia, hypochloraemia, hypokalaemia, metabolic alkalosis.
◆ Infections: chest and urinary tract.

Diagnosis

Clinical. Empty the stomach with a nasogastric tube. Test feed. Look for epigastric peristalsis and feel for the 'olive' tumour with the left hand. Typically firm, and intermittently palpable to the right of rectus sheath below the liver. If in doubt, ultrasound, Ba meal. See page 99.

Management

◆ Rehydrate and correct metabolic and electrolyte abnormalities. Half N saline in 10% dextrose water plus added potassium chloride over 24-36 hours. See Chapter 21.
◆ Treat infection.
◆ Give Vitamin K_1 1 mg IM.
◆ Pyloromyotomy once fully resuscitated.

Ranula

Single mucous-filled retention cyst in the floor of the mouth. Treat by deroofing and marsupialization.

Ranula: plunging (mucus extravasation syndrome)

Multilocular often bilateral mucous-filled cysts in the floor of the mouth extending posteriorly and occasionally into the neck. Not epithelial-lined. Requires sublingual gland excision for a cure.

Rectal bleeding

Aetiology

◆ Neonate: necrotizing enterocolitis, fissure, idiopathic colitis.
◆ Infant: fissure, intussusception, polyp, Meckel's diverticulum, enterocolitis.
◆ Child: juvenile polyp, fissure, Meckel's diverticulum, lymphoid hyperplasia. Dysentery (shigella, salmonella, campylobacter, amoebic, viral). From the upper GIT, e.g. peptic ulcer or variceal haemorrhage, haemangioma, duplication cyst.

Warning

Beware of underlying systemic illness (haematological, malignancy).

Management

◆ Exclude a bleeding diathesis and local anal cause. Identify the level of bleeding.
◆ Pass a nasogastric tube: the pathology is distal to the

duodeno-jejunal flexure if no blood is aspirated. Exclude a Meckel's diverticulum by technetium scan and enterocolitis by stool microscopy and culture. A colonic cause is confirmed by Ba enema and colonoscopy.
♦ A laparotomy may be necessary after negative investigation.

Rectal prolapse
Partial thickness

Most commonly due to a faulty bowel habit.

Management

Attend to constipation (See page 218).

Full thickness prolapse

Differentiate this from prolapsed intussusception which is characterized by a sulcus between the anal canal and intussusception, severe congestion and sausage shape, and the prolapse of a rectal polyp.

Identify a possible underlying cause such as cystic fibrosis, whooping cough, procto-colitis, trichuris infestation, neurologic causes, e.g. spina bifida; and anatomic causes, e.g. exstrophy of the bladder.

Management

♦ Emergency management requires sedation, reduction of the prolapse, and buttock-strapping for 48 hours.
♦ Definitive treatment is indicated after relapse with strapping.
♦ Sclerosant submucous injection of 5% PHENOL in almond oil.
♦ Thiersch circumanal suture using No. 1 gauge absorbable suture.
♦ Formal reconstruction or amputation is rarely required.

Scrotum (the acute scrotum)
Aetiology

♦ Torsion of the testes is the most common cause in all age groups.
♦ Other causes in order of frequency are:
  ◇ epididymo-orchitis;

◇ torsion of a testicular appendage;
◇ idiopathic scrotal oedema;
◇ funiculitis (infected material may descend into the scrotum via a patent processus vaginalis); or
◇ scrotal cellulitis.
◆ Always exclude a strangulated inguinal hernia by confirming scrotal rather than inguinoscrotal swelling.

Management

◆ A confident clinical diagnosis cannot be made. **Urgent surgical exploration is advocated.**
◆ When a torsion is found and, after correcting the torsion and fixing the testis, the opposite side must be explored and fixed.
◆ If inflammation is found, take a pus swab for culture and antibiotic sensitivity.
  ◇ If the testis is very swollen, a releasing incision in the tunica albuginea will alleviate pain and protect the testis from atrophy.
◆ Post-operatively an underlying genito-urinary abnormality should be sought.

Sternomastoid tumour
Infant

Presents with a firm mass in the sternomastoid muscle with the head turned away from, but tilted towards, the affected side.

Management

Passive stretching which, if performed diligently, is successful in nearly all cases.

Older child

Torticollis develops, which leads to facial hemi-hypoplasia and plagiocephaly due to persistent fibrosis and shortening of the muscle.

Exclude squints and cervical spine deformity which may also give rise to torticollis.

Management

Torticollis is treated by division of the sternomastoid muscle and deep fascia of the neck. Postoperative physiotherapy is essential to reorientate the plane of vision and to maintain the release.

Note: Postural torticollis that results from *in utero* positional moulding corrects itself in the first few months of life.

Tongue tie

Does not interfere with feeding or speech and seldom requires surgical correction.

Management

If at two years the child is unable to protrude the tongue beyond the incisors, and the tongue is indented in midline by frenulum tethering, perform release as a formal procedure under general anaesthetic.

Undescended testes

By definition this is a testis that has never been in the scrotum and cannot be manipulated to the bottom of the scrotum. This differentiates true undescended testes from retractile testes.

Management

◆ There is no place for hormonal therapy *per se*.
◆ Surgery is indicated: to improve fertility, prevent complications such as hernia and torsion; monitor for evidence of later malignant change (30-50 times greater incidence in intra-abdominal testes, ten times greater incidence in palpable testes); and for psychological reasons.
◆ Orchidopexy should be performed during the second year of life. Long-term follow-up is mandatory.

Umbilicus

Clinical presentation

◆ **Omphalitis:** See page 354.
◆ **Granuloma:** pale pink granuloma due to incomplete healing following separation of the cord. Treat with local excision or silver nitrate cauterization.
◆ **Polyp 'Cherry tumour':** vitelline mucosal remnant.
◆ **Faeculent discharge:** patent vitello-intestinal duct.
◆ **Purulent discharge:** treat as for omphalitis.
◆ **Watery discharge:** suspect a patent urachus.

Management

A sinogram will identify any deeper fistulous connection. Most require umbilical exploration to exclude an attached Meckel's band.

46 TUBERCULOSIS

M A Kibel

Primary infection

Infection with *Mycobacterium tuberculosis* that results in tuberculosis (TB) is generally derived from close contact with an adult who has active disease.

◆ Sites
  ◇ Common: lungs from inhalation of tiny droplets of secretions containing *M. tuberculosis*.
  ◇ Rare: oropharynx and tonsils, bowel (as a result of ingestion of non-pasteurized milk), and the skin and eyes, as a result of direct inoculation.
◆ Ghon focus
  Infection then develops at the primary site which is followed by spread along the lymphatics to the regional lymph nodes.
◆ Haematogenous spread
  Seeding of mycobacteria via the blood stream at this early stage may occur to areas with a high oxygen tension, e.g. the apices of the lungs, brain, bones and kidneys. Such foci may remain dormant and only become reactivated after many years.
◆ Hypersensitivity
  After six to eight weeks, the development of cellular immunity begins to contain the infection but this is associated with hypersensitivity to tuberculo-protein.

Clinical presentation

This clinical spectrum is remarkably varied. Any organ or part of the body may be involved by tuberculosis.

Silent infection

◆ 85% of cases.

Usual

◆ A reactive tuberculin skin test.

- Clinical evidence of hypersensitivity, i.e. mild fever and tiredness, or more rarely, erythema nodosum, phlyctenular conjunctivitis, and Poncet's arthritis.
- Failure to thrive is a general feature, and fever, lassitude and persistent cough are usually present.
- Palpable glands in the neck.
- Progression of the primary complex in the lung and/or regional glands may result in cough, wheezing and stridor.
- Miliary tuberculosis resulting from rapid haematogenous dissemination.

Less common

- Abdominal.
- Isolated haematogenous extension (brain, skeleton, kidneys etc.).
- Extension along lymphatics (cervical, abdominal or other nodes).
- Late reactivation (adult type TB). This is relatively common in older children and adolescents, and may even occur in toddlers with a depressed immunological system.

Diagnosis

A presumptive diagnosis is made, taking into consideration the history, clinical findings, tuberculin skin test, radiology and laboratory investigations.

History

- Suspicion is half-way to the diagnosis. Always enquire about possible contacts in the home.
- Think of TB when there is:
    ◇ weight loss or failure to gain;
    ◇ cough lasting longer than two weeks, especially when associated with a wheeze or stridor; or
    ◇ enlarged lymph nodes, liver or spleen.

Tuberculin skin tests

- Skin reactivity indicates either infection with the tubercle bacillus, vaccination with BCG, or infection with other mycobacteria.
- A positive test is not necessarily an indication of disease.
- The test is administered on the volar aspect of the left forearm.

Mantoux test

This is the most accurate test. A stabilized solution of 0,1 ml PPD is injected intradermally. A strength of 5 TU per dose is most generally used. Inject 5 TU PPD in 0,1 ml solution just beneath the skin surface with **the needle bevel facing upwards.** A skin weal of 6-10 mm in diameter should be produced.

Reading the Mantoux test

The test is read at 48-72 hours. **Measure the transverse diameter of palpable induration only.**

♦ Non-reactive (negative): 0-4 mm
♦ Doubtful: 5-9 mm
♦ Reactive and positive: 10-14 mm
♦ Strongly reactive and positive: 15 mm or more

Tine test

This is easy to administer, but less accurate, and doubtful results should be followed by a Mantoux test. It is a disposable test with dried PPD on four Tines which are pressed into the skin.

Reading the Tine test

This is done at 48-72 hours but the result can be read up to one week. Confluence of two or more papules with or without vesiculation is interpreted as strongly reactive and comparable to a Mantoux test induration of 15 mm or more. Any other reaction is regarded as doubtful and, where suspicion of TB is high, retesting by Mantoux is required **within one week** of the original test. The time limit is important in order to avoid boosting of the delayed hypersensitivity response.

Interpretation of skin tests

BCG vaccination, which induces a degree of skin reactivity, confuses the interpretation of the tuberculin skin test.

♦ **A strongly reactive** Mantoux or Tine test should be interpreted as indicating tuberculous infection. There may or may not be clinical evidence of disease (see pages 562-3).
♦ **A reactive** Mantoux test in a child who has not received BCG in the previous two years should be regarded as due to tuberculous infection. There may or may not be clinical

evidence of disease (see page 562). A **doubtful** or **non-reactive** test does not exclude tuberculosis.

> **Warning**
> ♦ Tuberculin tests are **contra-indicated** in phlyctenular conjunctivitis. Use only 0,5 TU if erythema nodosum is present.

Radiology

There are a variety of radiological presentations. See pages 468-9.

Laboratory investigations

♦ Gastric washings to identify the organism. Three consecutive early morning specimens should be obtained (sputum in older children). The acid in the gastric washings should be neutralized with bicarbonate before sending the specimen to the laboratory.
♦ The erythrocyte sedimentation rate (ESR) is usually elevated.
♦ Liver function tests should be done to obtain a baseline prior to commencement of drug therapy.
♦ Adenosine deaminase (ADA) levels in pleural aspirate may be elevated (>35 units/l).
♦ Biopsy of the liver, bone marrow, pleura or superficial lymph node for **histology and culture** may assist in making a diagnosis.

Management

Treatment

Highly effective therapy is available. There are, however, a number of practical difficulties associated with it:

♦ lengthy duration of the treatment;
♦ difficulty in ensuring compliance; and
♦ high costs of certain drugs, e.g. RIFAMPICIN.

General

Treatment is usually given in Local Authority Clinics and under supervision. Drugs other than ISONIAZID should never be issued unless compliance can be assured. At clinics, medications are given five times a week. See Table 46.1 for medicines (and their abbreviations) used in the treatment of TB.

Contacts

Infants and children (under two years) **of tuberculous mothers are at exceptional risk**, and should receive INH + PZA + RIF for three months. Mothers on therapy may continue to breast-feed. If supervision is possible, a child under the age of five years who has been exposed but is not infected (tuberculin test (TT) non-reactive) should be given INH + PZA + RIF for three months. Where supervision is not possible, give only INH for three months.

Table 46.1 Medicines used in the treatment of TB

Medication	Dosage (mg/kg/day)	Side-effects
RIFAMPICIN (RIF)	10	Hepatitis, rash, 'flu syndrome' pruritis, flushing of skin
ISONIAZID (INH)	10	Peripheral neuropathy, convulsions, hepato-toxicity
PYRAZINAMIDE (PZA)	20-40	Hepatotoxicity, fever photosensitivity, rash
STREPTOMYCIN	20-40	Vestibular damage, fever, rash
ETHAMBUTOL	15-20	Retrobulbar neuritis
ETHIONAMIDE[1]	10-20	Nausea, vomiting, abdominal pain
THIACETAZONE	2,5-3,5	Nausea, vomiting, rash

[1] ETHIONAMIDE. Only limited stocks exist. These should be reserved for tuberculous meningitis, or multiresistant cases.

Infected patients

Children under five years who are infected (strongly reactive tuberculin skin test) but who have no apparent clinical disease: INH + PZA + RIF should be given for three months under supervision. Otherwise, INH only for six months.

Patients with disease

Standard treatment of TB now consists of a four-month supervised regimen of INH, RIF and PZA given five times a week for 8 weeks followed by INH and RIF only for 8 weeks. The latter can be given either 5 times a week or twice weekly in high dosage (intermittent therapy). Advanced disseminated cases should receive a full six months of therapy with all three agents. When these drugs are used individually, the standard dosages are:

◆ **INH:** 10 mg/kg/day
◆ **PZA:** 25 mg/kg/day
◆ **RIF:** 10 mg/kg/day.

For miliary TB and TBM, higher dosages are given (INH 20, PZA 40, RIF 20 mg/kg/day) and ETHIONAMIDE (20 mg/kg/day) added. All drugs should be given in a single daily dose before breakfast. Standard dosages should be introduced after two months of therapy.

Notification

TB is a notifiable disease in terms of the Health Act No. 63 of 1977. It is the responsibility of the doctor who makes the diagnosis to notify the relevant local authority.

Categories that are notifiable are shown on page 277.

Prevention of tuberculosis

BCG, a live attenuated vaccine provides considerable protection against progressive and disseminated tuberculosis. It should be given at birth and repeated at three months if no visible scar is present. It was previously also repeated at pre-school and at school-leaving age but this practice has been discontinued. The normal reaction to BCG is a group of papules reaching a maximum size four to six weeks after vaccination. The development of a papule or ulcer within a week of administration should be interpreted as a strongly reactive tuberculin skin test. Such cases should be questioned regarding possible symptoms of tuberculous infection and investigated further.

Sterilization

Japanese Needle Planted Cylinder BCG Vaccinating Tool: sterilize in 2% solution of CYDEX between vaccinations to inhibit transmission of HIV and hepatitis B viruses. See sterilization instruction in every pack if CYDEX is not available.

Agents: Vaccina cc, PO Box 804, Gardenview.

APPENDIX 1
ANTIBIOTIC USAGE

D H Hanslo and P Roux

Notes on antibiotic usage

1. The availability of individual preparations may vary according to pharmacy coding or antibiotic policy. When in doubt consult with the local pharmacist or microbiologist.

2. Normal dosage, administration and length of therapy are implied, except where otherwise indicated. **Dosages of medication have been carefully checked, but the editor and publishers cannot take responsibility for inaccuracies. Always check product information. See page 315.**

3. For practical purposes the following have equivalent antimicrobial activity and can be regarded as interchangeable:
   ♦ GENTAMICIN = TOBRAMYCIN = NETILMICIN
   ♦ CEFOTAXIME = CEFTRIAXONE
   ♦ AMOXYCILLIN (for oral therapy) = AMPICILLIN (for parenteral therapy)
   ♦ Oral cephalosporins: CEFACLOR = CEFADROXIL = CEPHALEXIN = CEPHRADINE; but CEFUROXIME = CEPHRADINE; but CEFUROXIME, CEFPODOXIME and CEFIXIME are more active.

Condition	First choice	Alternate agents	Comments
CARDIAC or ENDOCARDITIS			
Endocarditis on prosthetic valve or material			
Early (under six months)	CLOXACILLIN 100 mg/kg/day IV + GENTAMICIN 5 mg/kg/day for six weeks		
Late	PENICILLIN 250 000 U/kg/day + GENTAMICIN for four weeks		
Enteric G-ve Bacillus/Haemophilus	CEFOTAXIME 100 mg/kg/day for four to six weeks	AMPICILLIN	Add GENTAMICIN 7,5 mg/kg/day in severe cases
Enterococcus	PENICILLIN + GENTAMICIN for four weeks		
Organism not known	PENICILLIN + GENTAMICIN for four weeks		Low serum levels of GENTAMICIN adequate for synergy. Add CLOXACILLIN if Staphylococcus a possibility

Condition	First choice	Alternate agents	Comments
Staphylococcus	CLOXACILLIN IV + FUSIDIC ACID 30 mg/kg/day oral for four weeks	CLOXACILLIN + GENTAMICIN VANCOMYCIN alone	
'Viridans' streptococcus	PENICILLIN + GENTAMICIN for two weeks, then AMOXYCILLIN 250 mg oral 3 x daily + PROBENECID for two weeks		
Rheumatic fever	PENICILLIN V	PROCAINE PENICILLIN ERYTHROMYCIN	
Prophylaxis			
Dental, low risk	AMOXYCILLIN 750 mg-3 g oral stat depending on age	ERYTHROMYCIN for two doses	Given one hour before procedure
Nondental or high risk or anaesthesia	AMOXYCILLIN four hours before + six hours after	AMOXYCILLIN + PROBENECID four hours before	
Cardiac surgery	CLOXACILLIN + GENTAMICIN for three doses	VANCOMYCIN + GENTAMICIN	

Condition	First choice	Alternate agents	Comments
Rheumatic fever	BENZATHINE PENICILLIN IM monthly	PENICILLIN V oral 2 x daily ERYTHROMYCIN oral 2 x daily SULPHADIAZINE 500 mg daily	
ENT INFECTIONS			
Diphtheria Case	PENICILLIN IV		IMMEDIATE ANTITOXIN
Carrier	BENZATHINE PENICILLIN FORTIFIED IM stat	PENICILLIN V or ERYTHROMYCIN for ten days	Immunize if immune status negative or unknown
Epiglottitis	CHLORAMPHENICOL IV then oral	CEFOTAXIME	Prepare for a respiratory emergency
Mastoiditis	IV AMPICILLIN + METRONIDAZOLE for 48 hours then AMOXYCILLIN		Drain post-auricular abscess ENT referral

Condition	First choice	Alternate agents	Comments
Otitis media			
Acute	AMOXYCILLIN for ten days	PENICILLIN AMOXYCILLIN with CLAVULANIC ACID (CO-AMOXICLAV) CO-TRIMOXAZOLE	AMPICILLIN resistance increasing Start PENICILLIN treatment with IM injection
Chronic	CO-TRIMOXAZOLE	AMOXYCILLIN CO-AMOXICLAV	Add aural toilet and antiseptic ear drops For Pseudomonas use acetic acid drops
Pharyngitis or sore throat	nil		Usually viral
Sinusitis	AMOXYCILLIN for ten days	CO-TRIMOXAZOLE CO-AMOXICLAV, oral CEPHALOSPORIN	Add decongestant nose drops or mucolytic
Tonsillitis	BENZATHINE PENICILLIN FORTIFIED IM stat	PENICILLIN V for ten days ERYTHROMYCIN CO-TRIMOXAZOLE	Usually viral in children under three years Full ten-day treatment essential

Condition	First choice	Alternate agents	Comments
EYE INFECTIONS			
Conjunctivitis			
Neonatal	See 'Neonatal infections'		
Older children			
Organism not known or uncomplicated	CHLORAMPHENICOL eye ointment		In severe cases, consult ophthalmologist
Pseudomonas or enteric bacilli	GENTAMICIN eye ointment + subconjunctival injection		Consult ophthalmologist immediately
Herpes	ACYCLOVIR eye ointment		
GASTROINTESTINAL INFECTIONS			
Antibiotic-associated or pseudomembranous colitis	METRONIDAZOLE (oral)	VANCOMYCIN (oral)	Stop offending antibiotic(s)

Condition	First choice	Alternate agents	Comments
Dysentery			
Amoebiasis	METRONIDAZOLE		
Organism not known	AMOXYCILLIN	CO-TRIMOXAZOLE CHLORAMPHENICOL	
Shigella	AMOXYCILLIN	CO-TRIMOXAZOLE	
Typhoid fever	AMOXYCILLIN	CHLORAMPHENICOL CO-TRIMOXAZOLE	AMOXYCILLIN better than CHLORAMPHENICOL in preventing carrier state
Gastroenteritis			
Campylobacter	ERYTHROMYCIN		Eradicates carriage, but does not affect clinical course
Cryptosporidium	nil		
Organism not known	nil		Exception: CEFOTAXIME in first week of life

Condition	First choice	Alternate agents	Comments
Rotavirus	nil		
Salmonella	nil		Unless systemic invasion Antibiotic prolongs excretion
Shigella	AMOXYCILLIN	CO-TRIMOXAZOLE CHLORAMPHENICOL	Shortens duration of diarrhoea and reduces spread
Necrotizing enterocolitis	CEFOTAXIME + METRONIDAZOLE	PENICILLIN + GENTAMICIN + METRONIDAZOLE	Multifactorial; cultures often sterile

IMMUNOSUPPRESSED PATIENTS

AIDS			
Suspected infection	CO-TRIMOXAZOLE	AMOXYCILLIN	
Severely ill	CEFOTAXIME	AMIKACIN + CO-TRIMOXAZOLE	Suspect tuberculosis and treat.
CMV infection	GANCYCLOVIR 5mg/kg/day IV		
Hypogammaglobulinaemia	CO-TRIMOXAZOLE	AMOXYCILLIN	Prophylaxis as alternative to intramuscular gammaglobulin

Condition	First choice	Alternate agents	Comments
Kwashiorkor			
Suspected infection	CO-TRIMOXAZOLE	PENICILLIN + GENTAMICIN	
Severely ill	CEFOTAXIME	AMPICILLIN + GENTAMICIN	
Neutropenia			
Suspected infection	CEFOTAXIME + AMIKACIN		Add CLOXACILLIN or VANCOMYCIN if *S. aureus* or *S. epidermidis* suspected
Pneumocystis pneumonia			
Treatment	CO-TRIMOXAZOLE (2,5 ml/kg/day)		Add ACYCLOVIR if varicella or herpes suspected
Prophylaxis	CO-TRIMOXAZOLE		Standard doses two days/week
INFECTIOUS DISEASES Notifiable: see pages 276-7			
Diphtheria	PENICILLIN IV		**Immediate antitoxin** Inform infection control and prepare for a respiratory emergency

Condition	First choice	Alternate agents	Comments
Measles (only if severe, with pneumonia)	CLOXACILLIN + GENTAMICIN		Give Vitamin A <1yr 100 000 IU/day for two days >1yr 200 000 IU/day for two days Do Adenovirus screen
Meningococcal septicaemia or meningitis	PENICILLIN		Add CHLORAMPHENICOL till proven. Other infections can mimic
Pertussis	ERYTHROMYCIN ESTOLATE for 14 days	CO-TRIMOXAZOLE for 14 days	
Scarlet fever	BENZATHINE PENICILLIN IM stat	PENICILLIN V for ten days ERYTHROMYCIN for ten days	
Tetanus	PENICILLIN IV	METRONIDAZOLE	**Immediate:** tetanus human immunoglobulin
Typhoid fever	AMOXYCILLIN 100 mg/kg/day	CHLORAMPHENICOL CO-TRIMOXAZOLE	AMOXYCILLIN better than CHLORAMPHENICOL in preventing carrier state

Condition	First choice	Alternate agents	Comments
MENINGITIS OR NEUROLOGICAL INFECTIONS			
Brain abscess	PENICILLIN + METRONIDAZOLE + CHLORAMPHENICOL		Consult neurosurgeon.
Meningitis			
Neonatal (<3 months)	See 'Neonatal infections'		
Children (>3 months)			
Enteric G-ve bacillus	CEFOTAXIME	GENTAMICIN IV or INTRAVENTRICULAR	
Haemophilus	CHLORAMPHENICOL	CEFOTAXIME	Approx 5% resistant to AMOXYCILLIN. CHLORAMPHENICOL resistance still rare
Meningococcus	PENICILLIN	CHLORAMPHENICOL CEFOTAXIME	Add RIFAMPICIN for two days before discharge

Condition	First choice	Alternate agents	Comments
Organism unknown	PENICILLIN + CHLORAMPHENICOL	CEFOTAXIME	Until sensitivities known.
Pneumococcus	PENICILLIN	CHLORAMPHENICOL CEFOTAXIME VANCOMYCIN	If PENICILLIN-resistant, change to CEFOTAXIME or VANCOMYCIN.
Tuberculous	ISONIAZID + RIFAMPICIN + PYRAZINAMIDE + ETHIONAMIDE		Treat for six to 12 months See page 116
Prophylaxis Meningococcus	RIFAMPICIN for two days Less than one month 5 mg/kg 2 x daily Over one month 10 mg/kg 2 x daily	CEFTRIAXONE 125 mg IM stat	Only for index case and intimate respiratory contacts
Haemophilus	RIFAMPICIN for four days 20 mg/kg/day		Only for households with children under four years

Condition	First choice	Alternate agents	Comments
NEONATAL INFECTIONS			
Arthritis or Osteitis	CLOXACILLIN/FLUCLOXACILLIN + AMPICILLIN	FUSIDIC ACID (if nosocomial, possible resistant Staphylococcus)	To cover staphylococcus + haemophilus. Stop one or other once culture known. See pages 44-6
Breast abscess – maternal	ERYTHROMYCIN	FLUCLOXACILLIN Oral Cephalosporins	See page 87
Breast abscess – neonatal	ERYTHROMYCIN	FLUCLOXACILLIN Oral Cephalosporins	See page 546
Congenital syphilis	PROCAINE PENICILLIN 50 000 U/kg/day IM for ten days	BENZYLPENICILLIN IV for ten days	
Conjunctivitis			
Chlamydial	TETRACYCLINE eye ointment + oral ERYTHROMYCIN 50 mg/kg/day for ten days	CHLORAMPHENICOL eye ointment + CO-TRIMOXAZOLE for ten days	Accounts for about 30% of cases locally

Condition	First choice	Alternate agents	Comments
Gonococcal	PENICILLIN eye drops + PROCAINE PENICILLIN 25 000 U/kg/day for seven days	CEFTRIAXONE 50 mg/kg IM once daily for three to five days	See page 353. Refer mother and her sexual partner(s) for treatment
Organism unknown	TETRACYCLINE eye ointment (1%)		
Prophylaxis	TETRACYCLINE eye ointment (1%)	ERYTROMYCIN* eye ointment (0,5%)	To cover Gonococcus + Chlamydia
Gastroenteritis	CEFOTAXIME		Only if aged under seven days or weight <2,5 kg
Meningitis	CEFOTAXIME 200 mg/kg/day IV	AMPICILLIN + GENTAMICIN	Covers Group B streptococcus + enteric bacilli
Necrotizing enterocolitis	CEFOTAXIME + METRONIDAZOLE	PENICILLIN + GENTAMICIN + METRONIDAZOLE	Multifactorial; cultures often sterile

* Not currently available in South Africa

Condition	First choice	Alternate agents	Comments
Pneumonia			
Inpatient	AMPICILLIN + GENTAMICIN		Alter treatment as indicated by culture results
Outpatient	AMOXYCILLIN		
Chlamydial	ERYTHROMYCIN for ten days	CO-TRIMOXAZOLE for ten days	
Nosocomial	CEFOTAXIME	AMIKACIN	
Scalded skin syndrome	ERYTHROMYCIN	CO-TRIMOXAZOLE FLUCLOXACILLIN	Drain primary septic focus
Septicaemia	CEFOTAXIME	AMPICILLIN + GENTAMICIN	
Umbilical sepsis	Topical drying/cleaning agents or antiseptics	CEFTRIAXONE	Antibiotic only for severe, toxic cases
RENAL INFECTIONS			
Lower urinary tract	NALIDIXIC ACID	NITROFURANTOIN, CO-TRIMOXAZOLE, AMOXYCILLIN	Depending on sensitivity. NITROFURANTOIN, NALIDIXIC

Condition	First choice	Alternate agents	Comments
		Oral CEPHALOSPORIN CO-AMOXICLAV	ACID inappropriate for systemic infections
Upper urinary or site unknown			
Catheter associated or post surgery	CEFOTAXIME	AMIKACIN	Often multiresistant enteric bacilli
Inpatient	GENTAMICIN	CEFOTAXIME	For seven to ten days.
Outpatient (oral)	NALIDIXIC ACID	CO-TRIMOXAZOLE, CO-AMOXICLAV Oral CEPHALOSPORIN	Treat for five to seven days. Resistance to AMOXYCILLIN and CO-TRIMOXAZOLE widespread.
Outpatient (parenteral)	GENTAMICIN IM	CEFTRIAXONE IM	

Condition	First choice	Alternate agents	Comments
Prophylaxis Urinary Tract Infection	NALIDIXIC ACID	CO-TRIMOXAZOLE NITROFURANTOIN	Choice depends on sensitivity. Half doses given at night
Nephrotic syndrome	PENICILLIN	ERYTHROMYCIN	
RESPIRATORY INFECTIONS			
Septic effusion see page 518			
Kerosene aspiration		CO-TRIMOXAZOLE	Steroids ineffective
Laryngotracheobronchitis/ croup	nil	AMOXYCILLIN	Usually viral. Antibiotic only in superinfection
Pneumonia			
Inpatient aspiration/ lung abscess/ bronchiectasis	CLOXACILLIN + METRONIDAZOLE + GENTAMICIN		

Condition	First choice	Alternate agents	Comments
Bronchopneumonia	AMPICILLIN *		*Add GENTAMICIN if severe and toxic, or if aged under three months
Lobar, community acquired	PENICILLIN *	AMOXYCILLIN	
Nosocomial	CEFOTAXIME + AMIKACIN		Often multiresistant enteric bacilli
Outpatient, community acquired	AMOXYCILLIN	CO-TRIMOXAZOLE	IM PROCAINE PENICILLIN if not feeding
Haemophilus	AMOXYCILLIN	CO-TRIMOXAZOLE	
Measles (severe)	CLOXACILLIN + GENTAMICIN		Give Vitamin A 200 000 IU/day for two days Do Adenovirus screen
Neonatal	see 'Neonatal infections'		
Pneumococcus	PENICILLIN	ERYTHROMYCIN	

Condition	First choice	Alternate agents	Comments
Pneumocystis	CO-TRIMOXAZOLE		2-4 x usual doses.
Staphylococcus	CLOXACILLIN then oral FLUCLOXACILLIN	ERYTHROMYCIN CO-TRIMOXAZOLE	Treat for four to six weeks
Recurrent infections see pages 254-7			
Tuberculosis see pages 562-7	RIFAMPICIN + ISONIAZID + PYRAZINAMIDE		Use Rifater if more than seven years old (1 tab/10kg/day)
RICKETTSIAL INFECTIONS			
Tick bite fever	TETRACYCLINE for five to seven days	CHLORAMPHENICOL	Consider the side-effects of TETRACYCLINE vs CHLORAMPHENICOL. DOXYCYCLINE is the preferred TETRACYCLINE

Condition	First choice	Alternate agents	Comments
SEPTICAEMIA			
Neonatal (less than three months)	See 'Neonatal infections'		
Children (over three months)			
Anaerobe	METRONIDAZOLE	CHLORAMPHENICOL	
Enteric G-ve	GENTAMICIN	AMIKACIN CEFOTAXIME	May be GENTAMICIN resistant
Enterococcus	AMPICILLIN (+ GENTAMICIN*)		*If life-threatening
Haemophilus	CHLORAMPHENICOL	CEFOTAXIME	
Meningococcus (suspected)	PENICILLIN + CHLORAMPHENICOL		Other infections can mimic
Organism not known in community	PENICILLIN + GENTAMICIN	CEFOTAXIME	CEPHALOSPORIN if renal function impaired

Condition	First choice	Alternate agents	Comments
nosocomial	CEFOTAXIME + AMIKACIN		Often multiresistant organisms
neutropenia	CEFOTAXIME + AMIKACIN		if WBC <2x10⁹/l or granulocytes <1x10⁹/l
Staphylococcus	CLOXACILLIN (+ FUSIDIC ACID*)		* If life-threatening
Streptococcus	PENICILLIN (+ GENTAMICIN*)		* If life-threatening

SEXUALLY TRANSMITTED DISEASES see pages 148 and 308

Condition	First choice	Alternate agents	Comments
Chlamydial vaginitis	ERYTHROMYCIN 50 mg/kg/day for ten days	CO-TRIMOXAZOLE for ten days	Exclude sexual abuse
Gardnerella vaginitis	METRONIDAZOLE 7,5 mg/kg/day for five days	AMOXYCILLIN	Exclude sexual abuse
Genital Herpes	ACYCLOVIR 5-10 mg/kg 3 x daily for seven days		Reduces symptoms if given early. Exclude sexual abuse

Condition	First choice	Alternate agents	Comments
Gonorrhoea	AMOXYCILLIN 50 mg/kg oral (max 3 g) + PROBENECID 25 mg/kg (max 1 g)	CEFTRIAXONE 50 mg/kg IM stat	Follow up to ensure eradication; exclude sexual abuse
Neonatal ophthalmia	See 'Neonatal infections'		
Syphilis Congenital	See 'Neonatal infections'		
Older children	BENZATHINE PENICILLIN 50 000 U/kg (max 2,4mU) IM stat	ERYTHROMYCIN 50 mg/kg/day for 15 days	
Trichomoniasis	METRONIDAZOLE 7,5 mg/kg/day for seven days		Exclude sexual abuse

Condition	First choice	Alternate agents	Comments
SUPERFICIAL INFECTIONS			
Abscess or boils or carbuncles or furuncles	ERYTHROMYCIN	FLUCLOXACILLIN PENICILLIN CO-TRIMOXAZOLE	Use pre-surgery. Continue only if marked cellulitis is present
Cellulitis	PENICILLIN	ERYTHROMYCIN CO-TRIMOXAZOLE	If no response, change to FLUCLOXACILLIN
Impetigo	FLUCLOXACILLIN	CO-TRIMOXAZOLE ERYTHROMYCIN	Staphylococci occur in 90% of cases
Skin ulcer/bed sores	Local antiseptics only		Swab cultures unreliable. Mixed flora usually obtained
SURGICAL INFECTIONS			
Arthritis	CLOXACILLIN/FLUCLOXACILLIN		If aged six months to two years, add AMPICILLIN to cover Haemophilus. See page 244

Condition	First choice	Alternate agents	Comments
Biliary tree surgery	PENICILLIN + GENTAMICIN	CO-AMOXICLAV	For five to seven days
Bites and scratches: dog cat, other animal or human	PENICILLIN	CO-AMOXICLAV DOXYCYCLINE ERYTHROMYCIN	For ten to 14 days
Bowel surgery prophylaxis (including appendicectomy)	PENICILLIN + GENTAMICIN + METRONIDAZOLE		Start at induction; continue for 24 hours only
Brain abscess	PENICILLIN + METRONIDAZOLE + CHLORAMPHENICOL		Consult neurosurgeon
Burn wounds	ERYTHROMYCIN		Used if beta-streptococcus suspected or proven. Topical antimicrobial treatment important adjuvant
Cervical adenopathy	ERYTHROMYCIN	FLUCLOXACILLIN PENICILLIN CO-TRIMOXAZOLE	

Condition	First choice	Alternate agents	Comments
Compound fracture	PENICILLIN + GENTAMICIN	CEFOXITIN	For 48 hours
Dental abscess	PENICILLIN + METRONIDAZOLE		Dental referral
Liver abscess			
Organism not known	CLOXACILLIN + GENTAMICIN + METRONIDAZOLE		For at least seven days
Staphylococcus	CLOXACILLIN		Common isolate at Red Cross War Memorial Children's Hospital
Entamoeba	METRONIDAZOLE		
Enteric G-ve bacillus	GENTAMICIN		
Streptococcus	PENICILLIN		
Necrotizing fasciitis	METRONIDAZOLE + GENTAMICIN		Debridement essential

Condition	First choice	Alternate agents	Comments
Osteomyelitis			
Acute	CLOXACILLIN IV 100 mg/kg/day for two days, then FLUCLOXACILLIN 100 mg/kg/day for six wks		Add FUSIDIC ACID if CLOXACILLIN-resistant staphylococcus suspected in previously hospitalized neonate
Chronic	CLOXACILLIN		Short course pre- and post-surgery
Peritonitis (including contaminated bowel surgery)	PENICILLIN + GENTAMICIN + METRONIDAZOLE		For five days
Post-operative wound infection	Nil (irrigate with topical antiseptics)		Await culture results
Scratches	See 'bites' page 284		
Superficial lesions	See 'Superficial infections'		

APPENDIX 2
PHARMACOPOEIA

A Allie and the Staff of the Pharmacy

CAUTION: Doses of medications have been carefully checked, but the editor and publishers cannot take responsibility for any inaccuracies. Always check product information. See page 315.

Table 1 General medications

Medication generic name (Trade name)	Paediatric dose	Route	Frequency	Availability and remarks
ACETOZOLAMIDE (Diamox)	10-15 mg/kg daily 5-10 mg/kg	O IV	Divided doses 3 x daily. Six-hourly.	Tab.: 250 mg Inj.: 500 mg/10 ml
ADRENALINE	0,01 ml/kg/dose Max.: 0,5 ml	SC	Repeat after 30 minutes.	Inj.: 1 ml amp (1:1000). Painful injection. Consider using FENOTEROL (Berotec) aerosol in bronchospasm or the following by nebulization using respirator.

Medication generic name (Trade name)	Paediatric dose	Route	Frequency	Availability and remarks
				Solution: FENOTEROL (Berotec), SALBUTAMOL (Ventolin). Sol.: 1:1000 (25 ml). Use in croup. See page 516. Use in cardio-pulmonary resuscitation. See page 6.
	1 ml with 1 ml normal saline	Nebulization	See page 516.	
ALBENDAZOLE (Zentel)	Children over two years 2 tablets	0	Once only.	Tabs: chewable 200 mg Broadspectrum anthelmintic (has been used long-term for Hydatid cyst).
ALFACALCIDOL (One Alpha)	<20 kg 0,05 µg/kg/day >20 kg 1 µg/kg/day	0	Once daily.	Caps.: 0,25 µg, 1 µg Drops 10 ml 5 µg/ml
ALGINIC ACID with ANTACID (Gaviscon)	½-1 sachet/120-240 ml feed 5-10 ml 1 tablet	Added to bottle 0 0	To each feed. 4 x daily. (After meals and bedtime)	Infant sachets Susp.: Tablets (six to 12 years) Not for prems.

Medication generic name (Trade name)	Paediatric dose	Route	Frequency	Availability and remarks
ALUMINIUM HYDROXIDE (Amphojel)	2,5-7,5 ml	O	With meals.	Suspension
AMILORIDE CO (Moduretic)	1-4 tabs./day	O	Divided doses – 1-2 x daily	Tabs: AMILORIDE 5 mg + HYDROCHLOROTHIAZIDE 50 mg
(Moduretic HS)	0,5-2 tabs./day	O	1-2 x daily	Tabs: AMILORIDE 2,5 mg + HYDROCHLOROTHIAZIDE 25 mg Half strength used in hypertension.
AMINOPHYLLINE	Load: 6 mg/kg then constant infusion: 0,5-1 mg/kg/hour	IV	Over 20 minutes.	Inj: (IV): 25 mg/ml (10 ml amp). Beware of ampoule for IM use with 250 mg/ml. Suppositories not recommended. Tabs: 100 mg, 200 mg Toxic symptoms: vomiting, thirst, agitation, convulsions, shock, death. See also THEOPHYLLINE, page 630.

Medication generic name (Trade name)	Paediatric dose	Route	Frequency	Availability and remarks
	Prevention of apnoea in immature preterm infant: 8 mg/kg/day	O	Divided doses - 4 x daily.	
ASPIRIN SOLUBLE (Disprin)	30-60 mg/kg/day (Max.: 900 mg/dose)	O	Divided doses – 3-4 x daily.	Tabs: 300 mg (scored) Tabs (Junior): 75 mg Contra-indicated in influenza and varicella. Avoid repeated doses especially when febrile and urinary output reduced See rheumatic fever, page 108.
ASTEMIZOLE (Hismanal)	Six to 12 years 5 mg >12 years 10 mg	O	Daily.	Tab.: 10 mg Susp.: 5 mg/5 ml Take one hour before evening meal.
ATENOLOL (Tenormin)	1-2 mg/kg/day	O	1-2 x daily.	Cardio-selective β-blocker. Avoid in asthma. Reduce dose in renal failure.

Medication generic name (Trade name)	Paediatric dose	Route	Frequency	Availability and remarks
BACLOFEN (Lioresal)	Commencing dose 15 mg/day Maximum two to seven years 30-40 mg Over eight years 60 mg Unless hospitalized	0	Divided doses – 4 x daily.	Tabs: 10 mg, 25 mg Titrate increase against response. Used in spastic cerebral palsy. Take with meals or milk.
BECLOMETHASONE (Becotide, Viarox)	2-3 puffs (aerosol) 1 Rotacap/disc 100-200 µg according to age and severity.	Inhalation Inhalation	3-4 x daily 3-4 x daily	Aerosol: 50 µg/inhalation Rotacaps: 100, 200 µg Used with Becotide Rotahaler Prevention of asthma
(Beconase, Viarox)		Nasal insufflation	3-4 x daily	For allergic rhinitis. Nasal spray and aqueous nasal spray.
BENZHEXOL (Artane)	Commencing dose 1-3 mg/day (adult) Titrate against response Maximum adult dose 15 mg/day	0	Divided doses – 3-4 x daily	Tabs: 2 mg, 5 mg Titrate increase against response For basal ganglia dysfunction

Medication generic name (Trade name)	Paediatric dose	Route	Frequency	Availability and remarks
BIPERIDEN (Akineton)	2,5-5 mg	IV	Dilute and give slowly in 5 % dextrose solution.	Tabs: 2 mg Inj.: 5 mg/ml (1 ml amp.) Used in PHENOTHIAZINE intoxication. Used for control of extrapyramidal symptoms.
BROMHEXINE (Bisolvon)	Up to one year: 1-2 ml Under ten years: 2,5-5 ml Over ten years: 5-10 ml	0 0 0	3-4 x daily. 3 x daily. 3 x daily.	Tabs: 4 mg, 8 mg Solution: 10 mg/5 ml A mucolytic agent
BROMPHENIRAMINE (Dimetapp)	2,5 - 5 ml	0	3-4 x daily.	Elixir. Only for children over three years. Decongestant.
BUDESONIDE (Pulmicort)	2 puffs (aerosol)	Inhalation	2-4 x daily.	Aerosol 50 µg, 100 µg, 200 µg/inhalation.

Medication generic name (Trade name)	Paediatric dose	Route	Frequency	Availability and remarks
CALCIUM	30 mg/kg/day Ca^{++} 1-2 ml/kg (Max. 2g) of CALCIUM GLUCONATE 10%	0 Slow IV	Divided doses.	Equivalents of Elemental Calcium. Calcium Sandoz Syrup 5 ml = 110 mg Calcium Efferv. Tab. = 500 mg CALCIUM CARBONATE Tab. = 168 mg CALCIUM GLUCONATE Tab. = 50 mg 1g CALCIUM GLUCONATE is equivalent to 100 mg Elemental Calcium.
CAPTOPRIL (Capoten)	0,5-1 mg/kg/day increasing up to 5 mg/kg/day	0	2-3 x daily.	Tabs: 25 mg, 50 mg, 100 mg Angiotension-converting enzyme inhibitor. Contra-indicated in bilateral renal artery stenosis.
CARBAMAZEPINE (Carpaz, Degranol, Tegretol)	20 mg/kg/day	0	Divided doses – 3 x daily. Sustained release 2 x daily.	Tabs: 200 mg Susp.: 100 mg/5 ml Tabs: CR 200 mg, 400 mg Therapeutic range: 16-50 µmol/l Drug of choice for complex partial seizures.

Medication generic name (Trade name)	Paediatric dose	Route	Frequency	Availability and remarks
CETIRIZINE (Zyrtec)	>12 years 10 mg	O	Single dose daily in evening.	Tab.: 10 mg
CHLORAL HYDRATE	Hypnotic: 50 mg/kg/dose (Max 1 g) Sedative: 25 mg/kg/day	O	Repeat 3 x daily when necessary. Divided doses 3 x daily.	Syrup – strength may vary with hospital – check label. See also TRICLOFOS.
CHLORHEXIDINE-NEOMYCIN (Naseptin nasal cream)		Nasal	2-4 x daily.	Prophylaxis against high nasal staph. carriage.
CHLORMETHIAZOLE (Heminevrin)		IV	See literature.	Vial: 192 mg with buffer solution READ DILUTION INSTRUCTIONS

Medication generic name (Trade name)	Paediatric dose	Route	Frequency	Availability and remarks
CHLOR-PHENIRAMINE CO (Demazin)	Under one year: 1,5-2 ml one to three years: 2,5-5 ml three to six years: 5-10 ml	O O O	Every four to six hours.	Syrup
(Rinex)	2,5 ml	O	3-4 x daily.	Syrup decongestants
CHLORPROMAZINE (Largactil)	2 mg/kg/day See also Pertussis page 275.	O, IM, IV	Divided doses – 4-6 x daily.	Syrup: 25 mg/5 ml Tabs: 10 mg, 25 mg (coated) Inj: 10 mg/ml (5 ml amp.) 25 mg/ml (1 and 2 ml amp.) Supp.: 100 mg For nausea following chemotherapy.
	0,5 mg/kg/dose	IM	Up to six-hourly.	
CLONAZEPAM (Rivotril)	0,05-0,3 mg/kg/day See literature.	O IV	3 x daily.	Drops: 2,5 mg/ml (0,1 mg/drop) Tabs: 0,5 mg, 2 mg (scored) Inj.: 0,5 mg/ml Therapeutic range:

Medication generic name (Trade name)	Paediatric dose	Route	Frequency	Availability and remarks
				0,095-0,190 μmol/l IV alternative to DIAZEPAM for seizure termination.
CYCLIZINE (Valoid)	6 mg/kg/day	Rectal	3 x daily.	Supp.: 50 mg, 100 mg.
DESFERRIOXAMINE (Desferal)	3-7 g in 50-100 ml water Then: 15 mg/kg	O IV	Single. Hourly, to a total of 80 mg/kg.	Inj.: 500 mg dry powder See literature.
DEXAMETHASONE (Decadron)	In cerebral oedema: 2-4 mg/dose In bacterial meningitis: 0,2 mg/kg/day	IV O, IV	Give every six hours for 48 hours. 4 x daily for 48 hours.	Inj.: 4 mg/ml (2 ml vial) 20 mg/ml (5 ml - Shock Pak vial) Tab.: 0,5 mg First dose prior to chemotherapy.

Medication generic name (Trade name)	Paediatric dose	Route	Frequency	Availability and remarks
DIAZEPAM (Valium)	0,5-1 mg/kg/day	O, IV	Divided doses – 3 x daily.	Syrup: 2 mg/5 ml Tabs: 2 mg, 5 mg, 10 mg
	Status Epilepticus: Children under three years 5 mg Children over three years 10 mg OR 0,3 mg/kg (Max. 10 mg)	Rectally IV	Single dose.	Inj.: 5 mg/ml (2 ml amp.) IV drug of choice for termination of seizures. See page 340 Poor preventative. Ampoule may be used by parents at home to give medication rectally
	Neonatal tetanus: 7,5 mg	O, IV	Two to four-hourly	
DICYCLOMINE (Colix, Merbentyl, Nomocramp)	5-10 mg/dose Infants: 2,5-5 ml/dose	O O	3 x daily 15 minutes before feed	Syrup: 10 mg/5 ml Dilute with equal volume of water Tabs: 10 mg (scored) Do not exceed 40 mg daily. **Caution:** Not to be used in infants under six months

Medication generic name (Trade name)	Paediatric dose	Route	Frequency	Availability and remarks
DIGOXIN (Lanoxin)	Initial dose: 0,005 mg/kg/dose	O	Eight-hourly x 3 doses only.	Elixir: 0,05 mg/ml Tabs: 0,25 mg
	Maintenance dose: 0,005 mg/kg/dose	O	12-hourly	Inj.: 0,25 mg/ml (2 ml amp.)
	Intravenous dose: 0,005 mg/kg/dose	IV	12-hourly	**Use only if severe GIT disturbance.**
DIHYDRALAZINE (Nepresol)	0,1–0,2 mg/kg/dose	IM or IV (slowly)	Single dose, repeat 3-4 x daily if necessary.	Inj.: 25 mg amp. Action: renin-independent direct vasodilator. May cause lupus-like syndrome.
DIPHENHYDRAMINE (Benadryl)	5 mg/kg/day	O	Divided doses— 3 or 4 x daily.	Elixir: 12,5 mg/5 ml Caps.: 25 mg

Medication generic name (Trade name)	Paediatric dose	Route	Frequency	Availability and remarks
DOMPERIDONE (Motilium)	Chronic: 0,3 mg/kg (double dose if response insufficient)	O	3 x daily before food and if necessary before sleep.	Suspension: 10 mg/ml. Supplied with dropper (1 drop = 0,3 mg) Tabs: 10 mg Anti-emetic. Also used in gastro-oesophageal reflex.
	Acute: 0,6 mg/kg	O	3 x daily	
	0,2-0,4 mg/kg	IM, IV	3-6 x daily	
		IV over 15-30 mins	Max. 1 mg/kg/day	
DOPAMINE (Intropin)	2-5 µg/kg/min increased gradually by 5-10µg/kg/min Up to 20-50µg/kg/min may be given.	IV infusion		Inj.: 40 mg/ml (5 ml amp) See septicaemia, page 587.
ENALAPRIL (Renitec)	0,2-1 mg/kg/day	O	1-2 x daily.	Tabs: 5 mg, 10 mg, 20 mg Contra-indicated in bilateral renal artery stenosis.

Medication generic name (Trade name)	Paediatric dose	Route	Frequency	Availability and remarks
ETHOSUXIMIDE (Zarontin)	15-50 mg/kg	O	Single dose at night or divided doses 2 x daily.	Syrup: 250 mg/5 ml Caps.: 250 mg Therapeutic range: 280-700 µmol/l
FENOTEROL (Berotec)	0,1 mg/kg/dose	O Aerosol	3-4 x daily if necessary. 3 x daily (single puff).	Syrup: 2,5 mg/5 ml Tabs: 2,5 mg (scored) Aerosol 200 µg/inhalation For relief of acute bronchospasm in asthma.
	Nebulizer: 1 ml	Nebulization	Three to four-hourly	Inhalant solution: 1 mg/ml. Mix with equal volume normal saline.
FERROUS LACTATE (Ferro drops)	0,3-0,6 ml	O	Daily	25 mg iron/ml

Medication generic name (Trade name)	Paediatric dose	Route	Frequency	Availability and remarks
FERROUS SULPHATE	Therapeutic: 3-6 mg elemental iron/kg/day	O	Divided doses – 3 x daily.	Syrup (BPC): 300 mg ferrous sulphate/5 ml Elemental iron content – 60 mg/5 ml syrup
	Prophylactic: 1 mg elemental iron/kg/day	O	Daily.	Red Cross War Memorial Children's Hospital: elemental iron content – 20 mg/5 ml syrup Tabs: 200 mg (coated) – contain 60 mg iron
FLUTICASONE (Flixotide)	Children over six years: 50-100 µg	Inhalation	2 x daily.	Inhaler: 250 µg, 125 µg. 50 µg or 25 µg per actuation. Discs: 500 µg, 250 µg. 100 µg or 50 µg per blister (for Diskhaler).
FOLIC ACID	1-2 mg	O	Daily.	Tabs: 1 mg, 5 mg for three to four weeks
	2 mg/kg in Kwashiorkor	O	Daily.	For five days

Medication generic name (Trade name)	Paediatric dose	Route	Frequency	Availability and remarks
FUROSEMIDE (Lasix)	1-3 mg/kg/day 0,5-1 mg/kg/dose	O IM, IV	Daily. Maximum 3 x daily.	Tabs: 20 mg, 40 mg (scored) Sol.: 10 mg/ml (100 ml) Inj.: 10 mg/ml (2 and 25 ml amps.) Maximum 5-10 mg/kg/dose in renal failure Give supplementary potassium
GRANISETRON (Kytril)	Adult dose: 40 µg/kg/dose	IV	Over five minutes as infusion or injection. Max. three doses in 24 hours.	Amp.: 3 mg Dilute in 20 to 50 ml infusion fluid and administer over five minutes by slow intravenous injection or infusion. Use 0,9% sodium chloride or 5% dextrose solution as diluent. May be repeated after ten minutes.
HALOPERIDOL (Serenace)	0,05 mg/kg/day Increase cautiously if necessary 0,1 mg/kg/day in chorea.	O O	Divided doses – 2 x daily. Divided doses – 3 x daily.	Liq.: 2 mg/ml (20 drops) Tabs: 1,5 mg (scored) Caps.: 0,5 mg Extra pyramidal toxic effects.

Medication generic name (Trade name)	Paediatric dose	Route	Frequency	Availability and remarks
HEPARIN	50–100 units/kg/dose	IV	6 x daily	Inj.:1 000 units/ml (5 ml vial) 5 000 units/ml (5 ml vial) 25 000 units/ml (5 ml vial) Titrate dose to give 20–30 minute clotting time Antidote: PROTAMINE SULPHATE
HEXOPRENALINE (Ipradol)	Three to six months: 5 ml 1 µg	O IV (drip chamber)	1–2 x daily. 3 x daily.	Syrup: 0,125 mg/5 ml Inj.: 2,5 µg/ml (2 ml amp.) β-stimulant, bronchodilator.
	Six to 12 months 5 ml 2 µg	O IV (drip chamber)	1–3 x daily. 3 x daily.	
	One to three years: 5–10 ml 2–3 µg	O IV (drip chamber)	1–3 x daily. 3 x daily.	

Medication generic name (Trade name)	Paediatric dose	Route	Frequency	Availability and remarks
	Over three years: 10 ml	O	1-3 x daily.	
	3-4 µg	IV (drip chamber)	3 x daily.	
	Nebulizer: 1 ml	Nebulization	3-4 x daily.	Inhalant solution: 250 µg/ml Mix with equal volume normal saline.
HYDRALAZINE (Apresoline)	1-5 mg/kg/day	O	Four to eight-hourly.	Tabs: 10 mg, 25 mg, 50 mg Direct vasodilator. May cause lupus-like syndrome.
HYDROCHLORO-THIAZIDE (Dichlotride)	2 mg/kg/day	O	Divided doses – 2 x daily.	May cause hypokalaemia.
HYDROCORTISONE SODIUM SUCCINATE (Solu-Cortef, Ef-Cortelan)	Depends on indication.	IV, IM		Inj.: 50 mg/ml (2 ml vial) Stronger solution: 125 mg/ml (4 ml vial)

Medication generic name (Trade name)	Paediatric dose	Route	Frequency	Availability and remarks
HYDROXYZINE (Aterax)	Drops: infants 0,5 mg/kg/day Syrup: 2 mg/kg/day	O O	Divided doses – 3-4 x daily. Divided doses – 3-4 x daily.	Drops: 7,5 mg/ml Syrup: 10 mg/5 ml Inj.: 50 mg/ml (2 ml amp.)
	Inj.: 1 mg/kg/dose	IM		
HYOSCINE BUTYLBROMIDE (Buscopan)	Under six years: 1 tab. Over six years: 1-2 tabs.	O O	3-5 x daily. 3-5 x daily.	Tabs: 10 mg Inj.: 20 mg/ml (1 ml amp.)
	Under three years: 5 mg Three to six years: 10 mg Over six years: 20 mg	SC, IM, IV SC, IM, IV SC, IM, IV	Single. Single. Single.	
IBUPROFEN (Brufen)	20 mg/kg/day	O	Divided doses 3 x daily.	Susp. 100 mg/5 ml Tab 200 mg, 400 mg, 600 mg Take with food.

Medication generic name (Trade name)	Paediatric dose	Route	Frequency	Availability and remarks
IMIPRAMINE (Tofranil)	Nocturnal enuresis: Six to 12 years 10-25 mg Over 12 years 25-50 mg	O	After evening meal.	Tabs: 10 mg, 25 mg Not recommended under six years of age.
IPECAC - Syrup of	10-15 ml/dose	O	Single dose.	Follow with 200 ml clear fluid. Repeat in 15 mins if no vomiting. **Warning** Don't confuse syrup of IPECAC with tincture or liquid extract which are **much stronger.**
IPRATROPIUM BROMIDE (Atrovent)	Five years and older Under two years 0,5 ml with 1 ml saline Over two years 1 ml with 1 ml saline see status asthmaticus page 19.	Aerosol Nebulization	4 x daily. Up to 4 x daily.	Aerosol: 20 µg per inhalation. Resp. sol.: 250 µg/ml. 10 ml. Useful in infants and young children who do not respond to β-stimulants.

Medication generic name (Trade name)	Paediatric dose	Route	Frequency	Availability and remarks
IRON DEXTRAN COMPLEX (Imferon)	Prophylactic in preterm infants: 1 ml/dose	IM (deep)	Daily for two days.	Inj.: 50 mg elemental iron/ml (2 ml amp.) Use oral preparations whenever possible unless follow-up difficult.
ISOPRENALINE (Imuprel)	0,2 mg 0,02 mg Intravenous infusion: 0,2 mg/200 ml 5% dextrose water.	SC, IM IV IV	Single dose. Single dose. Rate of fluid administration depends on size and response of patient.	Inj.: 0,2 mg/ml
KETOCONAZOLE (Nizoral)	3-5 mg/kg/day	O	Once daily.	Tabs: 200 mg
KETOTIFEN (Zaditen)	1,5-5 ml	O	2 x daily.	Syrup: 1 mg/5 ml Prophylactic for asthma.
LACTULOSE (Duphalac)	3-15 ml/day	O	Daily, after breakfast.	Syrup Larger doses required in hepatic encephalopathy.

Medication generic name (Trade name)	Paediatric dose	Route	Frequency	Availability and remarks
LAMOTRIGINE (Lamictin)	5-15 mg/kg/day	O	Once per day.	Tabs: 25 mg, 50 mg, 100 mg. Action potentiated by SODIUM VALPROATE – use half dose.
LOPERAMIDE (Imodium)	Initial dose: 5 ml/12,5 kg body weight Thereafter: 2,5 ml/12,5 kg after each loose stool	O	See dose. See dose and remarks.	Syrup: 1 mg/5 ml Tabs: 2 mg Not more than 15 ml per 12,5 kg body weight per day. Not recommended in medical paediatric practice but used by surgeons.
MAGNESIUM	50 mg/kg/day $MgCl_2$	O		S/R Tab. MAG. CHLORIDE 535 mg Equiv. 64 mgMg^{++} Sol.: 440 mg/5ml. Equiv. 53 Mg^{++}
MANNITOL	1-2 g/kg	IV		Sol.: 15-25%. Administer over 30-60 minutes. To reduce intracranial and ocular pressure.

Medication generic name (Trade name)	Paediatric dose	Route	Frequency	Availability and remarks
MEBENDAZOLE (Vermox)	All ages 5 ml (1 tab.)	O	2 x daily for three days.	Syrup: 100 mg/5 ml Tabs: 100 mg (chewable) Broad spectrum anthelmintic for tape-, thread-, round- and whip worms.
	Tapeworms: 1 tab.	O	2 x daily for six days.	
MEFANAMIC ACID (Ponstan)	Six to 12 months: 5 ml	O	3 x daily.	Susp.: 50 mg/5 ml
	One to four years: 10 ml	O	3 x daily.	
	Five to eight years: 10 ml	O	4 x daily.	
	Eight to 12 years: 15 ml	O	4 x daily.	
MEFLOQUINE (Larium)	Contra-indicated in children under two years. Two to four years, 15-19 kg: ¼ adult dose	O	Prophylaxis of malaria. Once per week (on same day). Start one week before and weekly while in the	Tab.: 250 mg Contra-indicated in pregnancy and lactation.

Medication generic name (Trade name)	Paediatric dose	Route	Frequency	Availability and remarks
	Five to eight years, 20–30 kg: $1/2$ adult dose Nine to 15 years, 31–45 kg: $3/4$ adult dose Over 15 yrs – over 45 kg: adult dose adult dose: 250 mg (prophylactic dose)		area. Continue weekly for four weeks after leaving the area. Restrict use to three months.	
METHYLDOPA (Aldomet)	10–60 mg/kg/day	O	Divided doses – 3–4 x daily	Tabs: 250 mg, 500 mg Inj.: 50 mg/ml (5 ml amp.) Titrate dose according to response. May cause postural hypotension, drowsiness. Action: Renin-lowering.

Medication generic name (Trade name)	Paediatric dose	Route	Frequency	Availability and remarks
METHYLPREDNISOLONE (Medrol) (Solu-Medrol)		O		Tab.: 4 mg Equiv. 5 mg PREDNISOLONE
		IV		Mix-o-Vial 40 mg, 125 mg, 500 mg, 1000 mg.
METOCLOPRAMIDE (Maxolon, Primperan)	Under one year: 1 mg	O	2 x daily.	Paed. Drops: 1 mg/ml Syrup: 5 mg/5 ml
	One to three years: 1 mg	O	2-3 x daily.	Tabs: 10 mg Inj.: 5 mg/ml (2 ml amp.)
	Three to five years: 2,5 mg	O	3 x daily.	Supp. Paed.: 5 mg Max. daily dose 500 µg/kg
	Five to 14 years: 5 mg	O	3 x daily.	
METOCLOPRAMIDE (Maxolon)	One to three years 0,5 mg	IV, IM	2 x daily	
	Three to five years 1,0 mg	IV, IM	2 x daily	
	Five to fourteen years 2,5 mg	IV, IM	2 x daily	

Medication generic name (Trade name)	Paediatric dose	Route	Frequency	Availability and remarks
METRONIDAZOLE (Flagyl)	Amoebiasis			Syrup: 200 mg/5 ml
	<15 kg - 200 mg	O	3 x daily for five days.	Tabs: 200 mg, 400 mg
	>15 kg - 200 mg	O	4 x daily for five days.	Inj.: 5 mg/ml (100 ml vials)
	Giardiasis:			Suppositories: 500 mg and 1 g
	<15 kg - 500 mg	O	1 x daily for five days.	
	15-22 kg - 800 mg	O		
	>22 kg - 1 000 mg	O		
	Anaerobic infections:			See also page 646.
	7,5 mg/kg/dose	IV	Eight-hourly intervals.	
	Five to 12 years 500 mg	Rectally	Eight-hourly.	
MORPHINE SULPHATE	14-21 µg/kg/hour	IV	Infusion	Inj.: 10 mg/ml (1 ml amp.)
	0,1-0,2 mg/kg/dose	SC, IM	1-2 x daily	15 mg/ml (1 ml amp.)
	0,4 mg/kg/dose	O	Four-hourly as needed.	
NALOXONE (Narcan)	0,01 mg/kg/dose	IM, IV	Single dose, repeat in three minutes, if necessary.	Neonatal inj.: 0,02 mg/ml (2 ml amp.) Inj.: 0,4 mg/ml (1 ml amp.) – for bigger children.

Medication generic name (Trade name)	Paediatric dose	Route	Frequency	Availability and remarks
NIFEDIPINE (Adalat)	0,25-1 mg/kg/day	O	Divided doses – six to eight-hourly	Caps: 5, 10 mg
NIRIDAZOLE (Ambilhar)	25 mg/kg/day	O	Divided doses – 2 x daily for five to seven days.	Tabs: 100 mg, 500 mg Occasional mental confusion.
NITRAZEPAM (Mogadon)	2,5-15 mg/day	O	Divided doses – 3 x daily.	Tabs: 5 mg
OBIDOXIME (Toxogonin)	4-8 mg/kg	IV	See literature.	Inj.: 250 mg/ml (1 ml amp.) Cholinesterase reactivator in organophosphate poisoning.
ONDANSETRON (Zofran)	5 mg/m^2 5 mg	IV over 15 mins. O	Eight-hourly up to five days.	Amp: 2 mg/ml (2 ml amp) IV: prior to chemotherapy. Tabs: 4 mg, 8 mg. Child over four years.

Medication generic name (Trade name)	Paediatric dose	Route	Frequency	Availability and remarks
OXYBUTININ (Ditropan)	Over five years 5 mg Maximum 5 mg	O	2 x daily. 3 x daily.	Tabs: 5 mg For frequency, urgency
PARACETAMOL (Panado)	Under one year: 2,5 ml/dose One to three years: 2,5-5 ml/dose Three to six years: 5 ml/dose Six to 12 years: half tab./dose	O	3-4 x daily.	Syrup: 120 mg/5 ml Tabs: 500 mg
PARACETAMOL CO (Asalen)	2,5 ml/dose increasing with age	O	3 x daily.	Syrup (Paed) contains/5 ml: PARACETAMOL 75 mg PHENYLEPHRINE 2,5 mg PHENYLDIAMINE HCl 3,75 mg CAFFEINE 7,5 mg

Medication generic name (Trade name)	Paediatric dose	Route	Frequency	Availability and remarks
(Syndette)	Birth to two years: 2,5-5 ml/dose Two to 12 years: 5-10 ml/dose	O O	4-6 x daily As above.	Syrup contains/5 ml: PARACETAMOL 120 mg DOXYLAMINE 5 mg
PARALDEHYDE	Anticonvulsant 0,15 ml/kg/dose			Not available in South Africa.
PENTAMIDINE ISETHIONATE	4 mg/kg	IM	Once daily for 14 days.	Amp.: 200 mg dry powder For pneumocystis.
PETHIDINE	1 mg/kg/dose Maximum 6 mg/kg/day	IM	Single, repeat if necessary.	Inj.: 25 mg/ml (1 ml amp.) 50 mg/ml (1 & 2 ml amp.)
PHENOBARBITONE	5-10 mg/kg/day (Adult dose: 90-180 mg/day) Never exceed 120 mg/day IV	O, IM	Single dose at night or divided doses 2 x daily.	Elixir: 15 mg/5 ml Tabs: 15 mg, 30 mg and 60 mg Inj.: 200 mg/ml (1 ml amp.) Newborn: IV load 20 mg/kg Serum PHENOBARBITONE - therapeutic range 45-130 µmol/l

Medication generic name (Trade name)	Paediatric dose	Route	Frequency	Availability and remarks
PHENYL PROPANO- LAMINE CO. (Eskornade)	Under 12 years: 1,25-5 ml/dose	O	3 x daily.	Syrup and spansule capsules
PHENYTOIN (Epanutin)	5-8 mg/kg/dose	O	Single dose or divided doses 2 x daily.	Susp.: 125 mg/5 ml and 25 mg/5 ml Caps. or tabs.: 50 mg, 100 mg Infatabs: 50 mg scored chewable tabs. Inj.: 50 mg/ml (5 ml amp.) **Never give IM.** Serum PHENYTOIN - therapeutic range 40-100 µmol/l
	For resistant convulsions 10-15 mg/kg	IV		If dilution is necessary use saline rather than DEXTROSE solution.
	Should not exceed 50 mg per minute	IV		
PHYTOMENADIONE (Konakion)	Prophylaxis: 1 mg Treatment: 5-10 mg	IM IM or IV	Single. Single.	Inj.: 1 mg/0,5 ml (0,5 ml amp.) 10 mg/ml (1 ml amp.)

Medication generic name (Trade name)	Paediatric dose	Route	Frequency	Availability and remarks
PIPERAZINE (Antepar, Helmezine)	120 mg/kg/dose up to maximum of 4 g (Average dose 2-3 g according to age)	0	Single.	Elixir: 750 mg/5 ml Give with evening meal for round worms.
PRAZIQUANTEL (Biltricide)	40 mg/kg	0	Single or two doses in one day.	Lacquered tablets 600 mg For Schistosomiasis.
PRAZOSIN (Minipress)	0,05-0,4 mg/kg/day	0	2-3 x daily.	Tabs: 1 mg, 2 mg, 5 mg α-adrenergic blocker and direct vasodilator. Give small test dose first to avoid postural hypotension. Use only in patients over 15 kg body weight
PREDNISOLONE (Meticortelone)	See literature	0		Tabs: 5 mg
PREDNISONE (Meticorten)	0,5-2 mg/kg/day depending on indications	0		Tabs: 1 mg, 5 mg

Medication generic name (Trade name)	Paediatric dose	Route	Frequency	Availability and remarks
PRIMIDONE (Mysoline)	10-20 mg/kg/day	O	Divided doses – 3-4 x daily.	Susp.: 250 mg/5 ml Tabs: 250 mg Partly converted *in vivo* to PHENOBARBITONE.
PROBENECID (Benemid)	Over two years 25 mg/kg initial dose, then 10 mg/kg	O	4 x daily.	Tabs: 0,5 g Ensure adequate fluid intake. For gonorrhoea. 50 mg/kg single dose with AMOXYCILLIN.
PROCATEROL (Normalin)	1,25 µg(0,25 ml)kg	O	2 x daily.	Susp. 0,025 mg/5 ml Tabs: 0,025 mg, 0,05 mg

Medication generic name (Trade name)	Paediatric dose	Route	Frequency	Availability and remarks
PROCHLOR- PERAZINE (Stemetil)	0,5 mg/kg/day	O	Divided doses – 3 x daily.	Syrup: 5 mg/5 ml Inj.: 12,5 mg/ml (1 ml amp.) Tabs: 5 mg Supp. paed.: 5 mg Supp. adult: 25 mg Extrapyramidal side-effects.
	0,25 mg/kg/day	IM		
PROMETHAZINE (Phenergan)	0,5 mg/kg/dose	O, IM	See remarks.	Elixir: 5 mg/5 ml Inj.: 25 mg/ml (2 ml amp.) Tabs: 10 mg, 25 mg Antihistaminic: full dose at night $1/4$ dose in morning or when necessary. Nausea/vomiting: half to full dose 4-6 x daily.
PROPRANOLOL (Inderal)	1-5 mg/kg/day May be increased if necessary to	O	Divided doses – 2-4 x daily.	Tabs: 10 mg, 40 mg Inj.: 1 mg/ml Contra-indicated in asthma and

Medication generic name (Trade name)	Paediatric dose	Route	Frequency	Availability and remarks
	10 mg/kg/day			heartblock. Action: adrenergic β-blocker Inhibits renin secretion.
PROTAMINE SULPHATE	1 mg/100 units of last dose of heparin	IV drip	Single.	Inj.: 10 mg/ml (5 ml amp.)
PYRANTEL (Combantrin)	Roundworm/pinworm: 10 mg/kg Hookworm: 10 mg/kg	0 0	Single dose. Daily x 3 days.	Susp.: 15 mg/ml Tabs: 125 mg
SALBUTAMOL (Ventolin)	0,15 mg/kg/dose	0	4 x daily.	Syrup: 2 mg/5 ml Tabs: 2 mg, 4 mg Tabs: (sustained action) 4 mg ,8 mg Metered inhaler: 100 µg/inhalation
	Metered aerosol: 1 puff	Inhalation	Repeated when necessary 4-5 x daily.	
	Rotacap <12 yrs 200 µg disc >12 yrs 400 µg Nebulization: 1 ml	Inhalation Nebulization	3-4 x daily. 3-4 hourly. Mix with equal volume normal saline.	Rotacaps: 200 µg, 400 µg Ventodisc 200 µg, 400 µg Respirator solution.

Medication generic name (Trade name)	Paediatric dose	Route	Frequency	Availability and remarks
SALMETEROL (Serevent)	Children four years and older: 50 µg	Inhalation	2 x daily.	Aerosol inhaler: 25 µg per metered dose. Discs and diskhaler 50 µg blisters.
SENNA standardized (Senokot)	1-2 tabs./dose	0	At night (see remarks).	Tablets. Usual time of action is eight to ten hours Titrate dose for desired effect.
SODIUM CROMOGLYCATE (Lomudal)	Halermatic or Spinhaler: 1 Spincap	Inhalation	3-4 x daily.	Spincap: 20 mg Halermatic or Spinhaler.
	Nebulization: 2 ml	Nebulization	3 x daily.	Nebulizer solution: 10 mg/ml (2 ml amp.)
	Inhaler: 2 puffs	Inhalation	4 x daily.	Inhaler: 1 mg, 5 mg Reduce frequency of administration on maintenance treatment.
(Rynacrom)	Nasal drops: 2 drops	Nose	4 x daily to each nostril.	Nasal drops: 0,8 mg
	Nasal spray: 2 squeezes	Nose	6 x daily to each nostril.	Nasal spray: 2,6 mg/squeeze

Medication generic name (Trade name)	Paediatric dose	Route	Frequency	Availability and remarks
SODIUM VALPROATE (Epilim) (Convulex)	All ages: 15-50 mg/kg/day	O	Divided doses – 3-4 x daily.	Syrup: 200 mg/5 ml (Epilim) 250 mg/5 ml (Convulex) Tabs: 200 mg, 500 mg enteric coated Caps: refer VALPROIC ACID – page 633. Petit mal, grand mal and mixed generalized epilepsy Serum SODIUM VALPROATE – therapeutic range: 50-100 µg/ml
SPIRONOLACTONE (Aldactone)	1-3 mg/kg/day	O	Divided doses – 1-2 x daily.	Tabs: 25 mg (scored) Contra-indicated in acute renal insufficiency.
SPIRONOLACTONE CO (Aldazide)	See literature	O	Divided doses – 1-2 x daily.	Tabs: SPIRONOLACTONE 25 mg + ISOBUTYLHYDROCHLOROTHIAZIDE 2,5 mg

Medication generic name (Trade name)	Paediatric dose	Route	Frequency	Availability and remarks
TERBUTALINE SULPHATE (Bricanyl)	2 puffs/dose	Inhalation	up to 4 x daily.	Aerosol For treatment of acute bronchospasm
THEOPHYLLINE Short-acting:	Elixir and syrup: 5 mg/kg/dose	0	4 x daily. divided doses	Short-acting preparations: Elixir: contains 30 mg THEOPHYLLINE/ 5 ml and 20 % alcohol Solphyllin Theophen Theostat Vernthol Syrup: 25 mg THEOPHYLLINE /5 ml (Nuelin)
	Tabs: 5 mg/kg/dose	0	4 x daily. divided doses	Nuelin tabs.: 50 mg, 125 mg
Long-acting:	10-12 mg/kg/dose	0	2 x daily.	Long-acting preparations: Euphyllin Retard: 350 mg AMINOPHYLLINE

Medication generic name (Trade name)	Paediatric dose	Route	Frequency	Availability and remarks
				Equiv. to 280 mg THEOPHYLLINE Microphyllin: 60 mg, 125 mg, 250 mg Nuelin SA tabs.: 250 mg (scored) Somophyllin: 100 mg, 250 mg Theodur: 200 mg, 300 mg (scored) tab. Cap 50 mg, 125 mg. THEOPHYLLINE therapeutic blood level: 10-20 μg/ml
THIORIDAZINE (Melleril)	0,5 mg/kg/day Increased if necessary to 4 mg/kg/day.	O	2-3 x daily	Sol.: 30 mg/ml (1 drop = 1 mg) Susp.: 0,5%: 5 mg/ml Tabs: 10 mg, 25 mg, 50 mg, 100 mg, 200 mg
TILIDINE (Valoron)	1 drop per each year of age	O	3-4 x daily.	Drops: 50 mg/0,5 ml (20 drops) Caps.: 50 mg An analgesic, see literature

Medication generic name (Trade name)	Paediatric dose	Route	Frequency	Availability and remarks
TINIDAZOLE (Fasigyn)	4 x 500 mg (adult dose)	O	Single dose.	Tabs: 500 mg
TRICLOFOS (Tricloryl)	Hypnotic: 50 mg/kg/dose Sedation: 25 mg/kg/day	O O	Repeat 3 x daily when necessary. Divided doses – 3 x daily.	Syrup (paediatric): 500 mg/5 ml Equiv. to 300 mg CHLORAL HYDRATE
TRIMEPRAZINE (Vallergan)	Pre-anaesthesia: 2–4 mg/kg/dose Antipruritic 7,5–15 mg daily (Up to 22 mg 3 x daily)	O O	Single. Divided doses 3–4 x daily.	Syrup: 7,5 mg/5 ml Syrup forte: 30 mg/5 ml Tabs: 10 mg
TRIPROLIDINE CO (Actifed)	Under one year: 2,5 ml/dose Over one to six years: 2,5–5 ml/dose Six to 12 years: 5–7,5 ml/dose	O O O	2–3 x daily. As above. As above.	Contents per 5 ml and per tablet: TRIPROLIDINE HCl 1,25 mg PSEUDOEPHEDRINE 30 mg

Medication generic name (Trade name)	Paediatric dose	Route	Frequency	Availability and remarks
VALPROIC ACID (Convulex)	All ages: 15-50 mg/kg/day	O	Divided doses 3-4 x daily.	Cap 150 mg, 300 mg See also SODIUM VALPROATE
VERAPAMIL (Isoptin)	Under one year: 0,1-0,2 mg/kg/dose Over one year: 0,2-0,3 mg/kg/dose	IV	Emergency use for tachyarrhythmias.	Inj.: 2,5 mg/ml (2 ml amp.) Repeat once after 30 mins if necessary. Tabs: 40 mg, 80 mg
	1-10 mg/kg/day increased gradually	O	3 x daily.	
ZINC	General deficiency 2 mg Elemental zinc/kg/day Suspected deficiency 1 mg Elemental zinc/kg/day Preterm infants 0,5 mg Elemental zinc/kg/day	O		

Table 2 Antimicrobials

Consult individual hospital's current antibiotic policy (see page 568.)

Medication Generic name (Trade name)	Paediatric dose	Route	Frequency	Availability and remarks
ACYCLOVIR (Zovirax)	5 mg/kg/dose Immunocompromised patients: 10 mg/kg/dose	IV	Eight-hourly.	250 mg per vial. Higher dose only if renal function is not impaired. Note: higher dose in encephalitis: 10 mg/kg/dose.
AMIKACIN (Amikin)	Preterm/neonates: Loading dose 10 mg/kg then 15 mg/kg/day Older children	IM, IV	Divided doses – 2 x daily.	Inj.: 100 mg, 250 mg, 500 mg (2 ml vials)
	15 mg/kg/day	IM, IV	2 - 3 x daily or total daily dose may be infused over one to two hours.	Oto- and nephrotoxic

Medication Generic name (Trade name)	Paediatric dose	Route	Frequency	Availability and remarks
AMOXYCILLIN (Amoxil)	Preterm: 30- 62,5 mg	0	Once daily for first one or two weeks, then 2 - 3 x daily.	Paed. drops: 125 mg/1,25 ml Syrup: 125 mg/5 ml and 250 mg/5 ml
	Infants to six months: 62,5 mg	0	2 - 3 x daily.	Caps.: 250 mg, 500 mg Inj.: 250 mg, 500 mg vials
	Six months – ten years: 125 mg	0	3 x daily.	
	See packet insert	IM, IV	Divided doses – 3 - 6 x daily.	
AMOXYCILLIN with CLAVULANIC ACID (Augmentin)	25-50 mg/kg/day of <u>AMOXYCILLIN</u>	0	3 x daily.	Susp.: 125 mg AMOXYCILLIN and 31,5 mg CLAVULANIC ACID/5 ml and 250 mg AMOXICILLIN and 62,5 mg CLAVULANIC ACID/5 ml.
	50-100 mg/kg/day of AMOXYCILLIN	IV	3 x daily.	Tabs: 250 mg AMOXICILLIN and 125 mg CLAVULANIC ACID. Vials: 0,6 g (AMOXYCILLIN 500 mg and CLAVULANIC ACID 100 mg) and 1,2 g (AMOXYCILLIN 1000 mg and CLAVULANIC ACID 200 mg).

Medication Generic name (Trade name)	Paediatric dose	Route	Frequency	Availability and remarks
AMPHOTERICIN B (Fungizone)	1 ml/dose:	O	4 x daily.	Susp.: 100 mg/ml Tabs: 100 mg for candidiasis
	Initial dose: 0.25 mg/kg/day Increasing to: 1 mg/kg/day	IV IV	Infuse over two to six hours. Infuse over two to six hours.	Inj.: 50 mg (20 ml vial) – dilute in 5% dextrose water for cryptococcal meningitis.
AMPICILLIN (Penbritin, Pentrex)	Normal dose: 50-100 mg/kg/day Severe infection: 200 mg/kg/day	O, IM, IV O, IM, IV	Divided doses – 4 x daily. As above.	Syrup: 125 mg/5 ml Syrup forte: 250 mg/5 ml Caps.: 250 mg, 500 mg Inj.: 250 mg, 500 mg, 1 g Bactericidal. Skin rashes common.
CEFACLOR (Ceclor)	20 mg/kg/day Severe infections 40 mg/kg/day	O	3 x daily.	Susp.: 125 mg/5 ml, 250 mg/5 ml

Medication Generic name (Trade name)	Paediatric dose	Route	Frequency	Availability and remarks
CEFADROXIL (Duracef)	Urinary tract infections: 25-50 mg/kg/day Other conditions: 20-80 mg/kg/day See literature	O O	2 x daily. 2 x daily.	Susp.: 250 mg/5 ml, 500 mg/5 ml
CEFAMANDOLE (Mandokef)	50-100 mg/kg/day 150 mg/kg if very severe infection	IM, IV	Divided doses – 3 - 4 x daily.	Vials: 1 g
CEFOTAXIME (Claforan)	50-100 mg/kg/day 200 mg/kg if very severe infection	IM, IV	Divided doses – 2 - 4 x daily.	Vials: 500 mg, 1 g
CEFOXITIN (Mefoxin)	Over two years of age: 80-160 mg/kg/day Severe infections: up to 200 mg/kg/day Maximum 12 g	IM, IV	4 - 6 x daily.	Vials: 1 g

Medication Generic name (Trade name)	Paediatric dose	Route	Frequency	Availability and remarks
CEFTAZIDIME (Fortum)	Over two months of age: 30 - 100 mg/kg/day Immunocompromised patients up to 50 mg/kg/dose	IM, IV	2 - 3 x daily. 3 x daily.	Vials 500 mg, 1g, 2g
CEFTRIAXONE (Rocephin)	20 - 80 mg/kg/day	IM, IV	Daily or 2 x daily.	Vials: 250 mg, 500 mg, l g, 2 g Use 1% LIGNOCAINE for IM.
CEPHRADINE (Cefril)	25 - 50 mg/kg/day Otitis media due to *H. influenzae*: 75 - 100 mg/kg/day	O O	4 x daily. 4 x daily.	Susp.: 125 mg/5 ml, 250 mg/5 ml
CHLOR- AMPHENICOL (Chloromycetin)	All newborn infants up to two weeks: 25 mg/kg/day Infants over four weeks: 50 mg/kg/day	O, IM IV O, IM IV	Divided doses – 4 x daily. As above.	Susp.: 125 mg/5 ml Caps.: 250 mg, 500 mg Inj.:1 g (Check dilutions carefully) Use Chloromycetin succinate for IM and IV.

Medication Generic name (Trade name)	Paediatric dose	Route	Frequency	Availability and remarks
	Children: 50 - 100 mg/kg/day	O, IM IV	As above.	Limit use – may be toxic. Measure blood levels.
CIPROFLOXACIN (Ciprobay)	7.5-15 mg/kg/dose Max.: 1500 mg/day 5-10 mg/kg/dose Max.: 800 mg/day	O IV	2-3 x daily. 2 x daily.	Tabs: 250 mg, 500 mg, 700 mg Vials: 2 mg/ml, 50 ml, 100 ml Not recommended <18 years. See literature.
CLINDAMYCIN (Dalacin-C)	8 - 25 mg/kg/day Over one month: 10 - 40 mg/kg/day Severe infections: not less than 300 mg/day regardless of weight	O IM, IV IM, IV	3 - 4 x daily. Divided doses – 2, 3 or 4 x daily. Divided doses – 3 - 4 x daily.	Susp.: 75 mg/5 ml Caps: 150 mg Inj.: 150 mg/ml (4 ml amp.)

Medication Generic name (Trade name)	Paediatric dose	Route	Frequency	Availability and remarks
CLOXACILLIN (Orbenin, Prostaphlin A)	50 - 100 mg/kg/day	O, IM, IV	Divided doses – 4 x daily.	Syrup: 125 mg/5 ml Caps: 250 mg, 500 mg Inj.: 250 mg, 500 mg (vials)
CO-AMOXICLAV (Augmentin)	As for AMOXYCILLIN with CLAVULANIC ACID See page 635.			
CO-TRIMOXAZOLE (Bactrim, Mezenol, Purbac, Septran)	six weeks to five months: 2,5 ml/dose	O	2 x daily.	Susp.: TRIMETHOPRIM 40 mg and SULPHAMETHOXAZOLE 200 mg/5 ml
	six months to five years: 5 ml/dose	O	As above.	
	Six to 12 years: 10 ml/dose	O	2 x daily.	Tabs Paed.: TRIMETHOPRIM 20 mg and SULPHAMETHOXAZOLE 100 mg
	Six weeks to five months: 1,25 ml	IV Infusion	2 x daily.	
	Six months to five years: 2,5 ml Six to 12 years: 5 ml Over 12 years: 10 ml			Septran for infusion: each ampoule of 5 ml contains: TRIMETHOPRIM 80 mg and SULPHAMETHOXAZOLE 400 mg.

Medication Generic name (Trade name)	Paediatric dose	Route	Frequency	Availability and remarks
				Not suitable for any other route or method of administration. Mix with GLUCOSE 5% or GLUCOSE 10% or sodium chloride 0,45% plus GLUCOSE 2,5%. Infuse over 60 – 90 minutes. Do not add sodium bicarbonate or any other medicament.
DOXYCYCLINE (Vibramycin)	Initial dose 4,4 mg/kg then 2,2 mg/kg	O	Once daily.	Susp.: 40 mg/5 ml Caps: 100 mg Less effect on tissues and teeth than other tetracyclines.

Medication Generic name (Trade name)	Paediatric dose	Route	Frequency	Availability and remarks
ERYTHROMYCIN (Erythrocin, Ilosone)	25 - 50 mg/kg/day	O	Divided doses – 4 x daily.	Syrup: 125 mg/5 ml (Erythrocin) 200 mg/5 ml (Erythrocin oral susp.)
	20 - 50 mg/kg/day (severe infections)	IV (over five minutes)	Divided doses – 3 - 4 x daily.	125 and 250 mg/5 ml (Ilosone) Inj. (IV): 300 mg: 1 g vial. Add 6 ml water to 300 mg or 20 ml water to 1g. Dilute to 1%. If using 5% dextrose add sodium bicarbonate 2,4 mmol/500 ml
ETHAMBUTOL (Myambutol)	15 - 20 mg/kg/day	O	Single dose, daily.	Syrup: 125 mg/5 ml Tabs: 100 mg, 400 mg Complication – optic neuritis.
ETHIONAMIDE	10-20 mg/kg/day	O	Single or divided doses after meals.	Use in TBM and miliary disease. See page 122.

Medication Generic name (Trade name)	Paediatric dose	Route	Frequency	Availability and remarks
FLUCLOXACILLIN (Floxapen)	25-50 mg/kg/day	O, IV	Divided doses 4 x daily.	Susp.: 125 mg/5ml Caps: 250 mg Inj.: 250 mg
FUSIDIC ACID (Fucidin)	25 - 40 mg/kg/day	O	Divided doses – 3 x daily.	Susp.: 250 mg/5 ml Caps: 250 mg
	6 - 7 mg/kg/dose	IV Infusion	3 x daily.	Dissolve the contents of one vial containing 500 mg sodium fusidic powder (equivalent to 488 mg of fusidic acid) in the 10 ml sterile phosphate-citrate buffer solution provided. Immediately after reconstituting add the fusidate-buffer solution to 250 to 500 ml of infusion fluid and infuse slowly over a period of not less than two to four hours. Infusions should be made into a wide bore vein with a good blood flow. The following IV solutions may be used: sodium chloride 0,9%, dextrose 5%, compound sodium

Medication Generic name (Trade name)	Paediatric dose	Route	Frequency	Availability and remarks
				lactate BP, sodium lactate BP, sodium chloride 0,18% and dextrose 4%, potassium chloride 0,3% and sodium chloride 0,9%, potassium chloride 0,3% and dextrose 5%. Fucidin-IV is incompatible with dextrose 40% and dextrose 50%. Fucidin is indicated in conjunction with other anti-staphylococcal agents in the treatment of several staphylococcal infections.
GENTAMICIN (Cidomycin, Garamycin)	50 mg/kg/day	O	Divided doses up to 6 x daily. Max. 360 mg/day or the total daily dose may be infused over 30 minutes.	Susp.: Make up from IV solution, dilute to required dose per ml. Not absorbed from GI tract. For persistent diarrhoea.

Medication Generic name (Trade name)	Paediatric dose	Route	Frequency	Availability and remarks
	3 - 6 mg/kg/day 6 mg/kg/day in neonatal septicaemia or meningitis	IM, IV IM, IV	Divided doses 2-3 x daily Divided doses – 2 x daily.	Inj.: 10 mg/ml, 40 mg/ml (2 ml vials) Monitor serum levels if possible Avoid prolonged concentration over 12 µg/ml Oto- and nephrotoxic.
GRISEOFULVIN (Fulcin, Grisovin)	10 mg/kg/day	O	Once daily or divided doses, with food.	Tabs: 125 mg, 500 mg For scalp – six weeks For nails – six months Not for other areas unless topical treatment has failed
ISONIAZID (INH)	10 - 15 mg/kg/day	O	Once daily.	Tabs: 50 mg, 100 mg (scored) Inj.: See literature
	15 - 20 mg/kg/day for miliary TB or TB meningitis Max. 300 mg/day	O	Once daily.	Complications: peripheral neuritis, hepatitis, hypersensitivity For neuritis, PYRIDOXINE 50 - 100 mg daily.

Medication Generic name (Trade name)	Paediatric dose	Route	Frequency	Availability and remarks
METRONIDAZOLE (Flagyl)	7 mg/kg/dose 7,5 mg/kg/dose	O IV	3 x daily. Eight-hourly.	Syrup: 200 mg/5 ml Tabs: 200 mg, 400 mg Inj.: 5 mg/ml (100 ml vials) Suppositories: 500 mg and 1 g **for anaerobic infections** For other uses, see page 619. Ineffective against pseudomonas.
NALIDIXIC ACID (Wintomylon)	Therapeutic: 50 mg/kg/day Maintenance: 25 mg/kg/day	O O	Divided doses – 4 x daily. As above.	Susp.: 250 mg/5 ml Tabs: 500 mg Not recommended under three months.
NEOMYCIN	100 mg/kg/day	O	4 x daily.	Elixir: 125 mg/5 ml Tabs: 500 mg Used in cases of liver failure and persistent diarrhoea.

Medication Generic name (Trade name)	Paediatric dose	Route	Frequency	Availability and remarks
NITROFURANTOIN (Furadantin)	5 - 7 mg/kg/day Contra-indicated under one month	O	Divided doses – 4 x daily.	Susp.: 25 mg/5 ml Tabs: 50 mg, 100 mg Caps: 50 mg, 100 mg Maintenance doses should be one half to one quarter of the therapeutic dose. Administer with food or milk.
NYSTATIN (Mycostatin)	Infants: 50 000 units/dose Children: 1 - 2 million units/day	O O	Divided doses – after each feed As above	Susp.: 50 000 units in 0,5 ml Tabs: 500 000 units
OFLOXACIN (Tarivid)	7,5 mg/kg/dose Max.: 800 mg/day	O	2 x daily.	Tabs: 200 mg
	5 mg/kg/dose Max.: 400 mg/day	IV	2 x daily.	Vials: 2 mg/ml, 100 ml Not recommended <18 years. See literature.

Medication Generic name (Trade name)	Paediatric dose	Route	Frequency	Availability and remarks
OXYTETRACYCLINE (Terramycin)	20 - 50 mg/kg/day	O	3 - 4 x daily	Susp.: 125 mg/5 ml for tick-bite fever Caps: 250 mg **Warning:** see TETRACYCLINE
PENICILLIN G or **CRYSTALLINE PENICILLIN** or **BENZYLPENICILLIN** or **SODIUM PENICILLIN** (Crystapen, Novopen)	Newborn: 60 000 iu/kg/day Older infants and children: 25 000-50 000 iu/kg/day Severe infection: 300 000-400 000 iu/kg/day	IM, IV IM, IV IV	Divided doses – 2 x daily. Divided doses – 4 x daily. As above.	Inj.: 500 000 iu (vial) 1 million iu (vial) 5 million iu (vial)
PROCAINE PENICILLIN (Novocillin)	25 000 iu/kg/day	IM	Single dose.	Inj.: 1 ml contains – PROCAINE PENICILLIN G 300 000 iu

Medication Generic name (Trade name)	Paediatric dose	Route	Frequency	Availability and remarks
BENZATHINE PENICILLIN FORTIFIED (Penilente Forte)	All purpose 600 000 - 1,2 million units	IM	As required.	Inj.:1,2 million iu (vial) 6 million iu (vial) BENZYLPENICILLIN 300 000 iu PROCAINE PENICILLIN 300 000 iu BENZATHINE PENICILLIN 600 000 iu per 1,2 million iu.
BENZATHINE PENICILLIN (Bicillin LA, Penilente LA)	Long-acting 600 000 - 1,2 million iu	IM	Monthly.	Inj.:1,2 million iu (vial) 6 million iu (vial)
PENICILLIN V PHENOXYMETHYL-PENICILLIN	50 - 1 000 mg/day	O	Divided doses – 4 x daily.	Syrup: 125 mg (250 000 iu)/5 ml 250 mg/5 ml Tabs: 125 mg, 250 mg
PIPERACILLIN (Pipril)	100 - 300 mg/kg per day	IV IM	3 - 4 x daily.	2 g vial 4 g vial

Medication Generic name (Trade name)	Paediatric dose	Route	Frequency	Availability and remarks
PYRAZINAMIDE (Pyran)	25 mg/kg/day 40 mg/kg/day in TBM and miliary TB. Max. 2 g	O O	Single daily dose. Single daily dose.	Tabs: 500 mg Complication: hepatitis.
RIFAMPICIN (Rifadin, Rimactane)	10 mg/kg/day 20 mg/kg/day in TBM and miliary TB Max. 600 mg/day 20 mg/kg/day	O O IV	Single daily dose. Single daily dose. Single daily infusion over three hours.	Syrup: 100 mg/5 ml Caps: 150 mg, 300 mg Complication: hepatitis. Inj.: 600 mg Complication: hepatitis.
STREPTOMYCIN	20 mg/kg/day up to 1 g	IM	Single or divided dose – 2 x daily.	Inj.: 1 g (vial) Do not exceed 1 g/day Complications: eighth nerve damage, nephrotoxicity.

Medication Generic name (Trade name)	Paediatric dose	Route	Frequency	Availability and remarks
TETRACYCLINE (See DOXYCYCLINE and OXYTETRACYCLINE)	20 - 50 mg/kg/day	O	Divided doses – 3 x daily.	Syrup: 125 mg/5 ml Tabs: 125 mg, 250 mg **Used only for mycoplasma, chlamydia and rickettsial infections.** N.B. Permanent staining of teeth if used for children under 12 years.
TOBRAMYCIN (Nebcin)	6 - 7,5 mg/kg/day	IM, IV	Divided doses – 3 x daily or total daily dose may be infused over 30 minutes.	Inj.: 10 mg/ml (2 ml vial) 40 mg/ml (2 ml vial)
	Prems and neonates up to 4 mg/kg/day	IM, IV	2 x daily.	Administer over 30- 60 minutes. Best aminoglycoside for pseudomonas infections. Monitor serum levels. Oto- and nephrotoxic.

Medication Generic name (Trade name)	Paediatric dose	Route	Frequency	Availability and remarks
VANCOMYCIN	Under one week: 15 mg/kg followed by 10 mg/kg/dose One week to one month: 15 mg/kg followed by 10 mg/kg/dose. Over one month: 40 mg/kg/day	IV	Every 12 hours. Every eight hours.	Inj.: 500 mg
		2 - 3 x daily.		

Table 3 Paediatric drugs in general use which contain phenothiazine derivatives or which can cause extrapyramidal symptoms

Drug	Active Ingredient
Actifed	TRIPROLIDINE HCl, PSEUDOEPHEDRINE HCl
Anthisan	MEPYRAMINE MALEATE
Demazin	CHLORPROPHENPYRIDAMINE MALEATE + PHENYLEPHRINE HCl
Eglonyl	SULPIRIDE
Eskornade	ISOPROPAMIDE IODIDE, PHENYLPROPANOLAMINE HCl + DIPHENYLPYRALINE
Maxolon	METOCLOPRAMIDE
Phenergan	PROMETHAZINE HCl
Sparine	PROMAZINE
Stelazine	TRIFLUOPERAZINE
Stopayne Syrup	PARACETAMOL, CODEINE, PROMETHAZINE
Stemetil	PROCHLORPERAZINE MALEATE
Syndette	PARACETAMOL, DOXYLAMINE SUCCINATE
Valoid	CYCLIZINE HCl
Vallergan	TRIMEPRAZINE TARTRATE

APPENDIX 3

CLINIC AND WARD SIDEROOM INVESTIGATIONS

M D Mann

Acid-base and blood gas parameters

If possible, arterial or arterialized capillary blood should be used for acid-base and blood gas analysis, though venous blood may be acceptable. Average differences between arterial and venous blood are: venous blood pH is approximately 0,03 units lower than arterial, venous PCO_2 is 6-7 mmHg higher and HCO_3 2,0-2,5 mmol/l higher. These differences will increase with stasis or shock. Changes on standing are: pH decreases at 0,014 units/hr at room temperature and 0,005 units/hr at 4 °C; PO_2 of fully saturated blood falls at 17 mmHg/hr at 4 °C; PCO_2 increases at 0,6 mmHg/hr at 4 °C.

Collection and transport of specimens on ice is always preferable and essential if there is any delay before analysis. Collection must eliminate airspace. For collection of venous or arterial blood into a syringe, first take up a small amount of heparin into the syringe, coat the walls, and squirt out the remainder. Then collect the sample, eliminate airspace, cork the end of the needle or cap the tube firmly, mix thoroughly by inversion and rapid rolling between the hands, label and send to the laboratory.

Arterialized capillary samples are taken into heparinized capillary tubes (200 µl), two tubes if possible. Seal one end, introduce an iron filing, seal other end eliminating air space and mix using a magnet. Transport in a marked labelled tube as above.

Bacteriological stains
Gram's stain

Make a smear in the centre of a glass slide and allow to dry. Fix by passing rapidly through a flame. Apply Crystal violet for ten seconds. Rinse briefly with water. Apply Gram's iodine for ten seconds. Decolorize with acetone (one to two seconds only) and rinse with water. Counterstain with dilute Carbol fuchsin for ten seconds. Rinse with water. Blot or air dry.

Identification of bacteria by Gram's stain

Bacteria	Gram's stain result	Appearance
Streptococci :	Gram-positive	Blue cocci in chains
Pneumococci :	Gram-positive	Blue cocci in pairs or short chains
Staphylococci :	Gram-positive	Blue cocci in clusters
Meningococci :	Gram-negative	Pink bean-shaped cocci in pairs
Haemophilus :	Gram-negative	Pink small coccobacilli
Enteric bacilli :	Gram-negative	Pink large rods

Methylene blue stain

♦ Scrapings of the buccal mucosa (for thrush), centrifuged deposit of CSF (for bacteria and leucocytes), faecal smear or pus smear is applied thinly to a slide.
♦ Dry and fix by passing through a Bunsen flame three times.
♦ Stain the slide with Methylene blue (0,5% aqueous solution) for one minute. Wash in water and dry.
♦ Examine under oil immersion.

Ziehl-Neelsen stain

Make a thin, even smear. Dry and fix by flaming rapidly. Cover the slide with concentrated Carbol fuchsin. Heat until steaming, do not boil. Stain for five minutes, heating intermittently. Rinse thoroughly with water. Decolorize with 3% HCl in 95% alcohol, till smear colourless or faint pink. Rinse with water. Counterstain with Methylene blue for 20 seconds. Rinse with water, then air-dry.

♦ AFB: red beaded bacilli.
♦ Cells and background: blue-green.

Blood counts

White blood cell count

Visual leucocyte count

◆ Prepare a 1:20 dilution of well mixed whole blood by adding 0,05 ml of blood to 0.95 ml of diluting fluid (2% acetic acid coloured pale violet with a drop of Gentian violet).
◆ Mix gently for at least two minutes to lyse red cells.
◆ Fill a Neubauer counting chamber, using capillary glass and tubing, taking care that excess fluid does not flow into the surrounding moat.
◆ Count the number of cells in each of the four corner squares (i.e. 4 x 1 mm^2) using a low power objective (x10).
◆ Calculation: number of cells counted x 50 = total leucocyte count (x 10^9/l)

Haematocrit (PCV) (micro method)

◆ Allow well mixed blood to enter a 75 mm capillary tube by capillarity, leaving at least 15 mm unfilled.
◆ Seal the tube by heating the dry end of the tube in a Bunsen flame or by using plasticine.
◆ Place the tube in a micro-haemotocrit centrifuge (sealed end against periphery) and centrifuge for five minutes. (10 000 rpm)
◆ Express the length of the red cell column as a percentage of the total length.

Erythrocyte sedimentation rate (Westergren method)

◆ Dilute venous blood with 3.8 % trisodium citrate in the proportion of one part citrate to four parts blood.
◆ Draw the well mixed sample up to the 200 mm mark in the Westergren tube.
◆ Place the tube in an exactly vertical position (special racks are commercially available).
◆ Read the fall in the column of sedimented cells to the nearest mm after one hour.

ESR is expressed in mm per hour (Westergren).

Mean corpuscular haemoglobin concentration (MCHC)

The MCHC refers to the percentage of haemoglobin in 100 ml of red blood cells as compared to the percentage of haemoglobin in 100 ml of whole blood.

It is calculated from

$$\frac{\text{Hb (g/100ml)}}{\text{Haematocrit \%}} \times 100$$

The normal range is 32-36% and the MCHC is low in iron deficiency anaemia.

Cerebrospinal fluid examination

Examine for colour, clarity, clots and xanthochromia.

♦ Cells: add one drop counting fluid (0,4% Methyl violet in 4% glacial acetic acid) to 0,5 ml CSF. Using a modified Fuchs-Rosenthal chamber, count five large squares to get total cell count (x 10^9/l).
♦ Globulin: add one drop CSF to 0,5 ml Pandy's reagent. Read immediately as nil or 1+ to 4+ according to turbidity. Globulin is normally absent. Presence of globulin is indicative of a raised CSF protein.
♦ Protein: add 0,5 ml CSF to 1,5 ml salicylsulphonic acid. Read after two minutes by comparing against standard opacity solutions. Normal = 0,1 – 0,4 g/l.
♦ Glucose: one drop CSF on Testape. Normal = a bright green colour change. Quantitative estimation desirable.

A Gram's stain and where appropriate a Ziehl-Neelsen stain should be performed on centrifuged deposits from hazy or purulent fluids. (See pages 654-5 for methods.)

Neonatal tests
Apt-test for fetal haemoglobin

To test blood-stained stool or vomitus, take equal parts of the blood-stained specimen and tap water. Shake and centrifuge. Add one part of supernatant to five parts of 1% NaOH. Read at one minute. Fetal Hb stays pink, whereas adult Hb denatures and turns brown.

Shake test

Place 0,5 ml gastric aspirate (collected within 30 minutes after delivery) in a clean, dry test tube. Add 0,5 ml normal saline and replace the cap. Shake well for 15 seconds. Add 1 ml 95% alcohol to the 1 ml mixture of gastric aspirate and saline. Again replace the cap, shake well for 15 seconds and read at 15 minutes.

Observation	Result	Risk of hyaline membrane disease
No bubbles	negative	very high
Incomplete ring of bubbles	intermediate	possible
Complete ring of bubbles	positive	very low

Stool tests

The bakkie test

A stool specimen is collected daily and placed in a clear plastic container. With a spatula, some stool is spread against the side of the container and observed for pigment, daily for seven days. Discoloration of the surface of the stool is ignored. A white to grey stool is indicative of complete cholestasis.

Microscopy

Preferably choose a portion of stool containing blood or mucus if present. Using an orange stick, emulsify in a drop of saline on a glass slide. Cover with a coverslip and examine under 100x and 400x magnification.

Apart from WBC's and RBC's, pathogens that may be seen include:

♦ *Entamoeba histolytica*: trophozoites have clear pseudopodia, are actively motile and ingest RBC's.
♦ *Giardia lamblia:* trophozoites are pear-shaped, flagellated, with typical 'falling leaf' motility. Cysts are oval, highly refractile, and contain two nuclei and 'whiskers'.
♦ *Ascaris lumbricoides:* ova are oval/rectangular with a thick frilly shell.

◆ *Trichuris trichiura:* ova are oval with plugs at either end ('tea-tray').

Reducing sugars

More than 0,5 g/dl reducing sugar in a stool suggests disturbed carbohydrate digestion or malabsorption. In infantile diarrhoea, reducing sugars in the stool are a marker of intestinal mucosal damage. Reducing sugars may not be the primary aetiological factor in persistent diarrhoea. It is essential to examine the fluid part of the stool. Collect stool in a polythene bag or reversed plastic-backed disposable nappy to avoid soaking away of liquid. Examine as soon as possible.

Clinitest

Add two parts of water to one part fluid portion of stool. Shake to mix. Take 15 drops of mixture and add one Clinitest tablet. After 60 seconds compare the resulting colour with colour chart. More than 0,5 g/dl is abnormal.

Test for sucrose (not a reducing substance)

Take great care in performing this test. Keep tube pointing away from operator. Do not pipette by mouth and perform in well-ventilated area. Add 1 part stool fluid (approximately 1 ml) carefully to 2 volumes concentrated hydrochloric acid and boil gently for 30 seconds. Add one Clinitest tablet to 15 drops of mixture and read as above. After 60 seconds compare the resulting colour with the colour chart. More than 0,5 g/dl is abnormal.

Urine tests
Microscopy

Decant 5 ml urine into a conical-bottomed test tube. Centrifuge at 1 500 rpm for three minutes. Pour off the supernatant and resuspend the deposit. Place a drop on a glass slide, cover with a coverslip, and examine under 400x magnification. The presence of >10 WBC's or >10 RBC's per field is abnormal and warrants further investigation. Other pathological elements such as casts or organisms may also be seen.

Reducing sugars

Reducing sugars detected in urine are abnormal and usually indicate disturbed carbohydrate metabolism.

Reagent strips based on the action of glucose oxidase upon glucose are specific for glucose. They are quick and convenient screening tests which have limitations. Bleach or hydrogen peroxide in the collecting container, homogentisic acid and drugs, e.g. CHLORAMPHENICOL, INH, NALIDIXIC ACID and TETRACYCLINES, may produce false positive results. Ascorbic acid, by retarding colour development, can give rise to false negative results. Benedict's test and Clinitest (Ames) based on the reduction of metallic ions (copper) are non-specific for glucose, detecting other reducing sugars, i.e. galactose and fructose. Study package inserts.

Glucose is the most commonly detected sugar in urine. Diabetes mellitus must be excluded where there is significant glycosuria. Other reducing sugars may indicate an inborn error of carbohydrate metabolism. Galactosaemia is suggested in an infant if the reagent strip is negative in the face of a positive Clinitest or Benedict's test. Definitive diagnosis depends on chromatography (to identify the specific sugars) and enzyme assay.

Testing urine

Reagent strips: dip into urine and remove excess by touching the side of the container with the strip. After ten seconds compare the colour with colour chart. Sensitive to glucose at 0,1 g/dl concentration.

Clinitest: to five drops urine add ten drops water in a test-tube. Add one Clinitest tablet and compare with the chart supplied with the test. Sensitive at the 0,2 g/dl level.

Benedict's test: add ten drops of urine to 5 ml Benedict's reagent in a test-tube. Mix and place in a boiling waterbath for five minutes. Allow to cool and read. The colour ranges from blue (no reducing substance present) through green, yellow, orange to brick-red colour (reducing substance present in significant amounts).

APPENDIX 4

USEFUL NORMAL VALUES, GRAPHS AND TABLES

M D Mann

Acid-base

Table 1 Normal values for acid-base (Astrup) and PaO_2 in arterial blood

Under two years

pH	7,34-7,46
$PaCO_2$	26,4-41,2 mmHg or 3,5-5,5 kPa
PaO_2	83-108 mmHg or 11,0-14,4 kPa
BE	−6,6-+0,2 mmol/l
SB	20-25 mmol/l

Over two years

pH	7,35-7,45
$PaCO_2$	32-48 mmHg or 4,3-6,4 kPa
PaO_2	80-105 mmHg or 10,6-14,0 kPa
BE	−2,3-+2,3 mmol/l
SB	22-26 mmol/l

Figure 1 Determining simple acid base disorders from measurements of pH, pCO₂, and serum bicarbonate

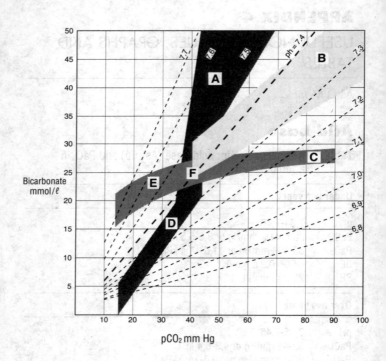

A = Acute and chronic metabolic alkalosis
B = Chronic respiratory acidosis
C = Acute respiratory acidosis
D = Acute and chronic metabolic acidosis
E = Acute respiratory alkalosis
F = Normal range

Adapted from Arbus GS in *Can Med Assoc J* 1973; 109:291 by permission of the Canadian Medical Association.

Body surface area

Figure 2 Normogram for determination of body surface area: adults

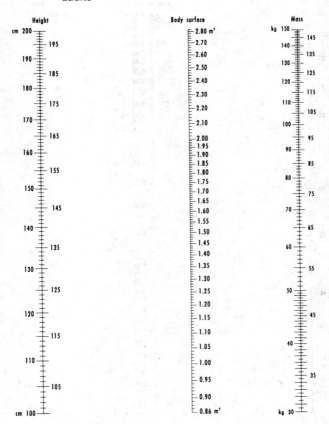

The body surface area is given by the point of intersection with the middle scale of a straight line joining height and weight.

From the formula of Du Bois and Du Bois, *Arch. intern. Med.*, 17:863 (1916):
$S = W^{0.425} \times H^{0.725} \times 71{,}84$, or $\log S = \log W \times 0{,}425 + \log H \times 0{,}725 + 1{,}8564$
(S = body surface area in cm², W = weight in kg, H = height in cm).
Reproduced by permission of Ciba-Geigy from Lentner C (Ed.) *Geigy Scientific Tables*
8th Edition Volume 1. Basel: Ciba-Geigy 1981:226-7.

Figure 3 Normogram for determination of body surface area: infants and young children

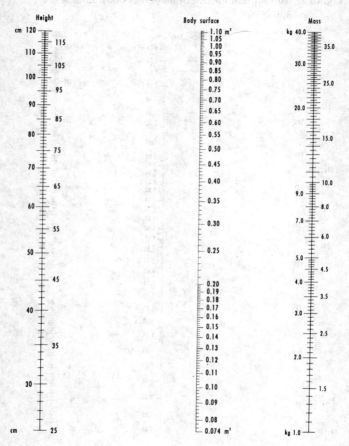

The body surface area is given by the point of intersection with the middle scale of a straight line joining height and weight.

From the formula of Du Bois and Du Bois, *Arch. intern. Med.*, 17:863 (1916):
S = W^0,425 x H^0,725 x 71,84, or log S = log W x 0,425 + log H x 0,725 + 1,8564
(S = body surface area in cm², W = weight in kg, H = height in cm).
Reproduced by permission of Ciba-Geigy from Lentner C (Ed.) *Geigy Scientific Tables* 8th Edition Volume 1. Basel: Ciba-Geigy 1981:226-7.

Coma

The Glasgow Coma Scale (GCS) is useful for identifying a high-risk patient for more invasive therapies. It is not an aid to deciding whether to withhold or withdraw therapy, nor is it a substitute for a good neurological assessment.

Scores less than 8 on admission suggest severe injury. A child with this score should have airway support and aggressive therapy to decrease ICP.

Table 2 The Glasgow Coma Scale

Age under one year	Over one year
Eyes opening	
4 Spontaneously	4 Spontaneously
3 To verbal command	3 To shout
2 To pain	2 To pain
1 No response	1 No response
Best motor response	
6 Obeys	6 Normal spontaneous movements
5 Localizes pain	5 Localizes pain
4 Flexion withdrawal	4 Flexion withdrawal
3 Flexor posturing	3 Flexor posturing (decorticate)
2 Extensor posturing	2 Extensor posturing (decerebrate)
1 No response	1 No response
Best verbal response	
Over two years	**Under two years**
5 Orientated, converses	5 Coos and babbles
4 Disorientated, converses	4 Irritable cries
3 Inappropriate words	3 Cries to pain
2 Incomprehensible sounds	2 Grunts
1 No response	1 No response

Total score = 3—15

Reproduced by permission of Butterworth-Heinemann Ltd from Harari MD *Paediatric pocket companion.* Oxford, Butterworth-Heinemann, 1991:161-2.

Decimal age

Table 3 Decimals of year

	1 Jan.	2 Feb.	3 Mar.	4 Apr.	5 May	6 June	7 July	8 Aug.	9 Sept.	10 Oct.	11 Nov.	12 Dec.
1	000	085	162	247	329	414	496	581	666	748	833	915
2	003	088	164	249	332	416	499	584	668	751	836	918
3	005	090	167	252	334	419	501	586	671	753	838	921
4	008	093	170	255	337	422	504	589	674	756	841	923
5	011	096	173	258	340	425	507	592	677	759	844	926
6	014	099	175	260	342	427	510	595	679	762	847	929
7	016	101	178	263	345	430	512	597	682	764	849	932
8	019	104	181	266	348	433	515	600	685	767	852	934
9	022	107	184	268	351	436	518	603	688	770	855	937
10	025	110	186	271	353	438	521	605	690	773	858	940
11	027	112	189	274	356	441	523	608	693	775	860	942
12	030	115	192	277	359	444	526	611	696	778	863	945
13	033	118	195	279	362	447	529	614	699	781	866	948
14	036	121	197	282	364	449	532	616	701	784	868	951
15	038	123	200	285	367	452	534	619	704	786	871	953
16	041	126	203	288	370	455	537	622	707	789	874	956
17	044	129	205	290	373	458	540	625	710	792	877	959
18	047	132	208	293	375	460	542	627	712	795	879	962
19	049	134	211	296	378	463	545	630	715	797	882	964
20	052	137	214	299	381	466	548	633	718	800	885	967
21	055	140	216	301	384	468	551	636	721	803	888	970
22	058	142	219	304	386	471	553	638	723	805	890	973
23	060	145	222	307	389	474	556	641	726	808	893	975
24	063	148	225	310	392	477	559	644	729	811	896	978
25	066	151	227	312	395	479	562	647	731	814	899	981
26	068	153	230	315	397	482	564	649	734	816	901	984
27	071	156	233	318	400	485	567	652	737	819	904	986
28	074	159	236	321	403	488	570	655	740	822	907	989
29	077		238	323	405	490	573	658	742	825	910	992
30	079		241	326	408	493	575	660	745	827	912	995
31	082		244		411		578	663		830		997

Reproduced by permission of Castlemead Publications from Tanner J M *Foetus into Man*, 2nd Edition. Herts: Castlemead Publications, 1989.

Growth assessment
Body proportions

Table 4 Ratio of upper segment to lower segment

Birth	1,7 : 1
10 years	1 : 1
14 years	0,9 : 1

Dentition

Calcification of deciduous teeth begins by the fifth month of gestation. Calcification of permanent teeth begins shortly after birth. The central incisors are the first to erupt.

Table 5 Age of eruption of teeth

Deciduous (20)	Usual age of eruption
Lower central incisors (2)	6-8 months
Upper central incisors (2)	7-9 months
Lower and upper lateral incisors (2+2)	8-11 months
Anterior molars (4)	10-16 months
Canines (4)	16-20 months
Posterior molars (4)	20-30 months

Permanent (32)	
First molar (4)	5-6 years
Incisors (8)	6-9 years
Bicuspids (8)	9-12 years
Canines (4)	9-12 years
Second molars (4)	12-13 years
Third molars (4)	17-22 years

Fontanelles

Table 6 Fontanelle closure

Posterior fontanelle:	closed by three months
Anterior fontanelle:	closed by nine to 18 months

Growth charts

Figure 4 Head circumference 0-36 months: boys

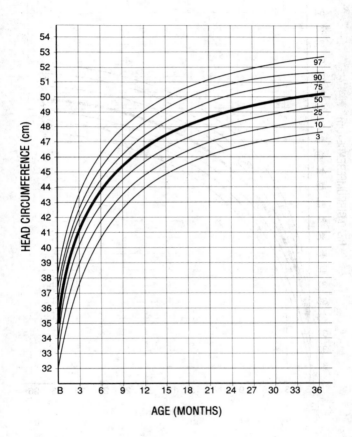

Figure 5 Head circumference 0-36 months: girls

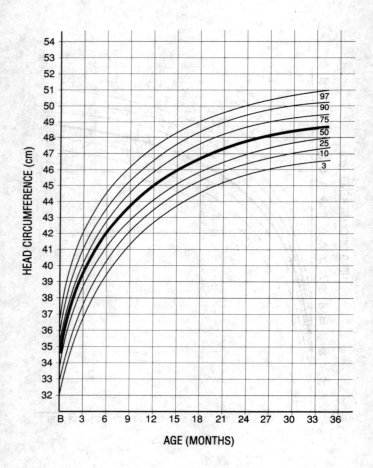

Based on *NCHS Growth Charts*, 1976. Monthly Vital Statistics Report. Vol 25, No. 3, Supp. (HRA) 76-1120. Reprinted with permission of Ross Laboratories, Columbus, OH 43216 from *NCHS Growth Charts*, – 1982 Ross Laboratories.

Figure 6 Weight and length 0-36 months: boys

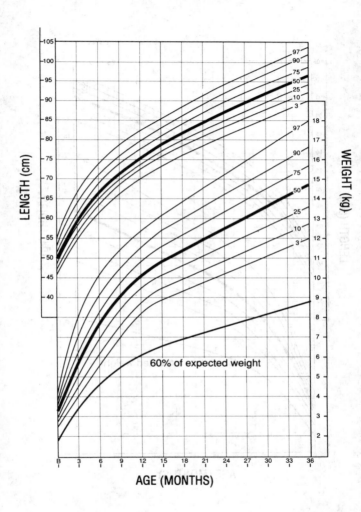

Based on *NCHS Growth Charts*, 1976. Monthly Vital Statistics Report. Vol 25, No. 3, Supp. (HRA) 76-1120. Reprinted with permission of Ross Laboratories, Columbus, OH 43216 from *NCHS Growth Charts*, – 1982 Ross Laboratories.

Figure 7 Weight and length 0-36 months: girls

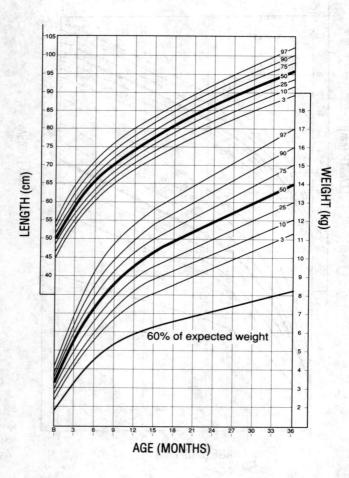

Based on *NCHS Growth Charts*, 1976. Monthly Vital Statistics Report. Vol 25, No. 3, Supp. (HRA) 76-1120. Reprinted with permission of Ross Laboratories, Columbus, OH 43216 from *NCHS Growth Charts*, – 1982 Ross Laboratories.

Figure 8 Weight and height 2-18 years: boys

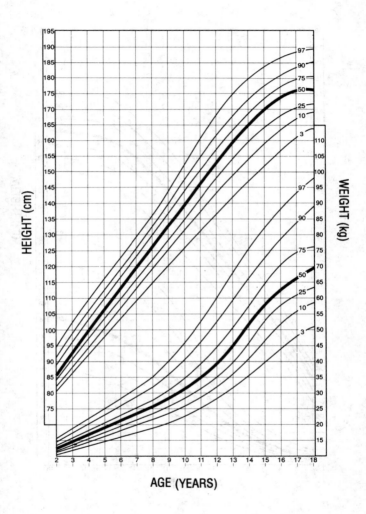

AGE (YEARS)

Based on *NCHS Growth Charts*, 1976. Monthly Vital Statistics Report. Vol 25, No. 3, Supp. (HRA) 76-1120. Reprinted with permission of Ross Laboratories, Columbus, OH 43216 from *NCHS Growth Charts*, – 1982 Ross Laboratories.

Figure 9 Weight and height 2-18 years: girls

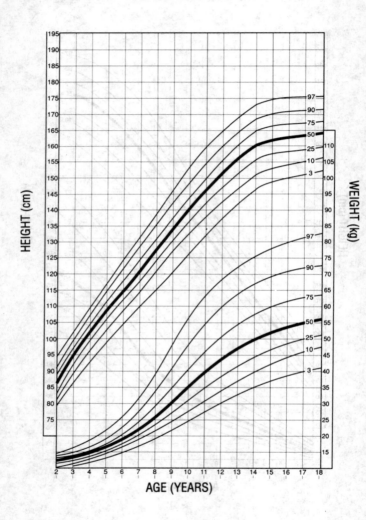

Intra-uterine growth charts

Figure 10 Head circumference 28-43 weeks: both sexes

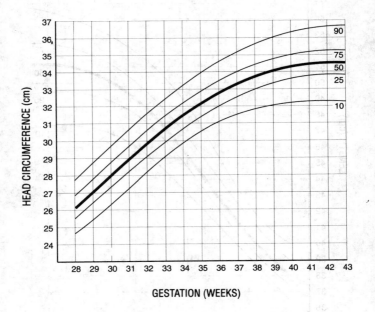

Figure 11 Standard infant length 28-43 weeks: both sexes

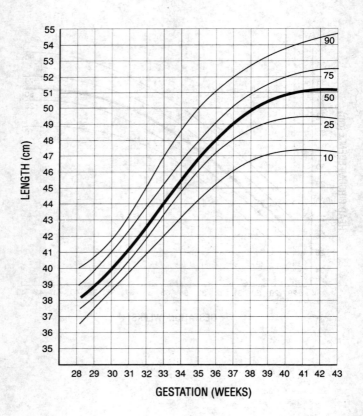

Reproduced by permission of the International Pediatric Research Foundation, Inc., from Naeye RL and Dixon JB 'Distortions in fetal growth standards' from *Pediatr Res* 12:987-91, 1978.

Figure 12 Standard infant weight 28-43 weeks: both sexes

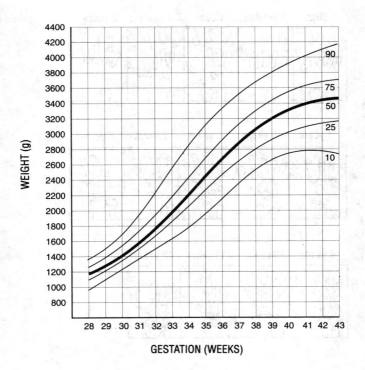

Reproduced by permission of the International Pediatric Research Foundation, Inc., from Naeye RL and Dixon JB 'Distortions in fetal growth standards' from *Pediatr Res* 12:987-91, 1978.

Ossification centres

Figure 13 Ossification centres of wrist and hand

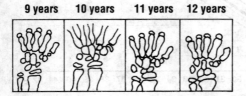

Centres present at:

Birth:	Distal femur and proximal tibia
One year:	Upper femur
One year:	Carpals – one in first year, thereafter, one additional per year

Reference values

Table 7 Body water: relative percentage

	ICF	ECF	TOTAL
Preterm	30	50	80
Neonate	30	40	70
Child	35	30	65
Adult	40	20	60

Table 8 CSF values

	Protein	Glucose*	Chloride	Cells/mm³
Normal				
Neonate	0,2-1,5	3-5	116-130	0-10 lymphocytes
Older	0,2-0,4	3-5	116-130	0-5 lymphocytes

*CSF glucose about 66% of blood glucose

Table 9 Percentiles of CSF white blood cell counts, polymorphonuclear leukocytes, and monocytes by age for total group*

	Total WBC/µl			Polymorphonuclear/µl			Monocytes/µl		
	25th	50th	75th	25th	50th	75th	25th	50th	75th
6 weeks	0,05	2,57	5,16	0,00	0,00	2,42	0,00	0,83	2,71
6 weeks to 3 months	0,34	1,86	3,75	0,00	0,00	0,66	0,00	0,96	2,78
3-6 months	0,00	1,11	2,31	0,00	0,00	0,40	0,00	0,43	1,64
6-12 months	0,41	1,47	3,25	0,00	0,00	0,52	0,03	0,93	2,32
12 months	0,00	0,68	1,82	0,00	0,00	0,00	0,00	0,25	1,45

*Units measured.
Reproduced by permission of *Pediatrics* Vol 75:484–487.

Eosinophil count

Up to 5% eosinophils or 40-440 eosinophils mm^3

Haematology normal values

Table 10 Neonate

The range of normal values is wider than at any other age. Neonates have a higher haemoglobin concentration, mean cell volume and reticulocyte count than older children and adults.

Polymorphs predominate at birth. After seven days a lymphocyte predominance develops and persists until five years of age.

Hb	13,5-21,5 g/dl
Haematocrit	54-68%
MCV	100-128 fl
Reticulocytes	3-6% (term); 3-10% (preterm)
Leucocytes	9-30 x 10^9/l
Platelets	100-300 x 10^9/l

Table 11 Lower limit of normal haemoglobin and red cell mean corpuscular volume*

Age	Hb g/dl	MCV** fl	MCH
Birth	13,5	100	32
6 weeks	9,5	80	26
3 months	10,0	72	25
6-12 months	10,5	70	
1-1,5 years	10,5	70	24
1,5-4 years	11,0	74	24
4-7 years	11,0	76	
7-12 years	11,5	78	
Post pubertal			
Boys	14,0	80	
Girls	12,0	80	

* Values below these indicate anaemia or microcytosis.

** For upper limit of MCV beyond the newborn period add 15 fl to lower limits given above.

Table 12 Differential white blood cell count

Age	WBC	Polymorphs	Lymphocytes
Birth	18 000	60%	30%
6-8 weeks	10 000	40%	60%
3 months			
1 year	8 000	30%	60%
1-4 years	8 000	40%	55%

Table 13 Heart rate per minute

Fetal	150
Birth	130-150
3 months	120-140
1 year	80-140
2 years	80-120
3 years	80-115
3 years	70-110

Table 14 Immunoglobulins in serum

Age	IgG g/l	IgA g/l	IgM g/l
Newborn	7,5-15,0	0-0,10	0-0,20
1-3 months	2,7-7,5	0,06-0,58	0,12-0,87
4-6 months	1,9-8,6	0,10-0,96	0,25-1,00
7-12 months	3,5-11,8	0,15-0,98	0,35-1,04
1-2 years	4,0-12,5	0,35-1,65	0,40-1,60
2-3 years	5,0-13,6	0,45-1,35	0,45-1,90
3-5 years	5,4-14,4	0,50-2,10	0,50-2,00
5-7 years	5,7-14,4	0,50-2,40	0,40-2,10
7-12 years	7,3-15,1	0,70-3,25	0,55-2,10
Adult	7,7-15,1	0,80-3,00	0,65-2,10

Table 15 Insensible water loss

	30 ml/kg/day (infant)
	12 ml/kg/day (child)
or	0,5-1 ml/kg/hr

Respiratory function

Figure 14 Forced vital capacity (FVC ±20%) and maximal mid-expiratory flow rate (FEF 25-75, ±20%)

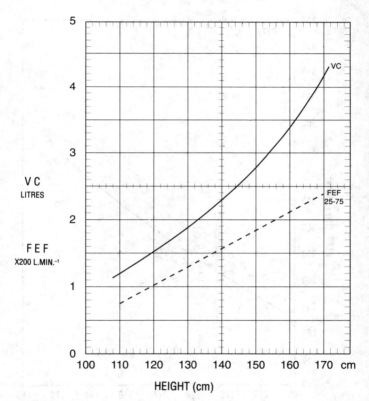

Reference values for vital capacity (VC)
Maximal mid-expiratory flow rate (FEF 25-75)

Note: sex and race-specific growth curves of pulmonary function vs height are available in Wang *et al.* Pulmonary function between six and 18 years of age. *Pediatric Pulmonology* 1993;15:75-88.

Reproduced by permission of WB Saunders Company and adapted from Polgar G and Promadahat V *Pulmonary Function Testing in Children*. Philadephia: WB Saunders 1971.

Figure 15. Peak expiratory flow rate (PEFR)

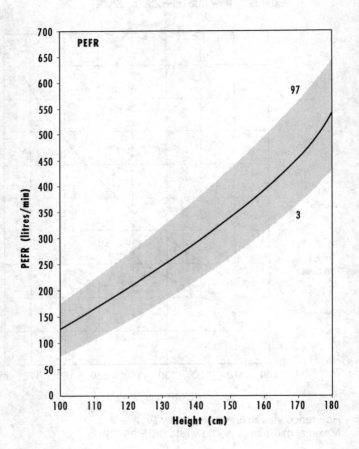

Table 16 Respiratory rate per minute

	Average		Upper limit
Newborn	35-50	<2 months	60
Infants	25-35		
12 months	25-30	2-12 months	50
4th year	25	1-5 years	40
8th year	14-20		
15th year	12-15		

Stools

Table 17 Time of passage of meconium after birth

	Cumulative
Delivery room	27,2%
12 hours	69%
12-24 hours	94%
24-48 hours	99,8%
48 hours	100%
First 48 hours of life	Meconium
2nd-3rd day	'Changing stools'
Number of stools	Varies in the individual infant from one after each feed to one daily: or in some breast-fed infants a stool may be passed every third or fourth day.

Temperature

Table 18 Normal temperatures

Site	Temperature
Abdominal skin (newborn)	26,5 ± 0,3 °C
Axillary	36,5 °C
Oral	37 °C
Rectal	37,5 °C

Trace elements

Table on page 687.

Urine

Table 20 Protein excretion

Normal protein excretion up to 150 mg/d/1,73m²

Table 21 Urine output

Time of passage of urine after birth:	Cumulative
Delivery room	17%
12 hours	67%
12-24 hours	92,4%
24-48 hours	99,4%
48 hours	100%

On normal fluid intake ±4 ml/kg/hour in infants to ±1 ml/kg/hour in adults.

or

First two days	15-50 ml/day
Next week	50-300 ml/day
End of first year	400-500 ml/day
Age seven to eight years	700-1000 ml/day
Age eight to 14 years	700-1500 ml/day
Polyuria	Urine output more than twice normal for age and size
Oliguria	In children <0,5-1,0 ml/kg/hour (±400 ml/1,73m²/day) In adults < 400 ml/1,73m²/day

---

Trace elements

Table 19 Reference values in serum*

| | Zinc (mol wt 65,37) | | Copper*** (mol wt 63,54) | | Caerulo-plasmin*** | Selenium (mol wt 78,96) | |
	µg/dl	µmol/l**	µg/dl	µmol/l	IU/ml	µg/dl	µmol/l
Birth	100 ± 17	15 ± 3	27 ± 13	4 ± 2	40 ± 13	5,9 ± 0,8	0,74 ± 0,1
Infants (1 month)	77 ± 13	12 ± 2	71 ± 17	11 ± 3	< 77	3,9 ± 0,8	0,49 ± 0,1
Infants (1 year)	78 ± 18	12 ± 3	158 ± 27	25 ± 4	—	7,4 ± 2,06	0,94 ± 0,26
Adults (> 14 years)	96 ± 14	15 ± 2	129 ± 44	20 ± 7	111 ± 28	7,3 ± 1,4	0,92 ± 0,17
Pregnancy	Progressive fall		Progressive increase			Little change	
Mothers (term)	66 ± 21	10 ± 3	212 ± 40	33 ± 6	212 ± 43	8,1 ± 1,8	1,02 ± 0,22
Females (on oral contraception)	96 ± 14	15 ± 2	168 ± 38	26 ± 6	181 ± 44	7,8 ± 1,5	0,98 ± 0,19

* These reference values were measured in the Western Cape and are generally similar to other reported values.

** Conversion µg/dl to µmol/l = $\frac{\text{µg/dl} \times 10}{\text{mol wt}}$

*** Values tend to be higher in coloureds and blacks compared to whites.

APPENDIX 5

USEFUL INFORMATION, ADDRESSES AND TELEPHONE NUMBERS

Accident prevention
Child Accident Prevention Foundation of South Africa

The Foundation collects and collates statistics on incidence, causes, patterns and effects of accidents of all kinds in childhood. Preventative programmes based on research findings are then set up and implemented within the community and at schools. Education and promotion of public awareness about the incidence and nature of childhood accidents and their prevention is achieved through the dissemination of information. Recommendations are also put forward to the relevant departments on safety standards and legislation sought to enforce these standards, e.g. child restraints, poisons, toys etc.

Cape Town branch

Contact person:	Mrs N du Toit
	Child Accident Prevention Foundation of South Africa
	Cnr Klipfontein and Harris Roads
	Rondebosch, 7700
Telephone:	(021) 685 5208
Fax:	(021) 685 5331

Johannesburg branch

Contact person:	Mrs J W Clarke
	P O Box 1001
	Bromhof 2154
Telephone:	(011) 7933149 or (011) 792 4332
Fax:	(011) 792 6623

Alcoholics Anonymous: area offices

Johannesburg	(011) 483 2471
East Rand	(011) 421 1992

Vaal Triangle	(016) 33 5341
Pretoria	(012) 322 6047
Cape Town	(021) 24 7559
Port Elizabeth	(041) 55 4019
Durban	(031) 301 4959

Allergy Society of South Africa

ALLSA Resource Centre
P O Box 88
Observatory 7925
Telephone: (021) 47 9019
Fax number: (021) 479019

Antivenom for bites and stings

South African Institute for Medical Research
P O Box 1038
Johanesburg, 2000
Telephone: (011) 882 9940
Fax number: (011) 882 0812

Arthritis and disabled

Arthritis Organization

709 Tulbagh Centre, Cape Town, 8001
Telephone: (021) 254738
              (021) 252344 – Juvenile branch
Fax number: (021) 217330

Association for the Physically Disabled

71 Klipfontein Rd, Rondebosch, 7700
Telephone: (021) 685 4153
Fax number: (021) 685 3438

Breastfeeding Association

Breastfeeding Association of South Africa
Sawkins Road
Rondebosch 7700
Telephone: (021) 686863

Centers for Disease Control

Atlanta
Georgia 30111, USA
Fax no: (091) (404) 332 4555

Cystic Fibrosis Association

c/o Mr P Van Niekerk
4 Gruythos Street
Somerset West 7130
Telephone: (home)   (024) 51 4601
                           (024) 429 2284

Diabetes
South African Diabetes Association

National Office
P O Box 3943
Cape Town, 8000
Telephone: (021) 461 3715 and (021) 4611166

Epilepsy
South African National Epilepsy League

2A Milton Road
Observatory 7925
Telephone: (021) 47 3014
Fax No: (021) 448 5053

Eye disorders
The South African National Council for the Blind

Ms Shirley Odendaal
Community Liaison Office
6 Dalmore Road
Tokai 7975
Telephone: (021) 75 3563
Fax No: (021) 951 5118

Bureau for the Prevention of Blindness

Director: Herman Kluever
OPTIMA Services
P O Box 11149, Brooklyn
Pretoria 0007
Telephone (012) 346 1171

Genetic services

The major providers of genetic services are the departments of Human Genetics at universities, and the Genetic Services

Division of the Department of Health and Population Development. They can be contacted through their regional offices in Cape Town, Kimberley, Port Elizabeth, Bloemfontein, Durban, Pietermaritzburg, Johannesburg and Pretoria (head office).

Information centres

There are a number of information centres available to parents, professionals and the general public. These have links with a large range of organizations and self-care groups dealing with specific childhood needs and disabilities. These centres provide some or all of the following:

◆ assessment, counselling and practical advice to families of children with handicaps;
◆ toy library facilities for preschool mentally and physically handicapped children;
◆ play groups at the Centre as well as in the community for preschool children with handicaps;
◆ information on preschool educare facilities;
◆ links with self-help groups and organizations that specialize in mental handicaps, physical handicaps, learning disabilities, childbirth, breast-feeding, single parenting, parenting twins, food allergies etc;
◆ a library of books and resource files of relevant articles, magazine and newspaper cuttings;
◆ a formal teaching programme on handicaps for health professionals and an informal programme for members or groups of lay persons;
◆ to gather and disseminate information on health, education and welfare services and facilities for children; and
◆ compilation of 'Directory of Services' on health, welfare and educational facilities for children with special needs living in a specific region.

Western Cape

Child Care Information Centre

Rondebosch and Mowbray Children's Centre
Corner of Liesbeeck and Sawkins Roads
Rondebosch, Cape Town.
Telephone: (021) 689 1519 and (021) 685 4103. There is a 24-hour answering service.

PWV

Child Information Centre

Transvaal Memorial Institute for Child Health and Development
Private Bag X 39
Johannesburg
2000
Telephone: (011) 642 7554 ext. 2193 mornings only

Child Referral Centre

Room G041
Munitoria
Vermeulen Street
Pretoria
0002
Telephone: (012) 313 7911 (08h00-16h15)

Orange Free State

Bloemfontein Child Information Centre

Department of Paediatrics and Child Health
Faculty of Medicine
University of the Orange Free State
P O Box 339
Bloemfontein 9300
Telephone: (051) 47 3548 ext. 592 mornings only.
(051) 47 3548 – direct line with a telephone answering service.

Medic Alert Foundation of South Africa

P O Box 4841, Cape Town, 8000.
Telephones: (021) 461 7328 (021) 461 0000 for information in
emergencies and after hours.

Fax Number: 461 6654 – Toll-free number: 08002 22366

Tragic and fatal mistakes can be made during emergency medical treatment if hidden disorders are not recognized. The Medic
Alert emblem worn as a bracelet or necklace is engraved on the
reverse with the specific medical condition. The most important
of these in childhood are: allergies and asthma, bleeding disorders, blindness, deafness, diabetes, heart disorders and epilepsy.
The records of the foundation contain further information which
may be of relevance to medical practitioners.

Poison Information Centres

☞ Name
⊘ Time available
☎ Telephone number
👤 Service available to
❷ Type of advice

Western Cape

Cape Town and environs

Red Cross War Memorial Children's Hospital

☞ Poison Reference Service
⊘ All hours
☎ (021) 689 5227 – direct line
👤 Medical, paramedical personnel, general public.
❷ Emergency advice on treatment of poisoning.

Red Cross War Memorial Children's Hospital

☞ Poison Information Centre
⊘ Monday – Friday 08h30-13h00
☎ (021) 658 5308
👤 Medical, paramedical personnel, general public.
❷ General information on poisoning.

Tygerberg Hospital

☞ Pharmacology and Toxicology Consultation Centre
⊘ All hours
☎ (021) 931 6129 – ask for Poison Centre
⊘ Monday – Friday 08h00-16h30
☎ (021) 938 6235 – direct line
(021) 938 6084 – direct line
👤 Medical and paramedical personnel, general public.
❷ Emergency advice on treatment poisoning. General information on poisoning and pharmacology during office hours only.
Special interest: animal and plant toxicology.

Groote Schuur Hospital

☞ Emergency Unit
⊘ All hours
☎ (021) 404 4450 – direct line
♀ Medical, paramedical personnel, general public.
❷ Emergency advice on treatment of poisoning.

UCT Medical School

☞ Medicines Information Centre (Department of
   Pharmacology)
⊘ Monday – Friday 08h30-17h00
☎ (021) 406 6291 – direct line
   (021) 406 6280 – direct line
   (021) 406 6427 – direct line
   (021) 448 3202 – direct line
♀ All members of health professions in southern Africa.
❷ Therapeutic drug information and adverse reactions.

East London

Frere Hospital

☞ Department of Paediatrics
⊘ Monday – Friday 08h00-17h00
☎ (0431) 49 1077 – direct line
⊘ After hours
☎ (0431) 49 1118 – casualty
   (0431) 49 1111 – hospital exchange – ask for duty
   paediatrician.
♀ Medical, paramedical personnel, general public.
❷ Emergency advice on treatment of poisoning.

Kimberley

Kimberley Hospital

☞ Pharmacy Department
⊘ Monday – Friday 07h30-16h15
   Saturday 08h30-11h00
☎ (0531) 802 2336 – direct line
   (0531) 802 2355 – direct line
☎ After hours for **emergencies** only
   (0531) 802 9111 – ask for duty pharmacist
♀ Medical personnel.
❷ Emergency advice on treatment of poisoning.

Mdantsane

Cecilia Makiwane Hospital

☞ Paediatric Intensive Care Unit
⊙ All hours
☎ (0403) 61 3111 ext 2330 and 2514.
🛉 Medical, paramedical personnel.
❓ Emergency advice on treatment of poisoning.

Port Elizabeth

Livingstone Hospital

☞ Intensive Care Unit
⊙ Monday – Friday 08h00 – 16h00
☎ (041) 405 2455 – direct line
🛉 Medical, paramedical personnel, general public.
❓ Emergency advice on treatment of poisoning.

Provincial Hospital

☞ Department of Pharmacy
⊙ Monday – Friday 07h45-16h15
   Saturday 08h00-11h45
☎ (041) 392 3220 – direct line.
🛉 Medical, paramedical personnel, general public.
❓ Emergency advice on treatment of poisoning.

Orange Free State

Bloemfontein

Universitas Hospital

☞ Casualty Department
⊙ All hours
☎ (051) 405 3503
   (051) 405 3506
   (051) 405 3507 – all direct lines
🛉 Medical, paramedical personnel, general public.
❓ Emergency advice on treatment of poisoning.

University of Orange Free State

☞ Department of Pharmacology, Poison Control and
   Medicine Information Centre
⊙ All hours

☎ (051) 475 353 – direct line
Office hours
(051) 405 3067 – direct line

👤 Medical, paramedical personnel, general public.

❷ Emergency advice and non-urgent information on treatment of poisoning. General information on toxicology and pharmacology.

PWV

Johannesburg

Johannesburg General Hospital

☞ Poison Information Centre
⊘ All hours
☎ (011) 642 2417
(011) 488 3108
👤 Medical, paramedical personnel, general public.
❷ Emergency advice on treatment of poisoning and non-urgent information

Medical Rescue International

⊘ All hours
☎ (011) 403 7080 – direct line
👤 Medical, paramedical personnel and general public.
❷ Emergency advice on treatment of poisoning.

Kempton Park

Emergency Medical Response

☞ ARWYP Medical Centre
⊘ All hours
☎ 0800 091911 – toll free
(011) 922 1145
👤 Medical, paramedical, personnel, general public.
❷ Emergency advice on treatment of poisoning.

Pretoria

Medunsa

☞ Department of Paediatrics
⊘ Monday – Friday 08h00-15h45
☎ (012) 529 4444
👤 Medical, paramedical personnel, general public.
❷ Emergency advice on treatment of poisoning.

Natal
Durban
St Augustine's Hospital

☞ St Augustine's Trauma and Poison Unit
⊘ All hours
☎ 0800 333 444
🚶 Medical, paramedical personnel, general public.
❓ Emergency advice on the treatment of poisoning.

Specimens and viral transportation

☞ Diagnostic Virology Laboratory
UCT Medical School
Anzio Road
Observatory, 7925
☎ (021) 406 6133/4/5
FAX (021) 448 4110

Tuberculosis

☞ Agents: Vaccina cc, P O Box 804, Gardenview 2047

INDEX